The
BUPA
manual of
FITNESS
and
WELL~BEING

The
BUPA
manual of
FITNESS
and
WELL~BEING

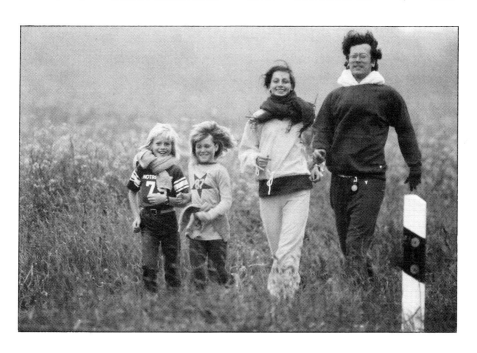

Macdonald

A *Macdonald* BOOK

First published in Great Britain 1984
by Macdonald & Co (Publishers) Ltd
London & Sydney
A member of BPCC plc
Reprinted in 1985

© 1984 Marshall Editions Limited

British Library Cataloguing in Publication Data
Wright, Beric
    The Bupa manual of fitness and well-being
    1. Health
    I. Title
    613   RA776
    ISBN 0-356-10165-7

Filmset by Filmtype Services Limited, Scarborough,
North Yorkshire
Origination by Gilchrist Brothers Limited, Leeds
Printed and bound in West Germany by Mohndruk
Graphische Betriebe GMBH

Macdonald & Co (Publishers) Ltd
Maxwell House
74 Worship Street
London EC2 2EN

Conceived, edited and designed by
Marshall Editions Limited,
71 Eccleston Square, London SW1V 1PJ

EDITOR   Ruth Binney
ART DIRECTOR   Mel Petersen
DEPUTY EDITOR   Rosanne Hooper
ASSISTANT EDITORS   Clare Badham
                        Gwen Rigby
DESIGN ASSISTANTS   Roger Boddy
                        Arthur Brown
PICTURE EDITOR   Zilda Tandy
PRODUCTION   Barry Baker
                        Janice Storr

About BUPA

BUPA — British United Provident Association — is a
non-profit making health insurance company, by far the
largest of its kind in Britain. Essentially, but with a
range of options, it pays for the cost of private hospital
and specialist treatment, for an annual premium.

But as well as its main insurance activity, BUPA also
operates health care facilities which include eight
screening centres for men and women, and a growing
chain of private hospitals in various parts of the
country. It was also originally instrumental in setting up
the Nuffield Nursing Home Trust — now Nuffield
Hospitals — the biggest private hospital chain in
Britain. There is also a Nursing Agency, supplying
nurses for hospitals and home care. A pilot scheme for
sheltered housing for the frail elderly is just starting.

BUPA thus covers both health insurance and
extensive health care facilities, which is why we are
pleased to be associated with this 'health promotion'
publication.

The publishers would like to thank the following people and
organizations for their invaluable help: Liz Anfield; Donald
Binney; Norman Ellis; Liv Lowrie; Peter McCullough; Tim
Newling; Bronwen Reynolds; Maggie Skiffington; Mike Snell;
Michelle Thompson; Alison Tomlinson; Joan White; Jane
Wilkie; Alison Williams; The Canada Fitness Survey; Central
Policy on Ageing; Daltons Sports/Fitness Industries; The
Disabled Living Group; The Health Education Council; Help
the Aged; Nautilus Fitness Centre, London SE 1; The
Pre-Retirement Association; The Vegetarian Society.

Consultant editor
H. Beric Wright MB, FRCS, MFOM
is chairman of the BUPA Medical Centre, and a
governor of BUPA in London. Until his recent
retirement he was medical advisor to the Institute of
Directors and president of the Pre-Retirement
Association. He is an expert on health problems of
executives and is the author of several books, including
Executive Ease and Dis-ease and
A Longer Life.

Consultants
Patricia Last FRCS, FRCOG
is head of the Women's Unit at the BUPA Medical
Centre, London, and lecturer in family planning at
St Bartholomew's Hospital, London.

Carolyn Ritchie PhD
is a nutritionist and head of research at BUPA Medical
Research, London.

Keith Stoll MSc, MPhil, PhD
is consultant clinical psychologist at the BUPA Medical
Centre, London, and in the Department of Psychiatry,
Guy's Hospital, London.

Clyde Williams BSc, MSc, PhD
is senior lecturer in the Department of Physical
Education and Sports Science at Loughborough
University of Technology. He is chairman of the
Society of Sports Sciences.

Peter Williams MA, BM, BCh
is head of the Fitness Assessment Unit at the BUPA
Medical Centre, London.

Authors
Gordon Jackson MB, MRCP
Judy Garlick BA
Thomas C. Kelly MA
Elizabeth MacFarlane MB, BS
Paulette Pratt
Arlene Sobel MA
Shelley Turner BA

CONTENTS

INTRODUCTION

More and more people, including doctors and health educators, now recognize that, to a considerable degree, your life is in your hands. This means that fitness and well-being have become matters for you and your family to promote and cultivate.

This is a book that has been specifically designed and written by a team of highly qualified consultants and authors to show you how fitness and well-being can be achieved. It is essentially a 'do it yourself' guide to fitness and well-being, not a book about illness and diseases. If you have the slightest doubt, on medical grounds, about adopting any of the advice given or activities recommended, your own doctor should be consulted.

It has become increasingly accepted that the mental may well largely determine the physical, which implies that if you are happily active and involved in living, you are less likely to be ill. Health is, because of its complexity, difficult to define, but it is certainly more than just the absence of disease. It must reflect a state of mental, social and physical well-being, which means that to be truly healthy you must be in reasonable tune with your environment. Health must be related to lifestyle, and this book is thus lifestyle-oriented.

The concept that well-being or mental tune may largely determine the physical state has come to be called 'holistic' or whole person medicine. Symptoms or upsets must then be assessed in relation to the whole person, their relationships and lifestyles, not just in terms of the symptoms or immediate complaint. Discovering *why* a person is ill is just as important as diagnosing the symptoms.

Another change of emphasis in medical thinking, which is also brought strongly into this book, is that many common and killing diseases, such as heart attacks and some forms of cancer, are either preventable or much better treated if discovered early. This again makes the point of personal responsibility for your health. It also reinforces the value of regular health screening.

Your life is in your hands, and by living sensibly, which is in no way miserably, you *can* largely determine your own destiny. And since we all live in family, social and cultural groups, the well-being of the group, particularly of the family, becomes of prime importance. Children tend to acquire both the best and the worst of their parents' lifestyle habits, which is why it is important to lead them by example. Similarly, the elderly and pregnant women have special needs.

As I said at the beginning, this is not a book about illness: it is a family guide to health and well-being, stressing the mental and physical aspects of both sets of factors. By adopting at least some of the advice given I am sure that you and your family will both feel and be much better for your revised lifestyle — and there is every chance that you will live longer.

H. B. Wright, *Consultant editor*

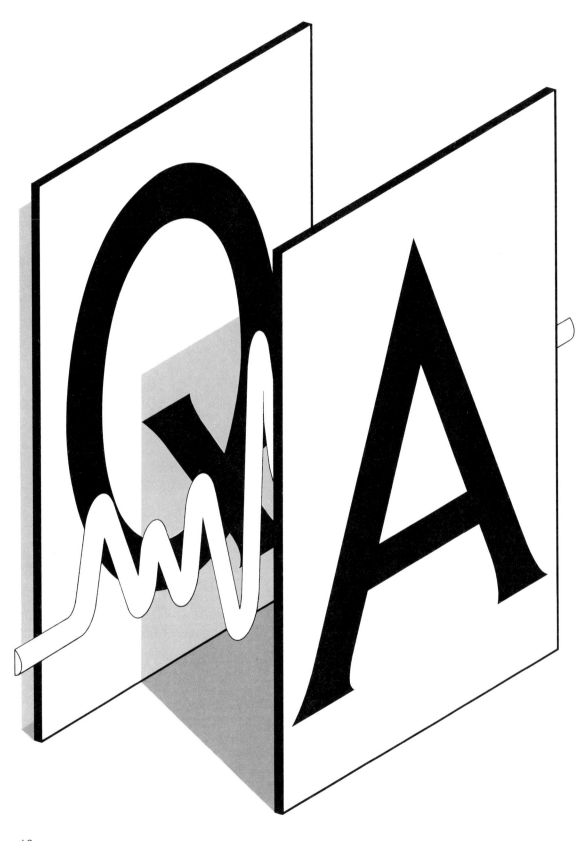

HOW ARE YOU?

Before you begin to think seriously about your fitness and well-being, there are a number of questions you must ask yourself. Do you know, for example, how fit you are, how well you cope or how you treat yourself and others? This chapter will not only help you to answer these and other questions but, more importantly, will enable you to identify those areas of your lifestyle that are impairing your fitness and need improvement.

However willing you may be to make changes in your daily routine, you are unlikely to arrive at the best solutions unless you first subject yourself to critical scrutiny. This preliminary self-assessment programme thus consists essentially of tests by which you can measure yourself. Your results will help you define your levels of fitness and flexibility, of external and internal stress, of private and social vitality. They will allow you to analyse your diet and enable you to calculate your projected life expectancy. Further back-up tests appear throughout the book.

Through analysis of your current levels of achievement and of your attitude toward yourself you will be able to use this book as fully as possible. As well as defining those parts of your life that would benefit from change, you will be able to identify those elements that cannot reasonably be changed and so begin to come to terms with them.

The quizzes and tests in this chapter are intended only as a guide. If, for any reason, you feel anxious about your physical or mental health, then you should consult a doctor. For a more detailed analysis of your current state of fitness, you need the facilities offered by a medically supervised health screen. Such a screen will provide scientific measurements of, for example, the working of your heart and respiratory system, will quantify your body fat percentage and analyse your blood and so give further insights into your metabolism and dietary needs.

Many people have an unrealistic idea of their level of fitness. Some take a lot of exercise without thinking about it, more take a little exercise and believe themselves ultra-fit. Fitness is a combination of heart and muscle capacity to use oxygen for energy production. To find out how you rate, try the tests on these pages and overleaf. Your scores will immediately reveal those areas in which you need to improve your performance.

Turn to Chapter 4, Getting Fit, Staying Fit pp. 86–133 for ideas about new sports and for information and exercise programmes for developing your fitness. After 6 weeks or when you are half way through an aerobic programme, retake these tests to measure your improved fitness. After a further 6 weeks, or at the end of an aerobic programme, try again — the results should be a great encouragement.

TEST 1

What is your resting pulse rate?
Your resting pulse is a simple and accurate gauge of cardiovascular fitness. As your fitness level increases, your resting pulse rate will become slower stronger and more regular. Take your pulse when you wake up in the morning because any form of emotional or physical exertion will affect it during the day. Individual rates vary but, as a general rule, women have a slightly higher pulse rate than men. If you find your resting pulse is over 100 beats a minute, consult your doctor immediately.

Take your pulse at your wrist (at the base of your thumb) or by feeling the artery in your neck, which is located below the ear and toward the jawbone.

TEST 2

What is your heart recovery time?
Try this simple step test to assess your aerobic fitness and stamina. The test reveals how efficiently your heart and lungs feed oxygen to your body by measuring the time it takes to slow down after it has speeded up for exercise. If your resting pulse rate is over 100 beats a minute, do not attempt this test. Step on to a stair about 20 cm (8 in) high then step down again, moving one foot after the other. Repeat 24 times a minute for 3 minutes. Stop and take your pulse. After resting for 30 seconds, take your pulse again and consult the chart. Repeat this test after a few weeks of participation in an aerobic exercise programme (see pp. 106-15) and see if your heart recovers more quickly. The heart's natural capacity declines with age, so beware of exceeding the safe limit as you grow older. If at any moment you feel dizzy, nauseated or painfully breathless, stop *immediately.*

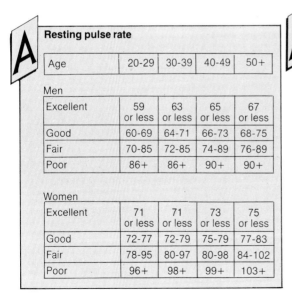

Resting pulse rate

Age	20-29	30-39	40-49	50+
Men				
Excellent	59 or less	63 or less	65 or less	67 or less
Good	60-69	64-71	66-73	68-75
Fair	70-85	72-85	74-89	76-89
Poor	86+	86+	90+	90+
Women				
Excellent	71 or less	71 or less	73 or less	75 or less
Good	72-77	72-79	75-79	77-83
Fair	78-95	80-97	80-98	84-102
Poor	96+	98+	99+	103+

Recovery pulse rate at 30 seconds

Age	20-29	30-39	40-49	50+
Men				
Excellent	74	78	80	83
Good	76-84	80-86	82-88	84-90
Fair	86-100	88-100	90-104	92-104
Poor	102+	102+	106+	106+
Women				
Excellent	86	86	88	90
Good	88-92	88-94	90-94	92-98
Fair	99-110	95-112	96-114	100-116
Poor	112+	114+	104+	118+

TEST 3
What is your safe maximum pulse rate?
During exercise, be sure not to exceed the following values:

Age	20-29	30-39	40-49	50+
Men	170	160	150	140
Women	170	160	150	140

TEST 4
How active are you?

How often do you take physical exercise (including keep fit classes and sport) that makes you out of breath?
a Four times or more a week
b Two to three times a week
c Once a week
d Less than once a week

How far do you walk each day?
a More than 5 km (3 mls)
b Up to 5 km (3 mls)
c Less than 1.6 km (1 ml)
d Less than 0.8 km ($\frac{1}{2}$ ml)

How do you travel to work/the shops?
a All the way by foot/cycle
b Part of the way by foot/cycle
c Occasionally by foot/cycle
d All the way by public transport or car

When there is a choice do you?
a Take the stairs —up and down—always
b Take the stairs unless you have something to carry
c Occasionally take the stairs
d Take the lift/escalator unless it is broken

At weekends do you?
a Spend several hours gardening/decorating/DIY/doing some sport
b Usually only sit down for meals and in the evening
c Take a few short walks
d Spend most of the time sitting reading/watching TV

Do you think nothing of?
a Doing the household chores after a day's work
b Rushing out to the shops again if you have forgotten something
c Getting other people to run your errands, even if you have time
d Paying for a telephone call when you could make a personal visit

Add up your score, allowing
4 points for every **a** answer
3 points for every **b** answer
2 points for every **c** answer
1 point for every **d** answer

20+
You are naturally very active and probably quite fit.

15–20
You are active and have a healthy attitude toward fitness.

10–15
You are only mildly active and would benefit from some more exercise.

Under 10
You are rather lazy and need to rethink your attitude toward activity. Try to reorganize your day to allow for some exercise.

TEST 5
What can you do?
How long does it take you to:
1 Walk 5 km (3 mls) on level ground
a 1 hr 15 min (or more)
b 50 min to 1 hr 10 min
c 45 min (or less)

2 Swim 1,000 m (1,000 yds)
a 50 min (or more)
b 40 min
c 20 min (or less)

3 Run 1.6 km (1 ml) on level ground
a 15 min (or more)
b 9-14 min
c 8 min (or less)

Scores:
a If you have covered the distance you have made a start. Now keep it up until the test feels easy.

b You are moderately fit. If you want to improve, increase the distance and speed up gradually.

c You have reached a good level of fitness and are ready to start a more vigorous fitness programme.

Strength and flexibility are two important adjuncts to all-round fitness. Similarly, being the correct weight for your size is also conducive to good health. Obesity and lack of flexibility can impair mobility; additionally obesity is associated with diabetes, with diseases of the gall bladder, heart and arteries, and with some kinds of cancer.

The tables on pp. 76-7 show you how to work out your body mass index and how to evaluate this in terms of obesity. The tests given here offer some quick ways of finding out what shape you are in. Retake all the tests regularly and chart your progress over a period of many weeks. You should be encouraged by your advancement as you look back at your early efforts.

Turn to Chapter 3, Eating for Health pp. 52-85 to find out how to revolutionize your eating habits with a view to losing fat. Chapter 4, Getting Fit, Staying Fit pp. 86-133, offers several exercise programmes, which are an important adjunct to any reducing schedule. It also gives ideas for improving your strength and flexibility.

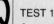

TEST 1

Are you carrying unwanted fat?

Pinch yourself at the waist and on your upper arm, grasping as much flesh as possible between your finger and thumb.

If you can pinch more than about 2.5 cm (1 in) of spare flesh, then this is an indication that you need to lose some fat. This may be a matter of merely toning up — replacing fat with muscle — or of losing weight. As a rule of thumb, every 0.6 cm ($\frac{1}{4}$ in) over 2.5 cm (1 in) on this test represents about 4.5 kg (10 lb) of body fat.

breathe in and measure the circumference of your chest when your lungs are at their fullest.

If the waist measurement is more than the chest one, then you are carrying too much fat around your waist. Repeat the measurements weekly.

If you are a regular swimmer, find a place in the pool where you have a clear view of the second hand on a clock, or enlist the help of a friend with a watch that measures in seconds. Float on your back, but do not paddle with your hands to keep you buoyant. Empty your lungs by breathing out as far as you can. Time how long it takes you to sink.

As you lose unwanted fat you will find that your buoyancy decreases. (This will not, incidentally, reduce your swimming efficiency.)

TEST 2

How am I changing?

Men and women tend to accumulate excess fat in different parts of their bodies. In men, flab is most likely round the waist, shoulders and upper arms. In women, waist, hips, thighs and bust are most prone to the build-up of unwanted fat.

TEST 3

How efficient are your lungs?

These quick tests give a rough guide to the efficiency with which your lungs are functioning. You need to have a laboratory test (see pp. 92-3, 98-9) to measure this accurately.

Take a deep breath in and time how long you can hold your breath. Breathe in and out as far as you can and measure your chest in each position.

Measure yourself with a tape measure. If you are a man, measure your waist, upper arm, forearm, hips. If you are a woman, measure your waist, upper arm, forearm, thighs, calves and bust. Make a note of your findings, along with the date. Measure in the same places each week and chart your progress.

If you are a man, breathe out then, keeping your muscles relaxed, measure (or get someone else to measure) your waist at the level of your navel. Then

If you can hold your breath for 45 seconds or more, and if the difference between the two chest measurements is 5-7.5 cm (2-3 in) cm or more, then it is likely that your lungs are working with adequate efficiency.

Test 4
How flexible are you?

Flexibility is an important attribute for *all* physical activities. In particular, tight leg and back muscles impede movement in many sports and can cause back pain and stiffness after exercise. Women tend to be more supple than men and peak at the age of 15 to 19, several years before men, and decline more gradually.

To test your flexibility, attach some string or a stick firmly to the ground and sit down with your heels touching this line and your feet comfortably apart. Keeping your legs straight, bend forward slowly from the waist and reach as far as you can without straining. Place a marker at this point and relax. Take a ruler or measuring stick and measure the distance between your marker and the line. Score a plus (+) figure if it lies *beyond* your heel line and a minus (−) figure if it does not.

TEST 5
How strong are you?

Muscular endurance is necessary for fitness because muscular effort has to be sustained without fatigue if aerobic fitness is to be maintained. Thus it is important for general fitness and a prerequisite for good performance in many sports and activities. One method of measuring strength is by your ability to do sit-ups.

How to do sit-ups
Lie on your back with your ankles firmly wedged beneath a solid object or held by another person. Put your arms behind your head and, **with knees bent**, pull yourself up to a sitting position, using the strength of your stomach muscles. See how many sit-ups you can manage within 60 seconds and consult the chart to measure your result. Men generally have greater muscular endurance than women, but reach a peak a few years later, usually between the ages of 15 and 19.

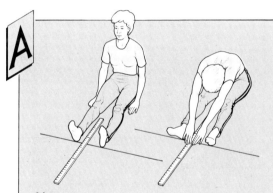

Men

Stretch rating	Age up to 35		Age 36-45		Age 45+	
	cm	in	cm	in	cm	in
Excellent	+6	$1\frac{1}{2}$	+5	2	+4	$1\frac{1}{2}$
Good	−3	$1\frac{1}{4}$	+2	$\frac{3}{4}$	+1	$\frac{1}{2}$
Fair	−5	2	−5	2	−6	$2\frac{1}{2}$
Poor	−8	$3\frac{1}{4}$	−10	4	−10	4

Women

Stretch rating	Age up to 35		Age 36-45		Age 46+	
	cm	in	cm	in	cm	in
Excellent	+8	$3\frac{1}{4}$	+7	$2\frac{3}{4}$	+6	$2\frac{1}{2}$
Good	+5	2	+4	$1\frac{1}{2}$	+3	$1\frac{1}{4}$
Fair	−1	$\frac{1}{2}$	−3	$1\frac{1}{4}$	−2	$\frac{3}{4}$
Poor	−4	$1\frac{1}{2}$	−5	2	−6	$2\frac{1}{2}$

Assess your performance

Men

Age	Muscular endurance		
	Excellent	Good	Poor
12-14	45	35	25
15-19	50	40	30
20-29	40	30	20
30-39	35	25	20
40-49	30	20	15
50-59	25	15	10
60-69	23	13	8

Women

Age	Muscular endurance		
	Excellent	Good	Poor
12-14	44	34	24
15-19	40	30	20
20-29	33	23	13
30-39	27	17	12
40-49	22	12	7
50-59	20	10	5
60-69	17	7	4

HOW'S YOUR DIET?

Eating is a pleasure and a habit, but many of us either eat more than we need, and put on excess weight, or become diet fiends. The questions on these pages are designed to allow you to analyse the way you eat and to assess whether your eating habits need improvement. It may help to ensure that your answers are accurate if you make a note of everything you eat, and the time and place in which you eat it, for a complete week. Remember, it is important to develop good eating habits, as much for your children's health as your own.

If your scores show that your diet and eating habits need improvement, or to find out more about healthy eating, turn to Chapter 3, Eating for Health pp. 52-85 and Chapter 9, The Whole Person pp. 224-61. You will also find facts about food in many other chapters of the book.

When you have revised your diet according to these guidelines, take the tests again.

TEST 1

Does your diet pass the test?

Answer **a**, **b**, or **c** to the following questions:

1 How many meals do you eat each day as a rule?
a Three or more
b Two
c One

2 Do these meals include breakfast?
a Always
b Once or twice a week
c Rarely

3 If you have breakfast, does it consist of:
a Cereals and toast, plus a drink?
b Fried foods such as bacon and eggs?
c Just a drink?

4 How many times a day do you eat snacks?
a Never or very rarely
b Once or twice
c Three or more times

5 How often do you eat red meat?
a Up to three times a week
b Three to six times a week
c More than six times a week

6 How often do you eat fresh fruit, vegetables and salads?
a Three times a day
b Once or twice a day
c Three or four times a week or less

7 How often do you eat fried foods?
a Once a week or less
b Three or four times a week
c Most days

8 Do you add salt to your food?
a Sparingly, if at all
b Moderately
c Liberally

9 How often do you eat creamy desserts or chocolate?
a Once a week or less
b One to four times a week
c Most days

10 To spread on bread do you use:
a Soft margarine made from polyunsaturated vegetable oil?
b A mixture of butter and soft and hard margarines?
c Butter or hard margarine only?

11 How many times a week do you eat fish?
a More than twice
b Once or twice
c Once or less

12 How often do you eat wholegrain cereals or wholemeal bread?
a At least once a day
b Three to six times a week
c Less than three times a week

13 Before cooking or eating meat do you:
a Trim off all the visible fat?
b Trim off some of the fat?
c Remove none of the fat?

14 How many cups of coffee or tea do you drink each day?
a One or two
b Three to five
c Six or more

15 How many alcoholic drinks do you consume each day?
a One or less
b Two or three
c More than three

Scoring: score yourself 2 points for every **a** answer, 1 for a **b** and 0 for a **c**, then add up your total:

25-30: You have an excellent diet, with little need for improvement.

20-25: You have a good diet, but it could improve a little.

15-20: You have a moderately good diet only, improvement is needed in some areas.

0-15: You have a poor diet, which needs considerable improvement.

TEST 2
How do you eat?

For you or your family, how many of the following statements are true?
1 Three-course meals are the rule.
2 Food is offered as a reward for good behaviour.
3 Sweets, potato crisps and other similar snacks are always available in the house.
4 Food is given to compensate for misfortune or disappointment.
5 Going without food is a punishment for poor behaviour.
6 Meals are eaten quickly, without conversation.
7 Eating results from tension or boredom.
8 Food is eaten standing up or 'on the run'.
9 Second helpings are the rule, not the exception.
10 Store cupboards are filled to overflowing.
11 Meals are served on large plates, amply filled.
12 The TV stays switched on during meals.

If you answer 'yes' to **3 or more** of these points, then you and/or the members of your family are probably eating more than you need — and not sensibly. You may thus risk being overweight.

TEST 3
Fat in your diet

On average, how many of the following foods do you eat or use in cooking each day?

Butter	Pies (sweet and
Margarine	savoury)
Cooking oil	Pastries/doughnuts
Sausages or frankfurters	Cream
Salami/other preserved	Potato crisps
meats	Nuts
Mayonnaise	Ice-cream
Salad (French) Dressing	Pâté
Fish canned in oil	Tongue
Bacon	Meat with fat
Avocado pears	Duck
Eggs	Chocolate
Cakes	Pancakes
Biscuits	Puddings
Hard cheese	
Cream cheese	
Fried foods of any kind	

If you regularly eat 3 or more of these foods each day, you are probably eating too much fat in your diet.

TEST 4
How much do you know about food?

Are the following statements true or false?
1 Potatoes, cereals and bread are fattening foods.
2 All but the best diets need supplementing with vitamins.
3 Vegetables do not contain proteins.
4 Liver is the only good source of iron in the diet.
5 Eating apples helps to clean your teeth.
6 Eating sugar is the best way to get 'instant' energy.
7 Skimmed milk contains less calcium and other minerals than whole milk.
8 Frozen vegetables are deficient in vitamins.

All these statements are false.

WHAT'S YOUR LIFESTYLE?

Your lifestyle has a great influence on your sense of well-being. It also reflects your personality and philosophy of living. Of course, not all aspects of life, such as your place of work and your home, are easily changed. However, you may be imposing unnecessary stresses on yourself by failing to recognize problem areas. Answer the questions on these pages to find out how much your way of life may be affecting your health and happiness.

For more advice and ideas about improving your lifestyle and sense of well-being, turn to:

Chapter 2, Whole Life Programmes pp. 24-51, Chapter 8, Growing Old Gracefully pp. 204-33, Chapter 9, The Whole Person pp. 224-61, Chapter 6, Your Sexuality pp. 158-85 and Chapter 10 Treats and Treatments pp. 262-97.

Having consulted the relevant pages and decided which elements of your lifestyle you want to change and how you can go about it, try putting your plans into action. Return to this quiz after three months and see if your score has improved and your lifestyle become more satisfying.

How are your living and working conditions?
Where and how you live and work can affect your physical health, your peace of mind, your achievements and your attitude to life. Take a fresh look at your life and see what change is desirable and possible. Work out a sensible list of priorities and stick to it.

TEST 1
Your working life

1 Can you improve the lighting by simple rearrangements?
2 Can you reorganize your office layout to create more space?
3 Can you do/say something to help improve the general cleanliness?
4 Can you improve the ventilation and heating?
5 Can you make the surroundings look more cheerful, with pictures/plants etc?
6 Are the people responsible for working conditions aware of any grievances?
7 Can you do anything to improve your job security/to earn more money in your present job?
8 Can you shield yourself from excessive noise?
8 Can you improve the seating?
10 Can you improve your interaction with colleagues?

TEST 2
Getting to work

1 Have you chosen the most suitable method of transport?
2 Is it worth leaving home half an hour earlier?
3 Can you reduce the cost, stress and pollution of your daily travelling?

4 Could you combine getting to work with taking exercise?

TEST 3
Home life

1 Could you reorganize the layout of any rooms to create more space?
2 Do you need to improve the lighting?
3 Should you consider alternative heating arrangements?
4 Does each member of the household have enough room and privacy ? If not, what can you do to improve matters?
5 Would one specific purchase, such as a more comfortable bed, help to improve your life?
6 Is it possible and practicable to move to a more suitable/convenient/pleasant home?
7 Can you block out any unnecessary noise?
8 Would it cheer you up to redecorate?
9 Could you streamline or share the housework?
10 Are you using any spare space to full advantage?

TEST 4
Emotional life

1 Is there room for improvement in your relationship with your children?
2 Can you do or say anything to improve your sex life?
3 What is lacking in your social life and how can you improve it?
4 Can you improve the quality of your interaction with your partner?
5 Do your loved ones feel loved?
6 Do you spend enough time with the people you care about?

TEST 5
Financial life

1 Are you living dangerously above your means?
2 Have you budgeted for future expenses?
3 Could you get a better deal from your employer and from any savings?
4 Are you claiming all the benefits due to you?

If you can be honest, your own answers to these questions will open up the solutions. Think each one through and act upon it.

TEST 6
How do you use your leisure time?

Do you remember that it takes an effort to use your leisure time well; an effort of planning to create time and an effort of will not to lapse back into bad habits? More important, do you enjoy your leisure time activities to the full?

Do you:

1 Watch TV for more than 2 hours, 4 or more evenings a week. (Score 0)
2 See friends at least twice a week. (Score 2)
3 Take the family out for some fresh air and exercise at week-ends. (Score 3)
4 Go to museums, theatres, cinemas. (Score 2)
5 Often wander around the shops for lack of anything else to do. (Score 1)
6 Tinker around at home. (Score 1)
7 Make time for exercise more than 3 times each week. (Score 4)
8 Spend 4 or 5 hours a week on an active hobby. (Score 4)
9 Spend 4 or 5 hours a week on a sedentary hobby. (Score 3)
10 Play sport for a team regularly. (Score 4)
11 Go out eating and drinking every night. (Score 0)
12 Go to a class or club every week. (Score 3)
13 Put aside a little time to relax/think/meditate alone. (Score 3)
14 Organize the rest of the family. (Score 0)
15 Do office work at home. (Score 0)
16 What leisure time? (Score −4)
17 Work on the home. (Score 3)
18 Enjoy your family. (Score 3)

Add up your score:
30 or over: You have a healthy, balanced lifestyle and deserve a sense of well-being.
20-30: You have a positive attitude toward leisure, but may benefit from some more physical exercise.
10-20: You may need to rethink your priorities. Your free time may not be evenly balanced, and you might benefit from introducing more variety and activity into your leisure time.
Under 10: You probably do not enjoy your free time much. If you often find yourself at a loose end, try to increase your circle of friends, take more exercise and cultivate a new interest. If you never have enough time to yourself, try to reorganize your life.

TEST 7
Are your holidays good for you?

1 Do you often end up working instead of going away?
2 Do you forget to take all your days off?
3 Do you leave it too late to shop around for the most suitable holiday?
4 Do you usually return home feeling exhausted by the family?
5 Do you always go to the same place out of habit?
6 Do you avoid 'active' holidays for the wrong reasons?
7 Do you spend your holidays doing up your house?
8 Do you always end up with the holiday you don't want but which suits your family/partner/friends?
9 Would you really prefer to go away with someone else?
10 Do you rarely get what you want from a holiday?

If you answered 'yes' to any of the above, ask yourself *why* this is true. Learn from past mistakes, decide what you really want from a holiday and explore all the possibilities. Discuss these with your intended companions and try to agree on a holiday that will give you all a massive injection of well-being.

WHO ARE YOU?

However physically fit and healthy you are, you will not enjoy a sense of well-being unless you are emotionally healthy. The quizzes on these pages will help to clarify your attitudes toward yourself, your life and other people.

To find out more about yourself and how to improve your self-image and lifestyle, turn to Chapter 2, Whole Life Programmes pp. 24-51, Chapter 6, Your Sexuality pp. 158-85, Chapter 9, The Whole Person pp. 224-61, Chapter 10, Treats and Treatments pp. 262-97.

Once you have identified problems, try to analyse the solutions, establish realistic courses of action and make sure you see them through. After three months, take the quiz again and see how you have changed for the better.

TEST 1
How are your loving relationships?

1. Do you have sexual problems in your relationship?
2. Do you find it hard to talk to your partner about personal matters?
3. Do you often snap at your loved ones and then regret it?
4. Do you think your relationship/marriage is emotionally one-sided?
5. Do you avoid visiting your parents if at all possible?
6. Do you dread going home?
7. Do you spend too much time arguing about money?
8. Do you feel jealous of your partner?
9. Do you feel trapped by your relationship?
10. Do you wish you had a relationship?
11. Do you feel your relationship is holding you back?

TEST 2
How are you coping with the world?

1. Do you find your emotions get out of control?
2. Do you try to avoid awkward situations and people?
3. Do you seek approval from everyone you meet?
4. Do you see yourself through others' eyes?
5. Do you dread being alone?
6. Do you feel unable to control your life pattern?
7. Do you think it is weak to feel grief, anguish, anxiety?
8. Do you believe that a perfect relationship is possible?
9. Do you feel detached from the rest of the world?
10. Do you dislike yourself?
11. Do you feel depressed and lonely?
12. Do you feel you have nothing to contribute?
13. Do you feel persecuted and talked about?
14. Do you avoid contact with other people?
15. Do you harbour regrets and resentments?

If *any* of the above is true, either your relationship or your attitude toward it needs some thought and effort. Analyse the good and bad points of your situation and try to come to a realistic conclusion.

Questions to ask yourself:

1. Can I see things from my partner's/relative's point of view? What is their perspective of life and of me? Is this why we always end up on opposite sides?
2. How can *we* change it? It's a problem, not a battle.
3. Have some of the solutions we've employed in the past produced more problems?
4. What is it that I may be doing to keep the problems going? After all, some of the responsibility *may* be mine.
   Try to identify the *pattern* that always leads to disaster in your relationship, discuss this with your partner or a close friend and try to change that pattern.

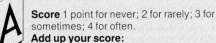

Score 1 point for never; 2 for rarely; 3 for sometimes; 4 for often.
Add up your score:
Under 20: You seem to have a rational view of life. Perhaps it is *too* rational and those around you might feel that you are a stable force but that sometimes life with you lacks a little sparkle.
20-30: You are lucky, you have a healthy, balanced outlook. You could, however, make life slightly easier for yourself by questioning some of your beliefs and expectations.
30-40: You suffer, as most people do, from some doubts and dissatisfactions. Accept who you are and make the most of yourself.
40-50: Look at your good points and take things less seriously. It's time for an overhaul of your ideas and actions.

TEST 3
Measure your self-esteem by answering the questions below and give yourself a score:

a = 1; b = 2; c = 3; d = 4

a Do you tend not to believe compliments?
b Do you like to be complimented?
c Do you know yourself and see compliments as irrelevant?
d Do you feel compliments are your due?

a Do you constantly criticize yourself?
b Do you feel most criticism of yourself justified?
c Do you welcome constructive criticism?
d Do you think a criticism is a jealous remark?

a Do you feel most at ease with people you consider inferior to you?
b Do you prefer to be with people like yourself?
c Do you enjoy meeting a variety of people?
d Do you prefer to mix with prestigious/powerful people?

a Do you need reassurance?
b Do you avoid disagreements?
c Do you trust your own judgement and capabilities?
d Are you *always* right?

TEST 4
What is your attitude to work?

a Do you feel over-tense at work?
b Do you see work as a means of self-fulfilment?
c Are you impatient to get back to work after a break?

a Do you blame yourself for every small mistake and feel angry or inadequate?
b Do you admit occasional failure and take it in your stride?
c Do you blame others for any mistakes?

a Do you always feel you are running to keep up and work overtime?
b Do you make sure you get enough breaks?
c Do you worry about tomorrow's tasks before you have completed today's?

a Do you work because you have to?
b Do you work to be useful/to learn/for mental stimulation/for enjoyment?
c Do you work for public recognition/prestige/power?

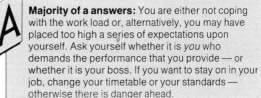

Majority of a answers: You are either not coping with the work load or, alternatively, you may have placed too high a series of expectations upon yourself. Ask yourself whether it is *you* who demands the performance that you provide — or whether it is your boss. If you want to stay on in your job, change your timetable or your standards — otherwise there is danger ahead.
Majority of b answers: You have a healthy, balanced attitude to work. You probably contribute a lot, derive satisfaction from your job and manage to lead a full life.
Majority of c answers: You are either an ambitious, but workaholic, employee, or you are extremely anxious about your performance. Be careful not to allow work to squeeze out your social life or your mental, physical and emotional well-being will suffer. Try to get your work into perspective.

Add up your score:
0-4: You seem to have an unnecessarily low opinion of yourself. Concentrate on your good points and try to take things less seriously. It's time to start doing things that will improve your self-confidence.
4-8: Start by selecting one aspect of yourself that you are least happy with and change it. Go on from there.
8-12: You are confident and seem to have a healthy and realistic view of yourself.
12-20: You probably disguise uncertainty behind arrogance. Try to find out how others see you and develop a greater understanding of yourself.

CAN YOU COPE?

All of us experience intense stress at certain periods in our lives. It usually occurs at times of change and is caused by events over which we do not always have control. However, many of us create our own psychological stresses, which, once identified, can be kept in check. Continual stress imposes a tremendous strain on the heart, it channels energy in unproductive directions and is extremely fatiguing. Resistance to disease, the ability to cope with even minor emotional and mental demands, and day-to-day performance are all severely impaired.

For more information on the causes, cures and side-effects of stress, see Chapter 9, The Whole Person pp. 224-61. For other advice about how to reduce stress, turn to Chapter 10, Treats and Treatments pp. 262-97 and Chapter 4, Getting Fit, Staying Fit pp. 86-133.

When you have pinpointed how best to control your own stress levels, put the ideas into practice and, after three months, retake these tests to see how effective you have been in resolving problem areas. If your stress ratings have not responded and you have not recently lived through a significant life crisis, turn again to the relevant pages for a different solution.

TEST 1
Is your personality stress-prone?

a Are you competitive and aggressive at work and in sports and games?
b If you lose a few points in a game, do you give up?
c Do you avoid any confrontation?

a Are you ambitious and anxious to achieve a lot?
b Do you wait for things to happen to you?
c Do you find excuses to put things off?

a Do you like to get things done quickly and often become impatient?
b Do you rely on other people to spur you into action?
c Do you often re-run the events of the day and worry about them?

a Do you talk fast, loudly and emphatically and interrupt a lot?
b Can you take 'no' for an answer with equanimity?
c Do you find it hard to express your feelings and anxieties?

a Do you get bored easily?
b Do you like having nothing to do?
c Do you always accommodate other people's wishes, not your own?

a Do you walk, eat and drink quickly?
b If you forget to do something do you not bother?
c Do you bottle things up?

For every 'yes' answer to an **a** question: score 6
For every 'yes' answer to a **b** question: score 4
For every 'yes' answer to a **c** question: score 2

Add up your score:
24-36: You live at a high-stress pace and may be prone to coronary heart disease, ulcers and so on. For your own sake, slow down, take time to relax. Look at your philosophy of life and perhaps take up a non-competitive hobby in your free time.
12-24: You are relaxed and free from stress. However, a certain amount of stress is healthy and a spur to positive achievement, and it may be an idea to be slightly more positive if you want to achieve more.
0-12: You create stress by inaction. First try to relieve any symptoms of stress, then start a campaign to build up your confidence, self-esteem and assertiveness. Make a list of your good points and concentrate on them.

Although there is a certain amount you can do to alter the way in which you react to situations and to those around you, it is difficult to change those aspects of your personality that have been present from an early age. Whether these aspects are determined by heredity or are a result of upbringing and environment is not clear, but their existence means that firmness of purpose is essential. It is well worth persisting in your attempts, however, especially if your personality puts your health at risk.

TEST 2
What is your stress score?

How many of the following life crises have you experienced in the last six months? Add up your score on this events table, worked out in America by Dr Richard Rahe, to find out how much 'stress cushioning' you need.

1	Death of a spouse	100
2	Divorce	73
3	Marital separation	65
4	Jail sentence	63
5	Death of a close family member	63
6	Personal injury or illness	53
7	Marriage	50
8	Sacking or redundancy	47
9	Marital reconciliation	45
10	Retirement	45
11	Change in health of a family member	44
12	Pregnancy	40
13	Sex difficulties	39
14	Gain of a new family member	39
15	Business readjustment	39
16	Change in financial state	38
17	Death of a close friend	37
18	Change to a different line of work	36
19	More or fewer arguments with a spouse	35
20	High mortgage or loan	31
21	Foreclosure of mortgage or loan	30
22	Change in responsibilities at work	29
23	Son or daughter leaving home	29
24	Trouble with in-laws	29
25	Outstanding personal achievement	28
26	Spouse beginning or stopping work	26
27	Beginning or ending school or college	26
28	Change in living conditions	25
29	Change in personal habits	24
30	Trouble with the boss	23
31	Change in work hours or conditions	20
32	Change in residence	20
33	Change in school or college	20
34	Change in recreation	19
35	Change in church activities	19
36	Change in social activities	18
37	Moderate mortgage or loan	17
38	Change in sleeping habits	16
39	More or fewer family get-togethers	15
40	Change in eating habits	15
41	Holiday	13
42	Christmas	12
43	Minor violations of the law	11

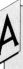

Add up your score:

100+: Your stress level has reached worrying proportions. You must change some aspect of your life to try and reduce that score.

80-100: You are over-stressed and your score is reaching the critical area. Look at the suggestions opposite to see if there is anything you can do to reduce your total. Learn to relax.

60-80: You are under the average amount of stress.

Up to 60: You are enjoying a particularly stress-free time. Make the most of it.

TEST 3
Do you display any of these symptoms of stress?

1 Do you often want to burst into tears?
2 Do you have any nervous tics/bite your nails/fidget/twiddle your hair?
3 Do you find it hard to concentrate and make decisions?
4 Do you feel you can't talk to anyone?
5 Do you often feel irritable, snappy and unsociable?
6 Do you eat when you aren't hungry?
7 Do you feel you can't cope?
8 Do you sometimes feel you'll explode?
9 Do you often drink/smoke to calm your nerves?
10 Do you sleep badly?
11 Do you rarely laugh/feel increasingly gloomy and suspicious of others?
12 Do you drive very fast?
13 Do you feel unenthusiastic/constantly tired?
14 Have you lost interest in sex?

If more than four of the above apply to you, you need to relax more and distract yourself. Identify the problem that you think may be leading to stress and do something about it. Also try some of the following:
— Listen to music — Take a break — Try meditation/yoga/relaxation — Exercise regularly — Buy a pet — Talk to a friend — Have a cuddle or a giggle — Make a list of the good things in life and enjoy some of them — Make time for other people — Buy yourself something new to wear — Smile at someone — Join a club.

HOW LONG MAY YOU LIVE?

The charts and questions on these pages will give you an idea of how long you can expect to live. Although there are a few fixed factors, most of us can take action to improve the quality and quantity of our lives. On average, for every person in the United Kingdom who is murdered, 6 die on the roads and 250 are killed prematurely by tobacco. In the USA, for every 6 people killed on the roads, 3 are murdered and nearly 200 die from smoking-related diseases. More information on improving life expectancy is to be found throughout this book.

TEST 1
Were you born with long life?

Your life expectancy is determined at birth by the time, the place and your genetic make-up. In developed countries, medical care, diet and preventive health care have improved conditions for life, so that a baby born in Europe in 1984 can expect to live 20 years longer than someone born in 1884. Statistics suggest that this trend will continue.

Famine and inadequate medical care in Third World countries keep life expectancy low, yet human greed, stress and laziness in the affluent nations still cause many premature deaths. In most countries, women live, on average, 5 to 8 years longer than men — and the gap is widening. Whites live, on average, 4 to 5 years longer than blacks, but in this respect the gap is beginning to narrow.

TEST 2
Have you inherited a long life?

If your mother and father lived, or are still living to a healthy old age, then you too stand the chance of a long life. If either of your parents died prematurely, this may affect your odds for survival.

Many of the diseases that shorten life to less than the average span have a hereditary element. Most obvious of these are diseases such as spina bifida, cystic fibrosis haemophilia and raised blood cholesterol (hyperlipidaemia) Although there is no way in which a genetic pathway can be traced for the inheritance of diseases such as diabetes, breast cancer and gall bladder disease, there is no doubt that a tendency toward these does run in families. With good preventive health care their onset can be delayed. And if they are detected early, successful treatment is often possible.

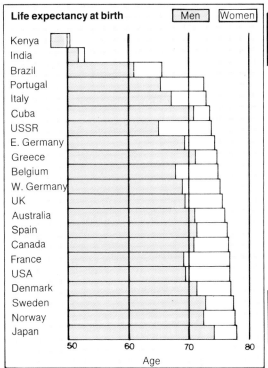

Life expectancy at birth | Men | Women

Kenya, India, Brazil, Portugal, Italy, Cuba, USSR, E. Germany, Greece, Belgium, W. Germany, UK, Australia, Spain, Canada, France, USA, Denmark, Sweden, Norway, Japan

50 60 70 80
Age

TEST 3
A matter of life and death: are you helping yourself?

1 Do you drink more than 2 pints of beer or 2 measures of spirits a day?
2 Do you have high blood pressure?
3 Do you regularly eat fried and high-fat foods?
4 Do you weigh more than the acceptable average for your height?
5 Do you ever smoke cigarettes?
6 Do you take little or no exercise?
7 Do you eat meat more than once a day?
8 Do you take drugs/sniff glue?
9 Do you live near a nuclear power station or waste dump?
10 Do you work in a dangerous environment?
11 Do you live in a violent neighbourhood?
12 Do you have a highly-stressed lifestyle?
13 Do you drive every day?

If you answered 'yes' to any of the above questions then you are risking an early death. If you are happy to take the risk and continue as before, it is your choice. If your aim is a long life, avoid *all* the above and take plenty of aerobic exercise.

TEST 4
What are the risks of smoking?

If you smoke cigarettes, refer to the chart *(right)* to see how it is reducing your life expectancy. If you have given up cigarette smoking, add a year for each five years since you stopped. The number of years lost from life expectancy through smoking is reduced as you get older because of the naturally shorter expectation of life. But the percentage of years lost through smoking *increases* with advancing age, so that a 65-year-old smoker stands to lose proportionally more years of those that remain than a 20-year-old.

The percentage of men aged 35 whose smoking habits will cause death before 65

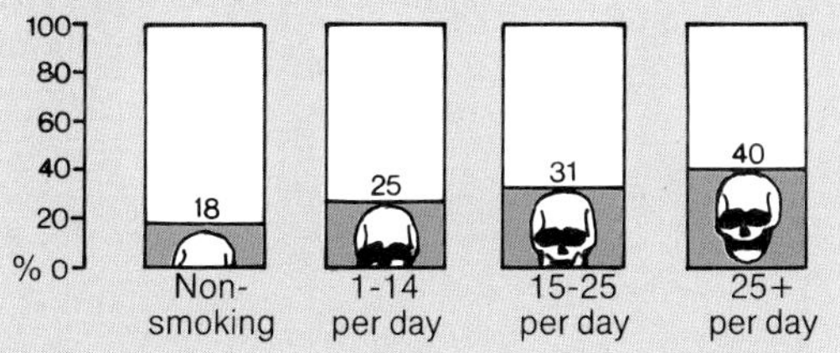

TEST 5
How will you die?

The cause of your death will depend, as the chart below indicates, on where you live. In the developed world (dark bands) deaths from heart disease and cancer predominate. In the developing world (lighter bands) respiratory and infectious diseases and are more common causes of death. The differences are due to lifestyle and medical care.

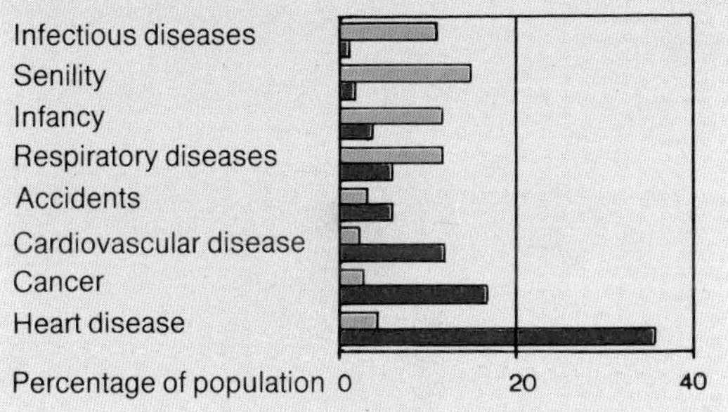

Present age	Cigarettes/ day	Years expected	Years lost
25 years	0	48·6	
	1 – 9	44·0	4·6
	10 – 19	43·1	5·5
	20 – 39	42·4	6·2
30 years	0	43·9	
	1 – 9	39·3	4·6
	10 – 19	38·4	5·5
	20 – 39	37·8	6·1
35 years	0	39·2	
	1 – 9	34·7	4·5
	10 – 19	33·8	5·4
	20 – 39	33·2	6·1
40 years	0	34·5	
	1 – 9	30·3	4·3
	10 – 19	29·3	5·2
	20 – 39	28·3	5·2
45 years	0	30·0	
	1 – 19	25·9	4·1
	10 – 29	25·0	5·0
	20 – 39	24·4	5·6
50 years	0	25·6	
	1 – 9	21·8	3·8
	10 – 9	21·0	4·6
	20 – 9	21·5	5·1
55 years	0	21·4	
	1 – 9	17·9	3·1
	10 – 19	17·4	4·0
	20 – 39	17·0	4·4
60 years	0	17·6	
	1 – 9	14·5	3·1
	10 – 19	14·1	3·5
	20 – 39	13·7	3·9
65 years	0	14·7	
	1 – 9	11·3	2·8
	10 – 19	11·2	2·9
	20 – 39	11·0	3·1

25

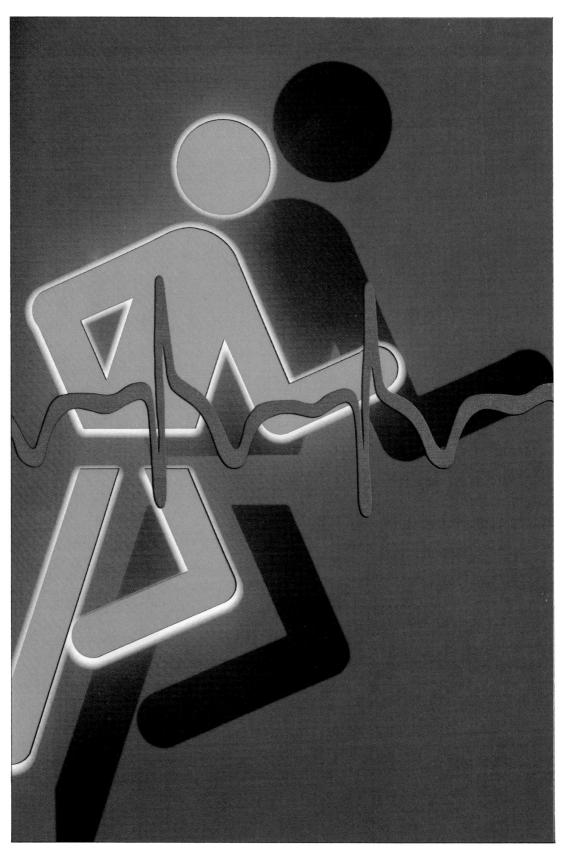

WHOLE LIFE PROGRAMMES

Whatever your age, positive thinking is one of the most important attributes to cultivate if you are to achieve and maintain a state of fitness and well-being. With improved quality and length of life as your aims, you need to work out the individual steps that make up the stairway to this achievement.

The whole life programmes which make up this chapter are constructed so as to help you work out those steps as they apply to your own life. At the same time, they will help you, by means of coded cross-references, to gain access to the wealth of informative and constructive material contained in the main part of this book. The programmes are devised to take account of the major changes that occur in our bodies and lifestyles as we get older and are grouped to account for the risks to fitness and well-being shared by people of a similar age and/or sex.

The goals that make up each programme are of two kinds. The first are specific goals related to various areas of your lifestyle and preventive health care. These are divided into five categories: emotional and mental health (including leisure); fitness and body care; work, finance and family; food and drink; and health checks. Following these, at the apex of each 'board game' are some general goals which, apart from the youngest age groups, are the same for all ages and sexes. These general goals apply to the central aspects of healthy living, namely diet, exercise, stress, smoking and drinking. Without regard to these general goals, it is impossible to reach the central goal of each programme — the achievement of fitness and well-being.

Before you make a start on the programme tailored to your own age group and, if appropriate, your sex, try the quizzes on pp. 10-25 and find out which areas of your life are in need of most attention. Then, with these in mind, work your way through your whole life programme, setting yourself new targets as you go. Of course there may well be some goals that you have already achieved — if so, well and good. But remember that to maintain fitness and well being you must keep up the improvement for life.

GROWING UP

In the formative years between birth and the age of 13, children change from babies into young people, who have, or who are about to acquire, a male or female sexuality. The childhood years are those in which habits of living are formed — habits which are hard to break in later life. This makes it especially important for parents to help and encourage children to aim for healthy goals in life, so that the foundations of fitness and well-being are secured. Parents should also help children establish a code of behaviour that will stand them in good stead as adult citizens.

Chapter references

Eating for Health pp.52-85

Your Sexuality pp.158-85

Getting Fit, Staying Fit pp.86-133

The Whole Person pp.224-61

Head to Toe pp.134-57

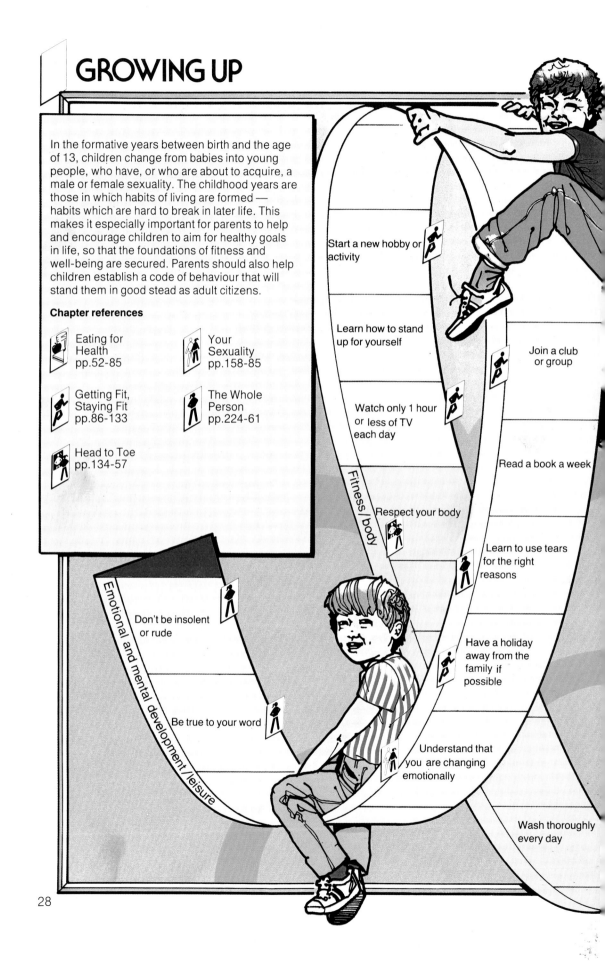

Start a new hobby or activity

Learn how to stand up for yourself

Watch only 1 hour or less of TV each day

Fitness / body

Respect your body

Join a club or group

Read a book a week

Learn to use tears for the right reasons

Have a holiday away from the family if possible

Emotional and mental development / leisure

Don't be insolent or rude

Be true to your word

Understand that you are changing emotionally

Wash thoroughly every day

CHILDREN 0-13

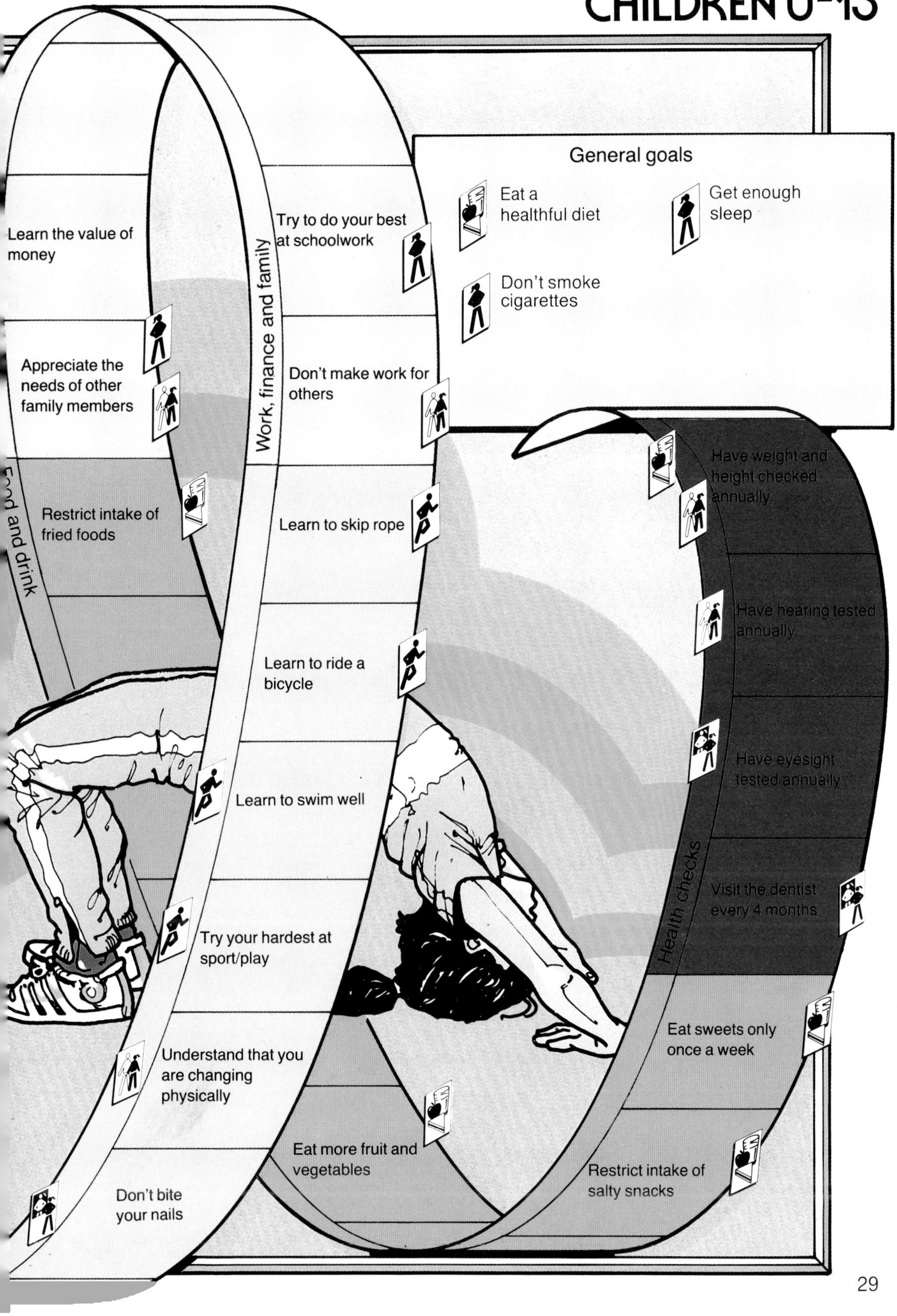

General goals

Eat a healthful diet

Get enough sleep

Don't smoke cigarettes

Work, finance and family

Learn the value of money

Appreciate the needs of other family members

Try to do your best at schoolwork

Don't make work for others

Food and drink

Restrict intake of fried foods

Learn to skip rope

Learn to ride a bicycle

Learn to swim well

Try your hardest at sport/play

Understand that you are changing physically

Don't bite your nails

Eat more fruit and vegetables

Health checks

Have weight and height checked annually

Have hearing tested annually

Have eyesight tested annually

Visit the dentist every 4 months

Eat sweets only once a week

Restrict intake of salty snacks

FINDING AN IDENTITY

The tempestuous teens, the years of rebellion, are those in which youngsters tend to reject — though often temporarily — the standards of their parents and teachers. These are the years of experimentation, but, under pressure from their peers, it is hard for many to resist high-risk temptations such as drugs. Parents should ease young people through these problem years sympathetically.

Chapter references

Eating for Health pp.52-85

Getting Fit, Staying Fit pp.86-133

Head to Toe pp.134-57

The Whole Person pp.224-61

Your Sexuality pp.158-85

Pregnancy and Birth pp.186-203

Treats and Treatments pp.262-97

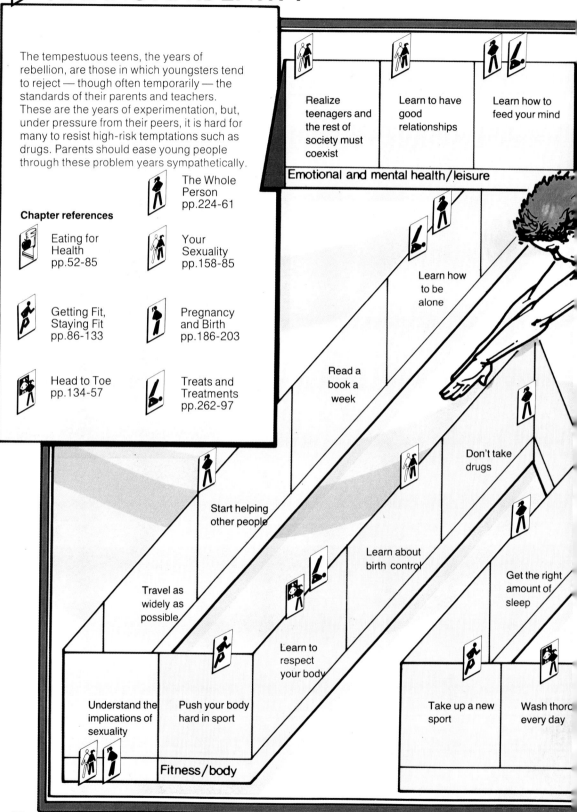

Realize teenagers and the rest of society must coexist

Learn to have good relationships

Learn how to feed your mind

Emotional and mental health/leisure

Learn how to be alone

Read a book a week

Don't take drugs

Start helping other people

Learn about birth control

Get the right amount of sleep

Travel as widely as possible

Learn to respect your body

Understand the implications of sexuality

Push your body hard in sport

Take up a new sport

Wash thoro every day

Fitness/body

TEENAGERS 14-18

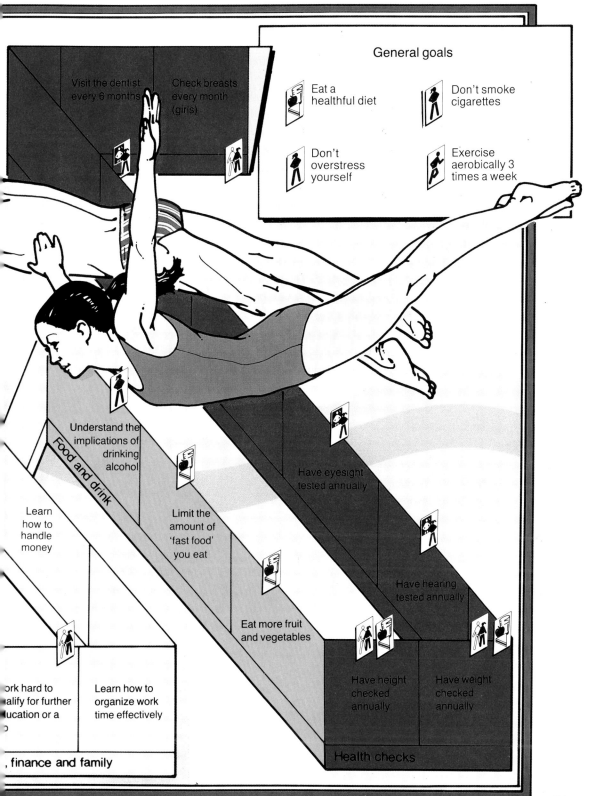

General goals

Eat a healthful diet

Don't smoke cigarettes

Don't overstress yourself

Exercise aerobically 3 times a week

Visit the dentist every 6 months

Check breasts every month (girls)

Food and drink

Understand the implications of drinking alcohol

Learn how to handle money

Limit the amount of 'fast food' you eat

Eat more fruit and vegetables

Have eyesight tested annually

Have hearing tested annually

ork hard to alify for further ucation or a

Learn how to organize work time effectively

Have height checked annually

Have weight checked annually

, finance and family

Health checks

31

YOUNG ADULTS

The early 20s are years of risk-taking —
car accidents are the greatest killers of
men in this age group. These years are
also ones of peak physical prowess, in
which the body should be pushed hard.
Both career and social goals are pursued
with vigour. In their jobs, young men find
themselves having to compete as adults
in an adult world for the first time — there
is no longer the licence allowed to
teenagers to fall back on. Socially, the
experimental phase started in the teens
continues for a while, but 24 is the
average age for 'first' marriage in the
USA and UK.

Chapter references

Eating for
Health
pp.52-85

Getting Fit,
Staying Fit
pp.86-133

Head to Toe
pp.134-57

Your
Sexuality
pp.158-85

Pregnancy
and Birth
pp.186-203

The Whole
Person
pp.224-61

Treats and
Treatments
pp.262-97

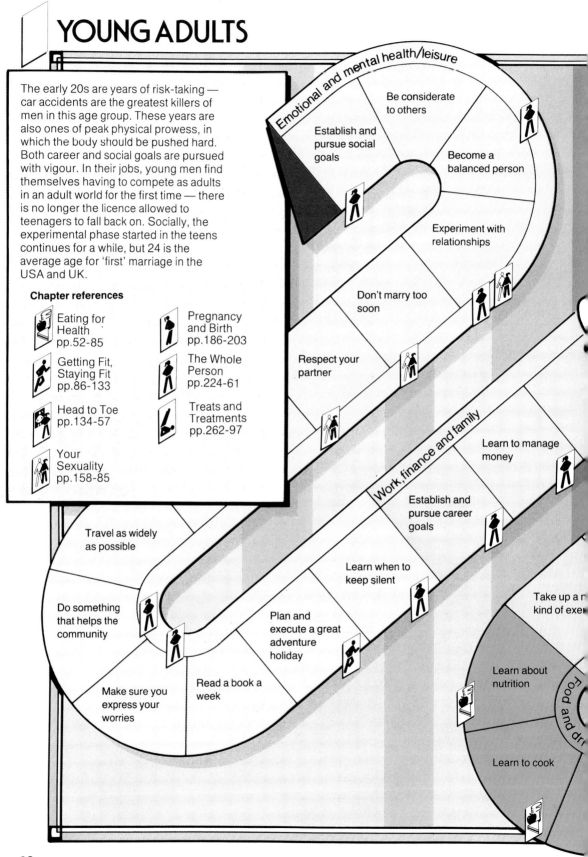

Emotional and mental health/leisure

Be considerate
to others

Establish and
pursue social
goals

Become a
balanced person

Experiment with
relationships

Don't marry too
soon

Respect your
partner

Work, finance and family

Learn to manage
money

Establish and
pursue career
goals

Learn when to
keep silent

Take up a new
kind of exercise

Travel as widely
as possible

Do something
that helps the
community

Plan and
execute a great
adventure
holiday

Learn about
nutrition

Make sure you
express your
worries

Read a book a
week

Learn to cook

Food and drink

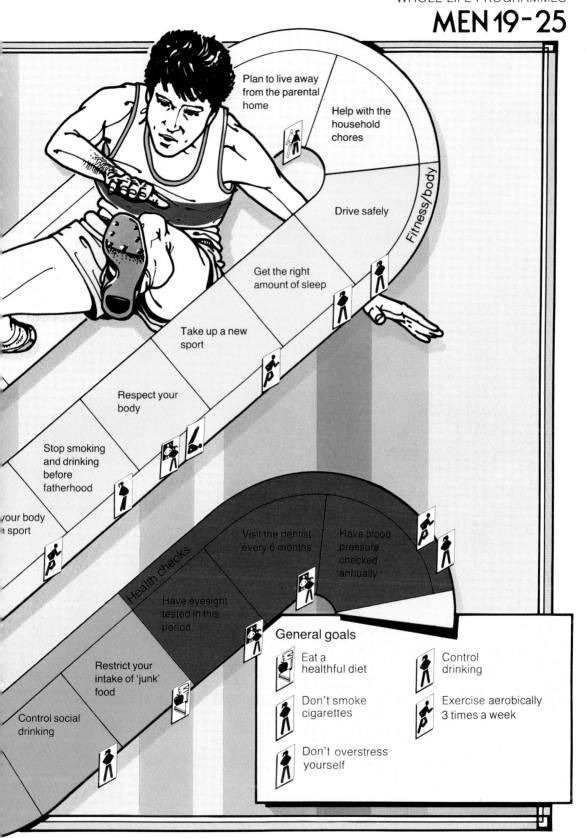

Plan to live away from the parental home

Help with the household chores

Drive safely

Fitness/body

Get the right amount of sleep

Take up a new sport

Respect your body

Stop smoking and drinking before fatherhood

your body n sport

Health checks

Visit the dentist every 6 months

Have blood pressure checked annually

Have eyesight tested in this period

Restrict your intake of 'junk' food

Control social drinking

General goals

Eat a healthful diet

Don't smoke cigarettes

Don't overstress yourself

Control drinking

Exercise aerobically 3 times a week

YOUNG ADULTS

For young women between 20 and 25, career and social goals tend to take equal priority. But while many will be preoccupied with establishing their careers, 20 is also the average age at which women in the USA and UK marry for the 'first' time. This fact underlines the difficult decision young women have to make in balancing career, partner and children. Although these are the safest years for childbearing, habits such as regular breast checks and cervical smears should become permanently established.

Chapter references

Eating for Health pp.52-85

Pregnancy and Birth pp.186-203

Getting Fit, Staying Fit pp.86-133

The Whole Person pp.224.61

Head to Toe pp.134-57

Treats and Treatments pp.262-97

Your Sexuality pp.158-85

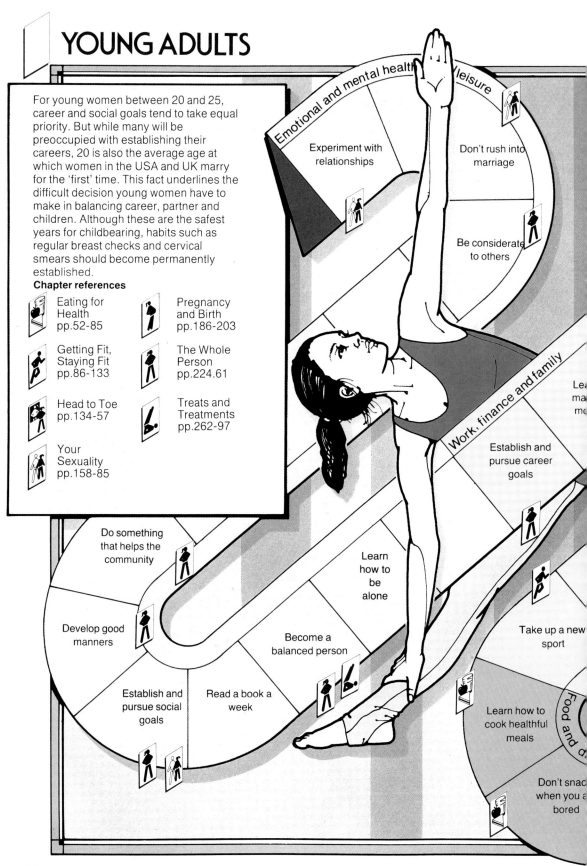

Emotional and mental health / leisure

Experiment with relationships

Don't rush into marriage

Be considerate to others

Work, finance and family

Le... ma... m...

Establish and pursue career goals

Do something that helps the community

Learn how to be alone

Take up a new sport

Develop good manners

Become a balanced person

Establish and pursue social goals

Read a book a week

Food and d...

Learn how to cook healthful meals

Don't snac... when you a... bored

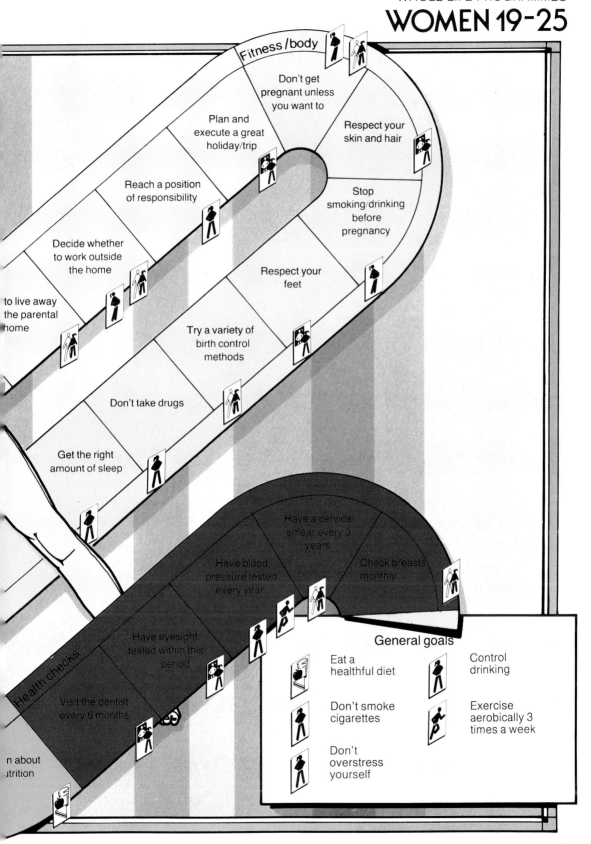

Fitness/body

Don't get pregnant unless you want to

Plan and execute a great holiday/trip

Respect your skin and hair

Reach a position of responsibility

Stop smoking/drinking before pregnancy

Decide whether to work outside the home

Respect your feet

to live away the parental home

Try a variety of birth control methods

Don't take drugs

Get the right amount of sleep

Have a cervical smear every 3 years

Have blood pressure tested every year

Check breasts monthly

Have eyesight tested within this period

Health checks

Visit the dentist every 6 months

n about utrition

General goals

Eat a healthful diet

Control drinking

Don't smoke cigarettes

Exercise aerobically 3 times a week

Don't overstress yourself

SETTLING DOWN

The years between 26 and 35 are those in which young men begin to 'sober up', a fact often related to the new duties of fatherhood and home ownership. In their careers, young men are, similarly, moving on and reaching positions of responsibility. However, these are years in which the risk of diseases of the heart and circulation in men begins to rise, and it is thus important that the goals of fitness and well-being include those specifically related to the prevention of heart and circulatory disease, including attention to diet and exercise, and not smoking cigarettes.

Chapter references

Eating for Health pp.52-85

Your Sexuality pp.158-85

Getting Fit, Staying Fit pp.86-133

The Whole Person pp.224-61

Head to Toe pp.134-57

Treats and Treatments pp.262-97

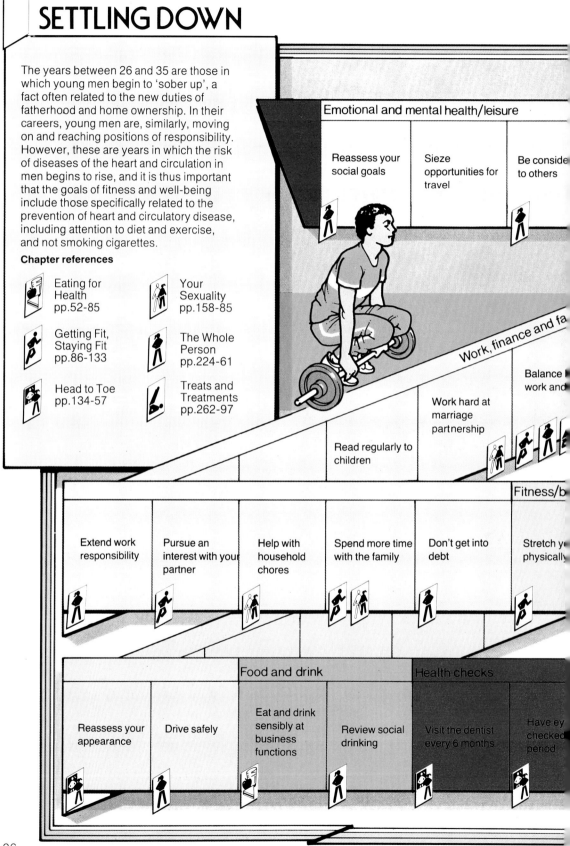

Emotional and mental health/leisure

Reassess your social goals

Sieze opportunities for travel

Be conside to others

Work, finance and fa

Work hard at marriage partnership

Balance work and

Read regularly to children

Fitness/b

Extend work responsibility

Pursue an interest with your partner

Help with household chores

Spend more time with the family

Don't get into debt

Stretch y physically

Food and drink

Health checks

Reassess your appearance

Drive safely

Eat and drink sensibly at business functions

Review social drinking

Visit the dentist every 6 months

Have ey checked period

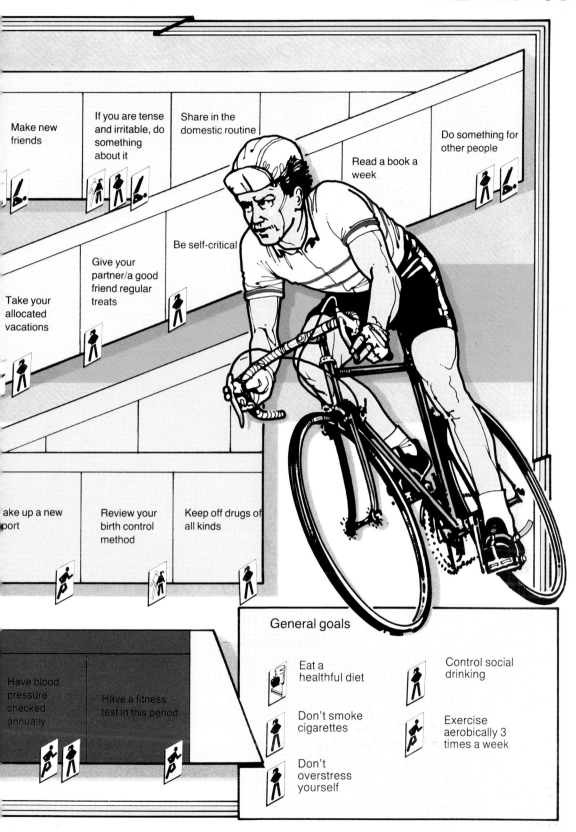

Make new friends

If you are tense and irritable, do something about it

Share in the domestic routine

Read a book a week

Do something for other people

Be self-critical

Give your partner/a good friend regular treats

Take your allocated vacations

ake up a new port

Review your birth control method

Keep off drugs of all kinds

Have blood pressure checked annually

Have a fitness test in this period

General goals

Eat a healthful diet

Control social drinking

Don't smoke cigarettes

Exercise aerobically 3 times a week

Don't overstress yourself

SETTLING DOWN

From their mid-20s to their mid-30s, the majority of women are concerned with completing their families. Childbearing now becomes increasingly risky, and in this age group the risk of death from cancer of the breasts and cervix also rises, making gynaecological health paramount. In their careers, women between 26 and 35 often change direction, a move commonly related to motherhood. For marriages, these are dangerous years, with divorce at its height. This is reflected by the fact that, in the USA, 34 is the average age at which a woman marries a second time.

Chapter references

Eating for
Health
pp.52-85

Pregnancy
and Birth
pp.186-203

Getting Fit,
Staying Fit
pp.86-133

The Whole
Person
pp.224-61

Head to Toe
pp.134-57

Treats and
Treatments
pp.262-97

Your
Sexuality
pp.158-85

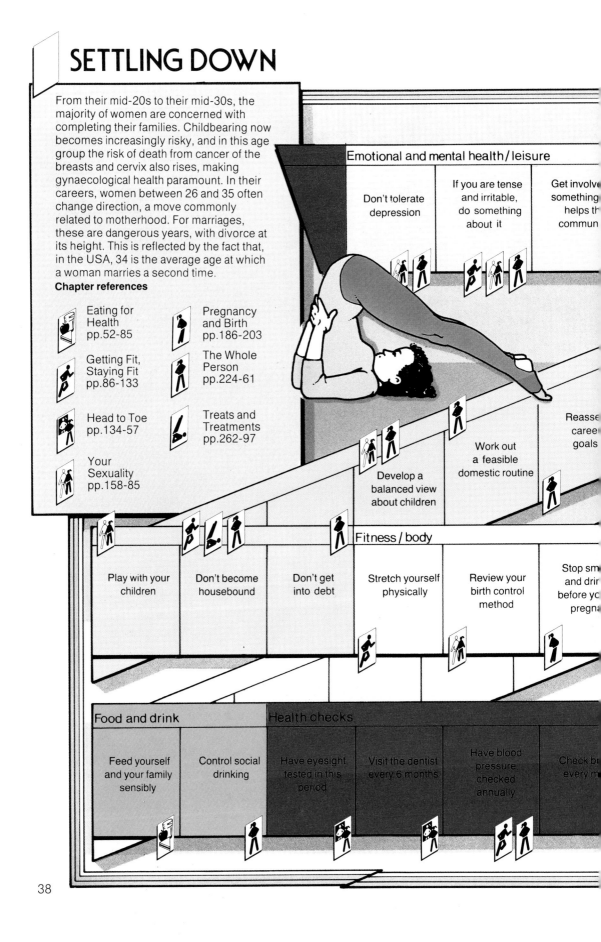

Emotional and mental health / leisure

Don't tolerate depression

If you are tense and irritable, do something about it

Get involve something helps th commun

Reasse caree goals

Develop a balanced view about children

Work out a feasible domestic routine

Fitness / body

Play with your children

Don't become housebound

Don't get into debt

Stretch yourself physically

Review your birth control method

Stop sm and drir before yc pregna

Food and drink

Feed yourself and your family sensibly

Control social drinking

Health checks

Have eyesight tested in this period

Visit the dentist every 6 months

Have blood pressure checked annually

Check br every m

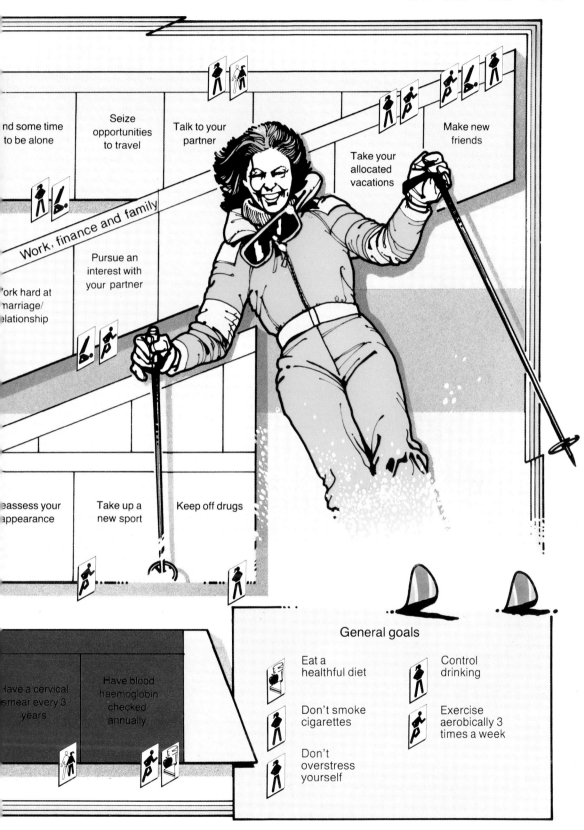

nd some time to be alone

Seize opportunities to travel

Talk to your partner

Take your allocated vacations

Make new friends

Work, finance and family

Pursue an interest with your partner

ork hard at marriage/ relationship

eassess your appearance

Take up a new sport

Keep off drugs

Have a cervical smear every 3 years

Have blood haemoglobin checked annually

General goals

Eat a healthful diet

Control drinking

Don't smoke cigarettes

Exercise aerobically 3 times a week

Don't overstress yourself

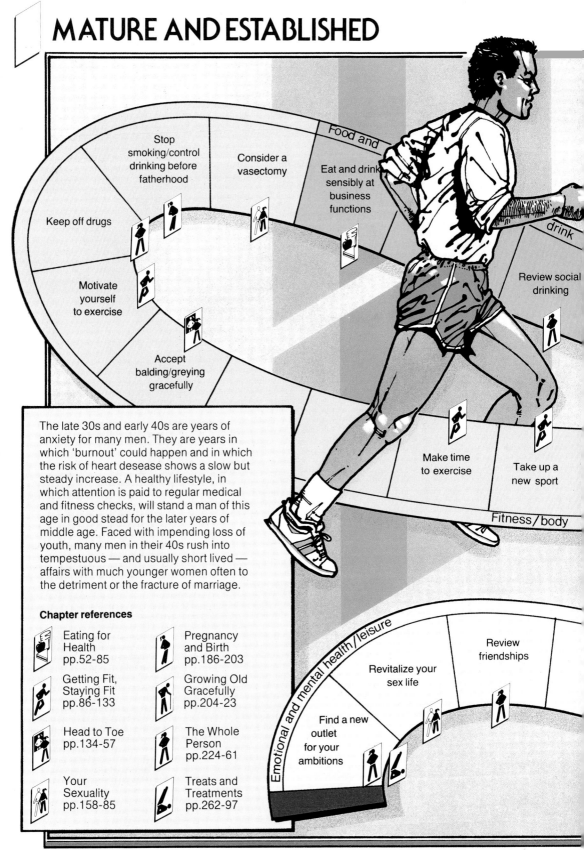

Stop smoking/control drinking before fatherhood

Consider a vasectomy

Eat and drink sensibly at business functions

Food and

Keep off drugs

drink

Review social drinking

Motivate yourself to exercise

Accept balding/greying gracefully

Make time to exercise

Take up a new sport

Fitness/body

The late 30s and early 40s are years of anxiety for many men. They are years in which 'burnout' could happen and in which the risk of heart desease shows a slow but steady increase. A healthy lifestyle, in which attention is paid to regular medical and fitness checks, will stand a man of this age in good stead for the later years of middle age. Faced with impending loss of youth, many men in their 40s rush into tempestuous — and usually short lived — affairs with much younger women often to the detriment or the fracture of marriage.

Chapter references

Eating for Health
pp.52-85

Pregnancy and Birth
pp.186-203

Getting Fit, Staying Fit
pp.86-133

Growing Old Gracefully
pp.204-23

Head to Toe
pp.134-57

The Whole Person
pp.224-61

Your Sexuality
pp.158-85

Treats and Treatments
pp.262-97

Emotional and mental health/leisure

Review friendships

Revitalize your sex life

Find a new outlet for your ambitions

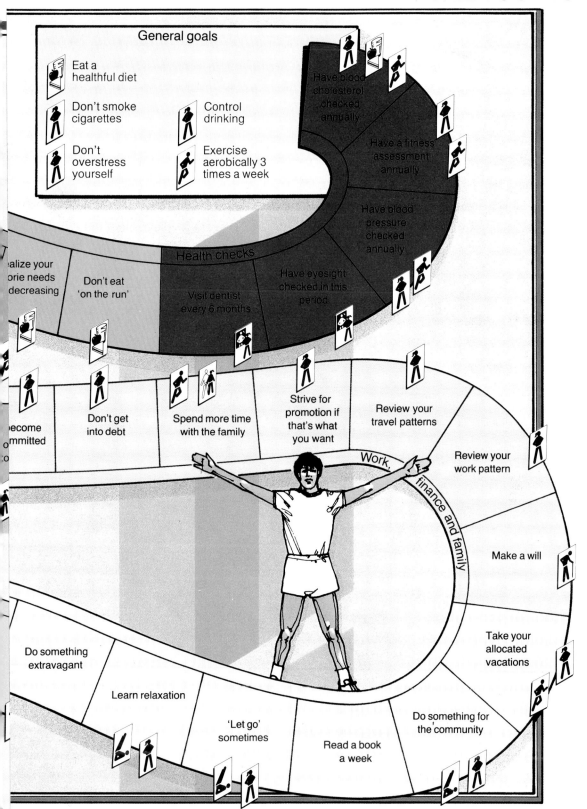

General goals

Eat a healthful diet

Don't smoke cigarettes

Control drinking

Don't overstress yourself

Exercise aerobically 3 times a week

Have blood cholesterol checked annually

Have a fitness assessment annually

Have blood pressure checked annually

Health checks

realize your orie needs decreasing

Don't eat 'on the run'

Visit dentist every 6 months

Have eyesight checked in this period

ecome ommitted o

Don't get into debt

Spend more time with the family

Strive for promotion if that's what you want

Review your travel patterns

Work, finance and family

Review your work pattern

Make a will

Take your allocated vacations

Do something extravagant

Learn relaxation

'Let go' sometimes

Read a book a week

Do something for the community

INTO MIDDLE AGE

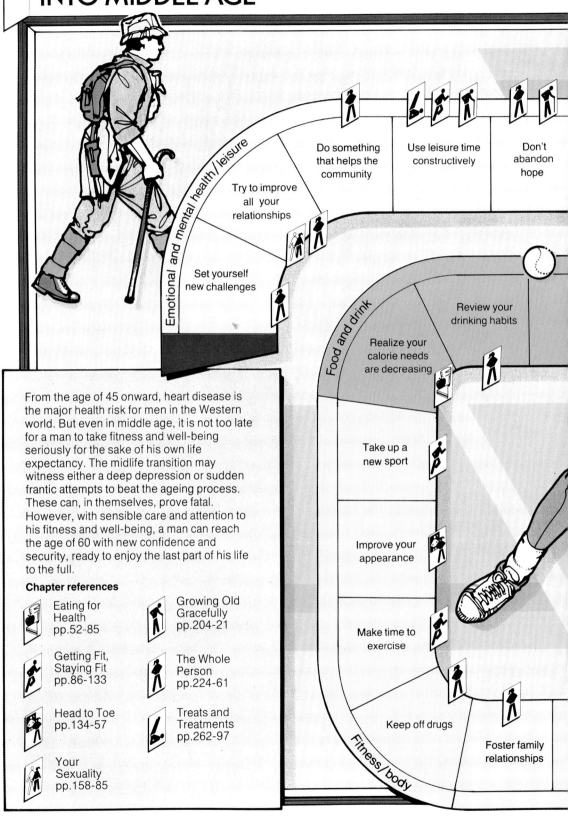

Emotional and mental health/leisure

Try to improve all your relationships

Do something that helps the community

Use leisure time constructively

Don't abandon hope

Set yourself new challenges

Food and drink

Realize your calorie needs are decreasing

Review your drinking habits

Take up a new sport

Improve your appearance

Make time to exercise

Keep off drugs

Foster family relationships

Fitness/body

From the age of 45 onward, heart disease is the major health risk for men in the Western world. But even in middle age, it is not too late for a man to take fitness and well-being seriously for the sake of his own life expectancy. The midlife transition may witness either a deep depression or sudden frantic attempts to beat the ageing process. These can, in themselves, prove fatal. However, with sensible care and attention to his fitness and well-being, a man can reach the age of 60 with new confidence and security, ready to enjoy the last part of his life to the full.

Chapter references

Eating for Health pp.52-85

Getting Fit, Staying Fit pp.86-133

Head to Toe pp.134-57

Your Sexuality pp.158-85

Growing Old Gracefully pp.204-21

The Whole Person pp.224-61

Treats and Treatments pp.262-97

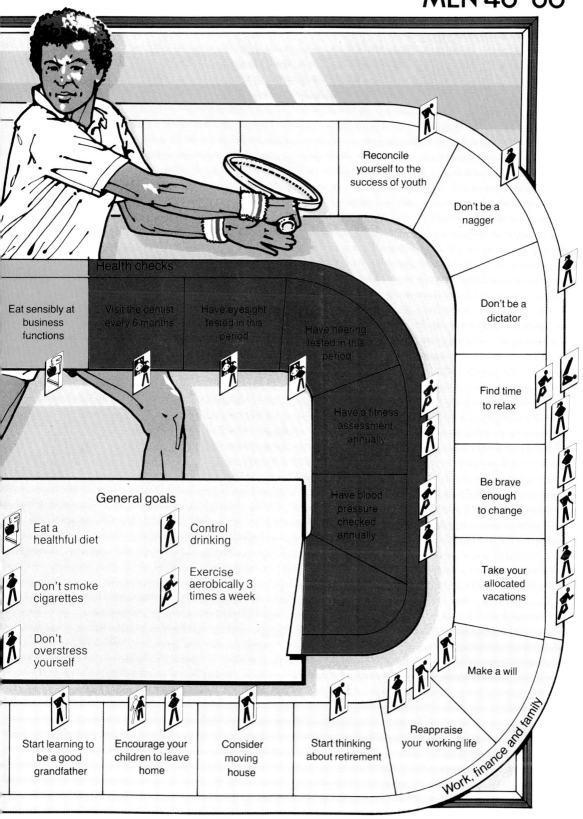

Reconcile yourself to the success of youth

Don't be a nagger

Don't be a dictator

Find time to relax

Be brave enough to change

Take your allocated vacations

Make a will

Health checks

Eat sensibly at business functions

Visit the dentist every 6 months

Have eyesight tested in this period

Have hearing tested in this period

Have a fitness assessment annually

Have blood pressure checked annually

General goals

Eat a healthful diet

Don't smoke cigarettes

Don't overstress yourself

Control drinking

Exercise aerobically 3 times a week

Start learning to be a good grandfather

Encourage your children to leave home

Consider moving house

Start thinking about retirement

Reappraise your working life

Work, finance and family

INTO MIDDLE AGE

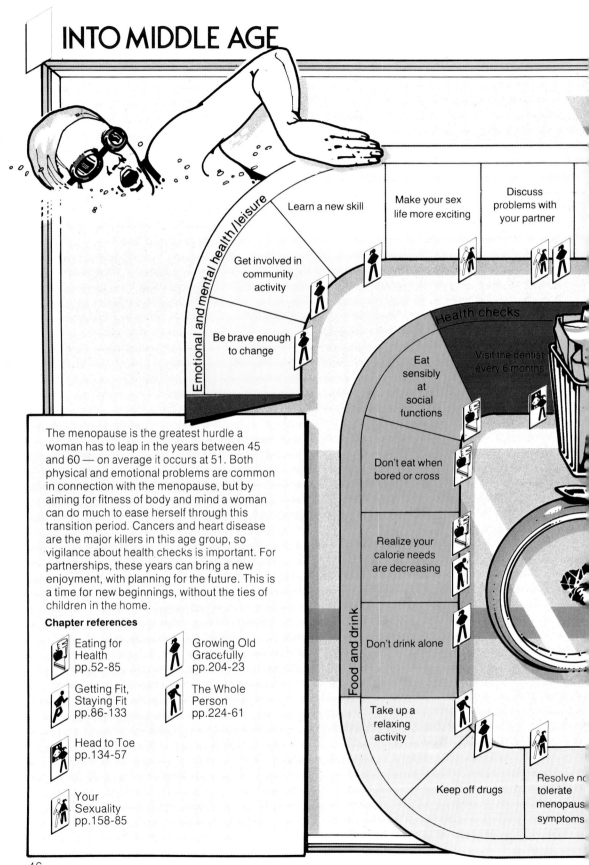

Emotional and mental health/leisure

Learn a new skill

Make your sex life more exciting

Discuss problems with your partner

Get involved in community activity

Be brave enough to change

Health checks

Eat sensibly at social functions

Visit the dentist every 6 months

Don't eat when bored or cross

Realize your calorie needs are decreasing

Food and drink

Don't drink alone

Take up a relaxing activity

Keep off drugs

Resolve no tolerate menopaus symptoms

The menopause is the greatest hurdle a woman has to leap in the years between 45 and 60 — on average it occurs at 51. Both physical and emotional problems are common in connection with the menopause, but by aiming for fitness of body and mind a woman can do much to ease herself through this transition period. Cancers and heart disease are the major killers in this age group, so vigilance about health checks is important. For partnerships, these years can bring a new enjoyment, with planning for the future. This is a time for new beginnings, without the ties of children in the home.

Chapter references

Eating for Health
pp.52-85

Growing Old Gracefully
pp.204-23

Getting Fit, Staying Fit
pp.86-133

The Whole Person
pp.224-61

Head to Toe
pp.134-57

Your Sexuality
pp.158-85

WOMEN 46-60

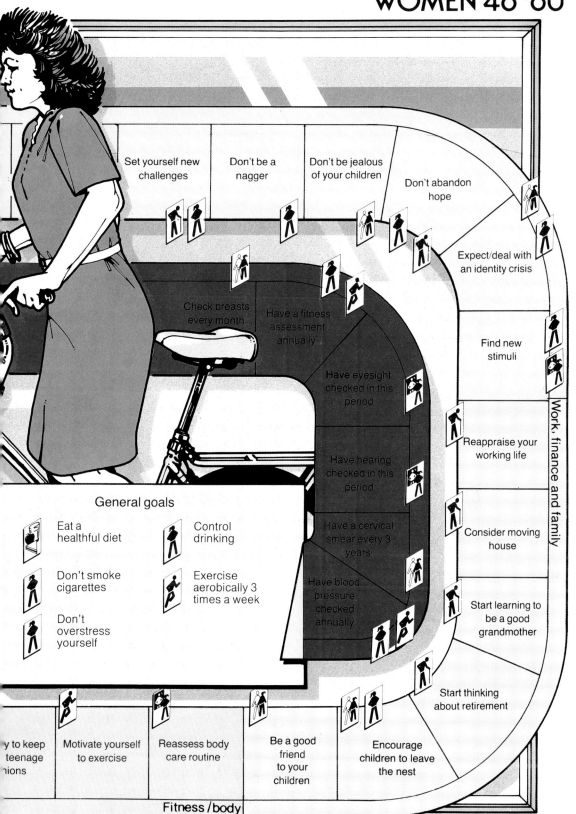

Set yourself new challenges

Don't be a nagger

Don't be jealous of your children

Don't abandon hope

Expect/deal with an identity crisis

Find new stimuli

Check breasts every month

Have a fitness assessment annually

Have eyesight checked in this period

Have hearing checked in this period

Have a cervical smear every 3 years

Have blood pressure checked annually

Reappraise your working life

Consider moving house

Start learning to be a good grandmother

Start thinking about retirement

Work, finance and family

General goals

Eat a healthful diet

Control drinking

Don't smoke cigarettes

Exercise aerobically 3 times a week

Don't overstress yourself

y to keep teenage nions

Motivate yourself to exercise

Reassess body care routine

Be a good friend to your children

Encourage children to leave the nest

Fitness / body

ADJUSTING TO RETIREMENT

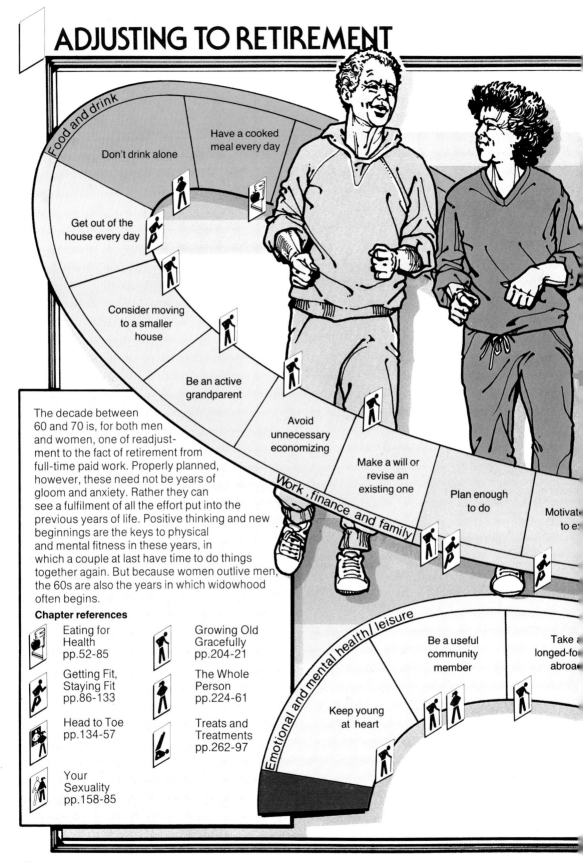

Food and drink

Don't drink alone

Have a cooked meal every day

Get out of the house every day

Consider moving to a smaller house

Be an active grandparent

Avoid unnecessary economizing

Work, finance and family

Make a will or revise an existing one

Plan enough to do

Motivate to e…

The decade between 60 and 70 is, for both men and women, one of readjustment to the fact of retirement from full-time paid work. Properly planned, however, these need not be years of gloom and anxiety. Rather they can see a fulfilment of all the effort put into the previous years of life. Positive thinking and new beginnings are the keys to physical and mental fitness in these years, in which a couple at last have time to do things together again. But because women outlive men, the 60s are also the years in which widowhood often begins.

Chapter references

Eating for Health pp.52-85

Getting Fit, Staying Fit pp.86-133

Head to Toe pp.134-57

Your Sexuality pp.158-85

Growing Old Gracefully pp.204-21

The Whole Person pp.224-61

Treats and Treatments pp.262-97

Emotional and mental health / leisure

Be a useful community member

Take a longed-fo… abroa…

Keep young at heart

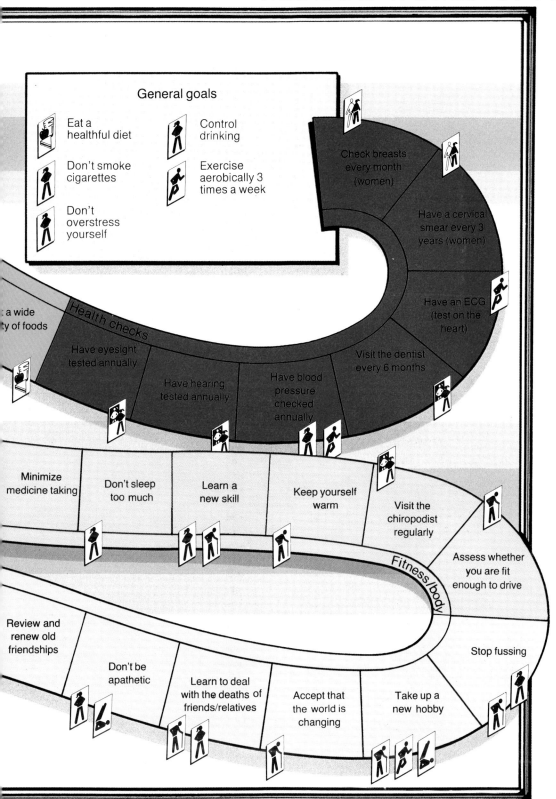

General goals

- Eat a healthful diet
- Don't smoke cigarettes
- Don't overstress yourself
- Control drinking
- Exercise aerobically 3 times a week

Health checks

- Check breasts every month (women)
- Have a cervical smear every 3 years (women)
- Have an ECG (test on the heart)
- Visit the dentist every 6 months
- Have blood pressure checked annually
- Have hearing tested annually
- Have eyesight tested annually
- a wide ty of foods

- Minimize medicine taking
- Don't sleep too much
- Learn a new skill
- Keep yourself warm
- Visit the chiropodist regularly
- Assess whether you are fit enough to drive
- Stop fussing

Fitness/body

- Review and renew old friendships
- Don't be apathetic
- Learn to deal with the deaths of friends/relatives
- Accept that the world is changing
- Take up a new hobby

OLD AND GRACEFUL

The years over the 'allotted' life span of 70 should be, above all, enjoyed to the full. History shows a staggering range of achievements by men and women over 70, and there is no need for anyone to shirk from reaching new heights in the last decades of their life. Of course these are years in which illness and the ageing process take their toll, but a youthful attitude to fitness and well-being will pay enormous dividends in terms of the quality and length of life.

Chapter references

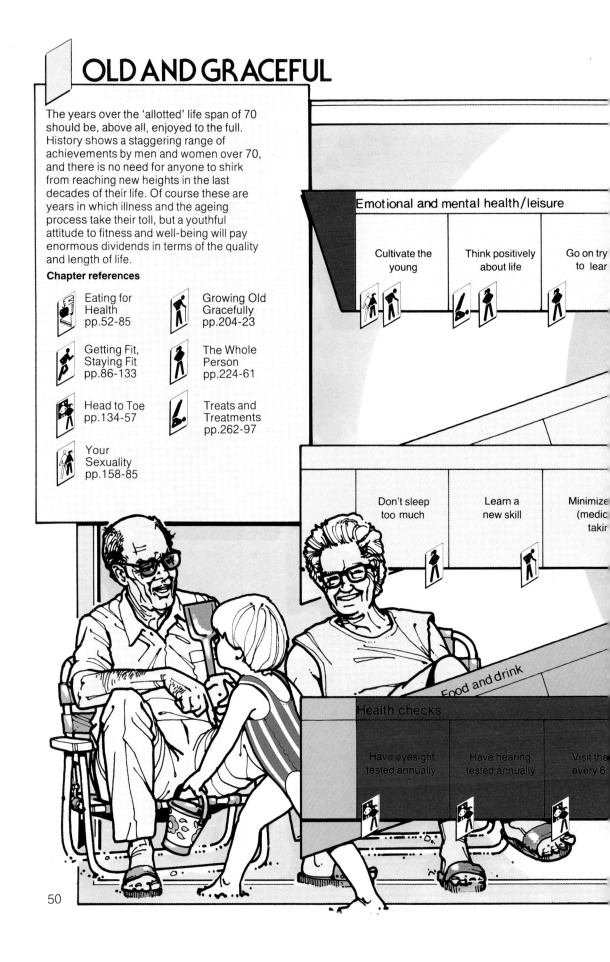

Emotional and mental health/leisure

Cultivate the young

Think positively about life

Go on try to lear

Don't sleep too much

Learn a new skill

Minimize (medic takir

Food and drink

Health checks

Have eyesight tested annually

Have hearing tested annually

Visit the every 6

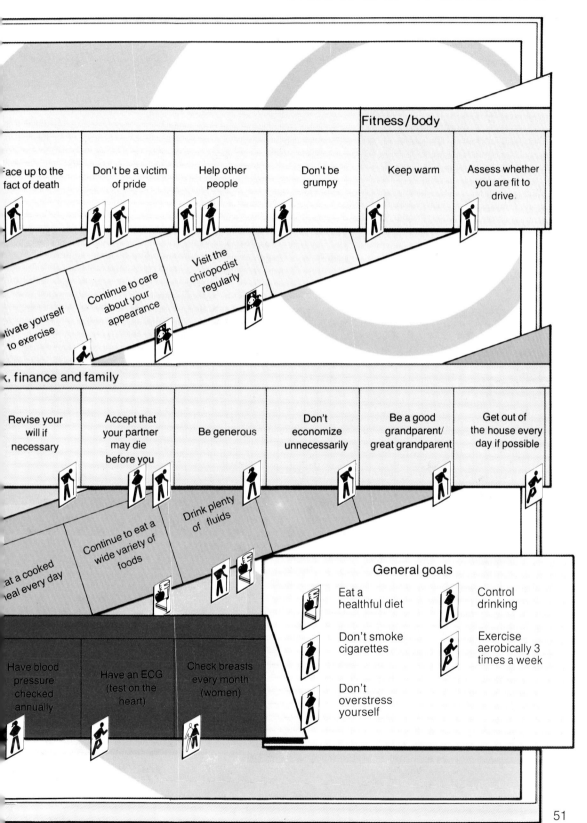

Fitness/body

Face up to the fact of death	Don't be a victim of pride	Help other people	Don't be grumpy	Keep warm	Assess whether you are fit to drive

Motivate yourself to exercise | Continue to care about your appearance | Visit the chiropodist regularly

Work, finance and family

Revise your will if necessary	Accept that your partner may die before you	Be generous	Don't economize unnecessarily	Be a good grandparent/ great grandparent	Get out of the house every day if possible

Eat a cooked meal every day | Continue to eat a wide variety of foods | Drink plenty of fluids

Have blood pressure checked annually	Have an ECG (test on the heart)	Check breasts every month (women)

General goals

Eat a healthful diet

Don't smoke cigarettes

Don't overstress yourself

Control drinking

Exercise aerobically 3 times a week

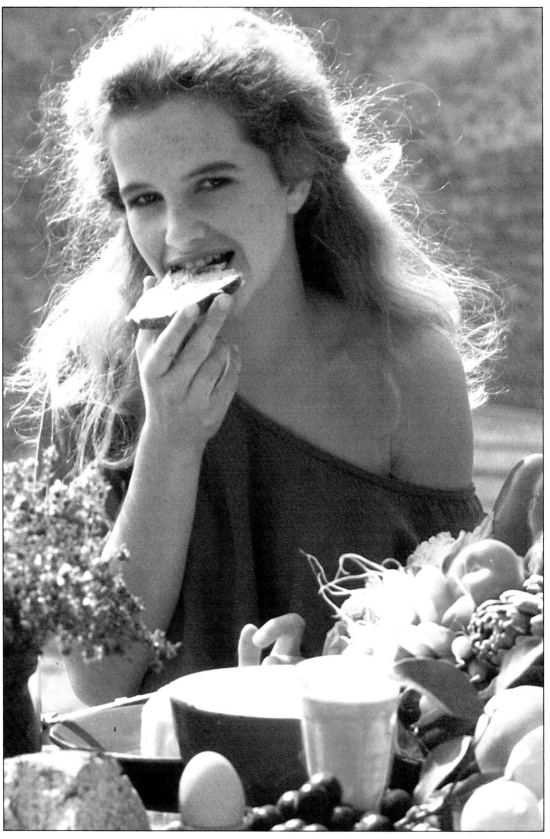

EATING FOR HEALTH

Food is fun. The wonderful variety of food in shops and markets throughout the year, the world's tempting range of restaurants and the huge advertising budgets of food companies, are all powerful testaments to the importance of food as a source of pleasure and contentment.

Food is the fuel that keeps the body alive, and provides building blocks for growth and repair, but the main aim of eating for health is to make eating enjoyable while, at the same time, reducing or eliminating those elements of the more traditional approach to food that work against your long term health and well-being. By exploiting the huge range of foods available you will find that healthy eating involves much less 'giving up' than you would expect. Rather the emphasis is on eating more of some foods and less of others, and extending the range of foods you eat.

Armed with knowledge of food and how the body uses it, rather than being swayed by the latest food fad, you can set yourself and your family new nutritional standards to aim for. This is not to say that the guidelines set out in these pages should be followed in rigid detail. They are a guide to help you toward healthier eating within a framework you and your family can follow and enjoy for life.

One of the great advantages of a healthy style of eating is that it tends to take care, automatically, of weight and calorie control. But for those who feel that they need to lose weight, the chapter also contains sensible help for slimmers.

Food is the mixture of nutrients that the body needs, not just for fitness and well-being but for life itself. The body's energy supply, and the basic building blocks needed for its growth and maintenance, come from the three main classes of foods — proteins, fats and carbohydrates. These are the 'macronutrients', the foods we must eat in considerable quantities each day.

If you are to eat a healthful diet, you must choose your macronutrients wisely. The problem with this is that most of us have been reared with ideas about food which now have to be modified or even overturned completely. The probability is that many developed societies need to alter their eating habits in order to live longer.

Until recently, it was universally accepted, for example, that meat is an ideal source of 'first class' protein and that a perfect diet contains substantial quantities of red meat. In many ways this notion is sound, since protein is essential and red meat contains plenty of high-quality protein, hence the 'first class' label.

The problem with eating red meat is, however, that it is impossible to eat large amounts of meat without eating much harmful animal fat at the same time. And nutritionists have found that there is no virtue in providing the body with more protein than it needs. The quality of proteins in vegetables such as pulses is, in fact, just as good as that in red meat; so, all in all, it seems healthier to eat more vegetable proteins and to relegate red meat, which is also expensive, to a more occasional place in your diet.

Proteins

Essentially, every human being is made of protein: the structural parts of the body that stop it dissolving into a puddle are all based on protein. The working parts of all body cells are also protein based, so there can be no doubt that proteins are macronutrients vital to the diet. Every protein consists of a string of building blocks, known as amino acids. Twenty-four different amino acids, all of which contain nitrogen, are found in the living world, and much of the chemical activity of the human body consists in extracting these amino acids from food sources, such as meat, fish, dairy products and vegetables, and rearranging them into new proteins, which the human body needs for the growth, repair, and replacement of tissues.

Underrated carbohydrates

Carbohydrates are the most underrated of the three macronutrients the body needs. The basic chemical that fuels the body is the carbohydrate, glucose. All the energy-producing chemical reactions of body cells are geared to using glucose, although they can use other fuels, including fats.

Glucose is one of a group of carbohydrates known as monosaccharides. The substance we call 'sugar' is sucrose, which consists of two monosaccharides, glucose and fructose, joined together. Starches, or polysaccharides, are made up of many monosaccharide molecules. Because the body is geared to digesting starches and eventually breaking them down into glucose for fuel, starches thus make the ideal staple food. Starches all come from vegetables, and there are healthful advantages in eating starches that have not been treated or refined in any way, since they contain a high proportion of vegetable fibre, which is now known to be important to the diet. Because complex carbohydrates take longer to digest than simple ones, they are more effective in staving off hunger.

The problem fats

Fats are the problem macronutrients and the ones which, rightly, cause most concern to consumers. Most relevant to a healthful diet is the amount of animal fat food contains, since eating animal fat seems to increase the level of harmful cholesterol circulating in the bloodstream (see p.63) and cholesterol is often found at higher than normal levels in people with heart disease.

All the fats we eat are composed of fatty acids, which are no more than long, stringy molecules made up of carbon and hydrogen. Weight for weight, they produce more than twice as much energy as carbohydrates. Fats are also needed by the body cells for growth and repair, so it is dangerous to eliminate them from your diet altogether.

From the healthful viewpoint, the most important aspect of fats is their degree of saturation. A saturated fat is one in which each carbon atom of a fatty acid is surrounded by the maximum possible number of hydrogen atoms. While animal fats are generally highly saturated, vegetable fats tend to contain unsaturated fatty acids and seem less likely to lead to a potentially life-threatening rise in the level of harmful cholesterol.

How much food does a body need?

Many countries, including Britain and the USA, have formed committees and agencies to propose recommended daily allowances of proteins, carbohydrates and fats, and to suggest how much alcohol men and women should consume. Worldwide, the figures published are similar to those given below.

The total food energy needed each day, which is measured in calories (kilojoules) depends on your age, sex and body size, and on the amount of exercise you take. For easy reference, the following data are based on average allowances of 2,000 calories (8,373 Kj) a day for women and 2,500 calories (10,467 Kj) a day for men.

Food	Percentage of total daily energy allowance	Weight in grams (oz)	
		Men	Women
Protein	11%	69g (2.4oz)	55g (1.9oz)
Carbohydrates	52%	325g (11.4oz)	260g (9.2oz)
All fats	32%	89g (3.1oz)	71g (2.5oz)
saturated fat		28g (1.0oz)	22g (0.8oz)
Alcohol	5%	18g (0.6oz)	14g (0.5oz)

PROTEIN	100g (3.5oz) CONTAINS
Baked white fish is 20% protein	36% total daily protein allowance
Baked beans in tomato sauce are 5% protein	9% total daily protein allowance
CARBOHYDRATE	**70g (2.5oz) CONTAINS**
Wholemeal bread is 45% carbohydrate	12% total daily carbohydrate allowance and about 20% of total daily fibre requirement
Chocolate chip cookies are 70% carbohydrate	19% of total daily carbohydrate allowance, a little fibre and 30% of total daily saturated fat allowance
FAT	**10g ($\frac{1}{4}$oz) CONTAINS**
Butter is 81% fat, of which 46-60% is saturated	11% total daily fat, but 20% total daily saturated fat allowance
Safflower oil is 100% fat, of which 25% is saturated	14% total daily fat allowance, but only 6% of total daily saturated fat allowance
TRADITIONAL 'FIRST CLASS' PROTEIN	**100g (3.5oz) CONTAINS**
Steak with lean and fat (e.g. sirloin steak) is 24% protein and about 30% fat	44% total daily protein allowance and 73% of total daily saturated fat allowance
Trimmed steak with all visible fat removed is 28% protein and only 10% fat	51% of total daily protein allowance and 20% of total daily saturated fat allowance
Cheddar cheese is 25% protein and about 38% fat	45% of total daily protein allowance, but 75% of the total daily saturated fat allowance

Did you know?

● The oils associated with fish proteins are probably less harmful than those associated with red meat.

● Brown sugar is chemically almost identical to white sugar.

● Butter and hard margarine contain about the same amount of saturated fat.

● Non-dairy creamers are made from coconut oil, which is high in saturated fat.

The table shows some of the ways in which you might eat a proportion of your daily allowance of proteins, carbohydrates and fats. It also shows how easy it is to exceed these allowances by injudicious eating.

The comparison between fish and baked beans shows that, while the beans are a reasonable protein source, they have to be eaten in large quantities to make up the daily protein allowance.

Wholemeal bread is an excellent source of carbohydrates and fibre. The chocolate chip cookies have the disadvantage of being high in saturated fat.

The figures clearly show the advantages of using an oil high in polyunsaturates rather than butter.

By eating steak without the fat trimmed off or a high-fat cheese, you can consume your daily allowance of saturated fat in a few mouthfuls.

As well as the fuel and building blocks the body needs, the healthful diet must also contain minute amounts of minerals and vitamins. These micro-nutrients are largely used as catalysts in essential chemical processes, but some minerals, such as the calcium in bones, are a structural part of the human body.

Any ordinary Western diet containing bread, cereals, fresh fruit and vegetables contains an adequate supply of vitamins. Except in special cases, such as pregnancy, there is absolutely no virtue in taking more than the daily allowance. And some vitamins, such as vitamins A and D can even cause disease if they are eaten in excess (see pp.82-3).

For best vitamin value, eat food in its freshest possible state, since storage, particularly in daylight, can destroy some vitamins. Careless cooking can also break down vitamins. Long exposure to high temperatures inactivates vitamin C. The

Vitamin	Best sources	Role	Recommended daily intake
Vitamin A (retinol)	Liver; milk; eggs; butter; dark green or yellow fruits and vegetables. The body converts the pigment carotene in yellow and green fruit and vegetables to vitamin A.	Needed by body membranes, including the retina of the eye, linings of lungs and digestive system. Also needed by bones and teeth.	about 1 mg
Thiamin (Vitamin B_1)	Pork; whole grains; enriched flour and cereals; nuts; pulses	Ensures proper burning of carbohydrates.	1.0-1.4 mg
Riboflavin (Vitamin B_2)	Milk; cheese; eggs; liver; poultry	Needed by all cells for energy release and repair.	1.2-1.7 mg
Nicotinic acid	Whole grains; enriched flour and cereals; liver; poultry; lean meat	Needed by cells for proper use of fuel and oxygen.	13-19 mg
Pyridoxine (Vitamin B_6)	Liver; lean meat; whole grains; milk; eggs	Needed by red blood cells and nerves for proper functioning.	about 2 mg
Pantothenic acid	Egg yolk; meat; nuts; whole grains	Needed by all cells for energy production.	4-7 mg
Biotin	Liver; kidney; egg yolk; nuts; most fresh vegetables	Needed by skin and circulatory system.	100-200 micrograms
Vitamin B_{12}	Eggs; meat; dairy produce	Needed for red blood cell production in the bone marrow. Also needed by nervous system.	3 micrograms
Folic acid	Fresh vegetables; poultry; fish	Needed for red blood cell production.	400 micrograms
Vitamin C (ascorbic acid)	All citrus fruits; tomatoes; raw cabbage; potatoes; strawberries	Needed by bones and teeth and by tissues for repair.	60 mg
Vitamin D	Oily fish and fish liver oils; dairy produce; eggs	Required for maintenance of blood calcium levels and thus for bone growth. Some vitamin D can be made in the skin in the presence of sunlight.	5-10 micrograms
Vitamin E (tocopherol)	Vegetable oils and many other foods	Needed for tissue handling of fatty substances and for making cell membranes.	8-10 mg
Vitamin K	Made by intestinal bacteria; found in leafy vegetables	Needed for normal blood-clotting.	70-140 micrograms

Mineral	Best sources	Role	Recommended daily allowance
Calcium	Dairy produce; green vegetables	Essential for blood-clotting and the structure of bones and teeth. Needed for working of nerves and all other electrically active body tissues.	about 800 mg in adults but more during growth
Phosphorus	Meat; dairy produce; pulses and cereals	Basic cell energy store; key element in cell reactions.	about 800 mg in adults but more during growth
Potassium	Avocados; bananas; apricots; potatoes and many other foods	Major mineral within body cells. Essential to fluid balance and for many cell reactions.	about 3 g
Magnesium	Pulses; nuts and cereals; leafy green vegetables	Needed by all cells. Important in electrical activity of nerves and muscles.	up to 500 mg
Iodine	All seafood; iodized salt Liver; meat; eggs; enriched cereals	Needed by thyroid gland. Needed in manufacture of haemoglobin, the oxygen-carrying compound in blood.	about 0.1 mg 10-15 mg
Fluorine Copper Zinc	Water; fluoride toothpaste Liver; seafood; meat Seafood; meat; wholewheat; pulses; nuts	Helps protect teeth from decay. Needed by cells to utilize oxygen. Needed in the structure of cell enzymes.	– about 1.5 mg 15 mg
Chromium Selenium Molybdenum Manganese	Trace elements in many foods	Minor roles in body chemistry.	minute amounts

B vitamins tend to wash out of food, so do not discard them with the cooking liquid.

Minerals are not destroyed by cooking, and mineral deficiencies are rare. The only ones common in Western countries are iron-deficiency anaemia and, in some areas, fluorine deficiency, which is known to be associated with a high incidence of tooth decay.

The role of fibre
There is nothing new about the idea of dietary fibre. In the past it was called 'roughage' and accepted as helpful in preventing constipation. Certainly a high-fibre diet produces bulkier, softer stools, and there is now good evidence that this helps give protection from a number of diseases of the large intestine, but it has more recently become apparent that fibre may have other important roles in maintaining health. It seems, for example, that increasing the fibre in the diet leads to a fall in blood cholesterol.

All dietary fibre comes from plants. It consists of those parts of them that the body cannot digest. Bran, for instance, comes from the outer part of wheat grains, while the main fibre in fruits is pectin. Different fibres may have different effects on the digestive system, and research is currently under way to assess these.

Ideally, you should consume fibre from all its best sources, that is, from bran and from unprocessed grains, pulses and fruit. Your minimum daily intake should be 25 g (0.8 oz) and your maximum about 50 g (1.8 oz). As a rough guide, you can obtain 5 g (0.2 oz) fibre in 2 slices of wholemeal bread, a large jacket potato or about 70 g (2.5 oz) of baked beans.

When you first increase the fibre in your diet, you may suffer from flatulence, but this should subside within about a month. Large amounts of fibre may also impair mineral absorption from the gut, but this is usually only a problem in people already poorly nourished.

FLUIDS AND THE FLUID BALANCE

Water is one of the essentials of the diet. All body functions use water and, in fact, about 60 per cent of the body is composed of this vital fluid. However, fat cells contain little water, so the fatter your body, the smaller its proportion of water. This also means that you lose little real weight by losing body water.

The chief task of the physical and chemical mechanisms that keep us alive is to ensure that all the body water, and the minerals dissolved in it, remain in the right place. Sodium, the mineral component of salt, is kept almost exclusively outside the cells, while nearly all the body's potassium is inside the cells. The body water will stay where it should be provided that the proper mineral balance is maintained across the body's internal barriers; and considerable body energy is expended in this maintenance.

Input and output

The other balancing act\that is needed is to match input with output. While output is looked after by the kidneys, the hunger and thirst mechanisms control input of water and minerals. Most food contains a high percentage of water. In fruit and

vegetables, for example, it is around 80 per cent, in cooked rice and pasta, 70 per cent and in bread about 35 per cent. Although water is lost as sweat and moist air breathed out through the lungs, the kidneys are able to monitor and alter the amounts of water, sodium and potassium in the urine as appropriate.

The fundamental mechanisms for controlling the body's total fluid balance are so sophisticated and so basic to life that normally it is unnecessary to give any thought to the amount you 'should' be drinking; but, on average, you should aim to consume 1 to 1.5 litres ($1\frac{3}{4}$ to $2\frac{1}{2}$ pints) of fluid a day. The body will see to it, however, that the more salty, sodium-rich food you eat, for example, the more thirsty you will become and the more you will drink to correct the imbalance.

When you experience a sudden change to a hot climate, it takes the body some time to acclimatize to the new, higher, temperatures, and considerable water will be lost as sweat. You should thus make a considerable effort to drink plenty of water for at least a week after you arrive in a place with a hot climate. In the tropics, it may be advisable to take extra salt to increase water

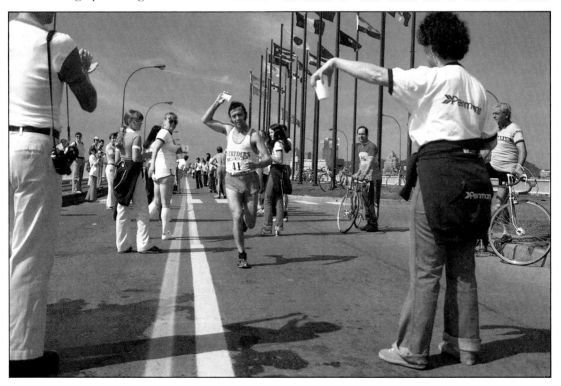

retention. When people undertake unusually heavy exercise — even in temperate climates — they, too, may need to make themselves drink.

Some people worry that if they drink too much water, especially with meals, they will put on weight. In fact, increasing or reducing your water intake has no effect on the amount of fat that is stored. Crash dieting may result in the loss of some body water over the first few days, but this is of no long-term benefit. Indeed, the amount of water in your body may vary from time to time, especially in women, who tend to retain fluid and feel bloated just before the onset of menstruation.

Some substances taken in with dietary fluids can, however, lead to excessive fluid loss through the kidneys. This diuretic effect is brought about by alcohol and by the caffeine in coffee, tea and cola. If taken in excess, such drinks can cause dehydration. Far from quenching the thirst, alcohol actually uses body water. It takes 225 ml (8 fl oz) of water, for example, to metabolize 57 ml (2 fl oz) of a spirit such as gin or vodka.

When you choose which fluids to drink, remember that while water is calorie-free, other drinks may be offering many unwanted 'empty' calories. Both alcohol and soft drinks are high in calories. Coca Cola, for example, contains about 40 cal (168 Kj) per 100 ml (3.5 fl oz), which is about average for fizzy drinks, and beer has about the same calorie level. Even the same volume of unsweetened orange juice, which has the advantage of providing vitamin C to the diet, contains about 35 cal (147 Kj). For anyone with a weight problem, low-calorie drinks are recommended.

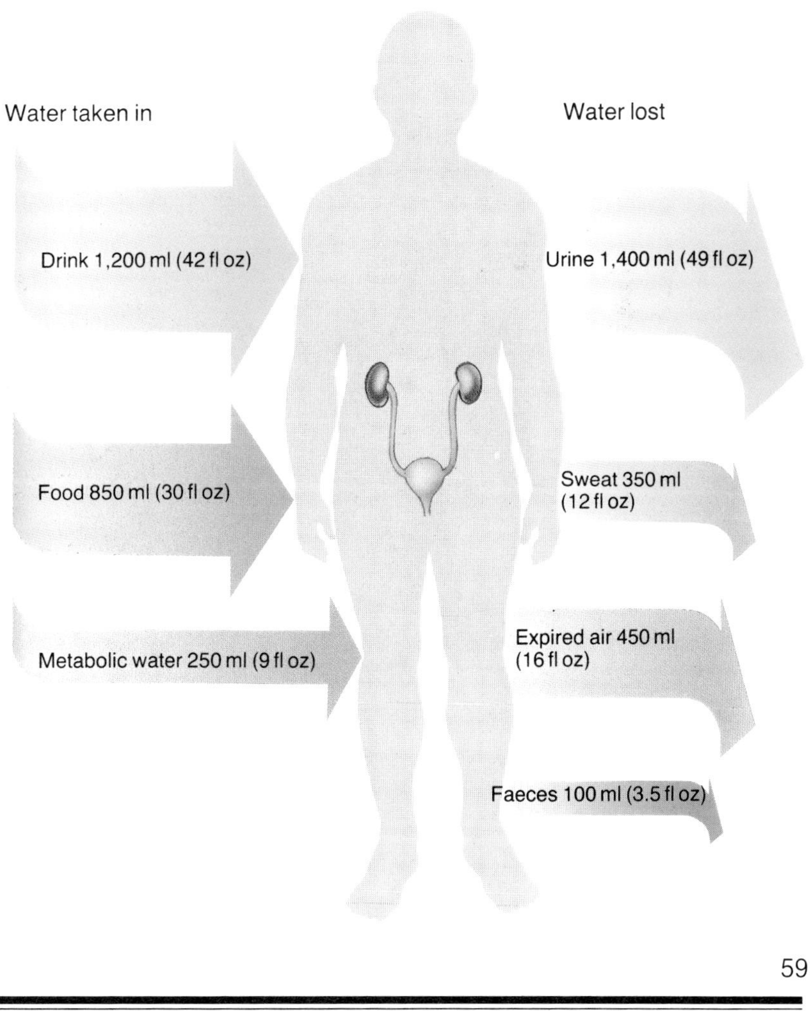

All body cells are bathed in a watery fluid similar in composition to the sea water in which life evolved. Of all the fluid in the body, about 37.5% is made up of this extracellular fluid. Some 55% is inside the cells; the remaining 7% is in circulation in the bloodstream. The diagram shows average daily water intake and loss for an adult man living in a temperate climate. In hotter climates water drunk and sweat produced both increase markedly. Metabolic water is that made by body cells as a result of their functioning.

A marathon runner loses 4.5 to 5.6 l (8 to 10 pt) of water during a race, which makes it important to replace lost fluid at feeding stations along the course (left). Runners are usually offered a choice between pure water and water with added glucose and vitamins.

Water taken in

Water lost

Drink 1,200 ml (42 fl oz)

Urine 1,400 ml (49 fl oz)

Food 850 ml (30 fl oz)

Sweat 350 ml (12 fl oz)

Metabolic water 250 ml (9 fl oz)

Expired air 450 ml (16 fl oz)

Faeces 100 ml (3.5 fl oz)

Snacks to avoid

- Crisps/chips

- Chocolate

- Ice-creams

- Candies

- Sweet biscuits

- High-calorie soft drinks

- Peanuts

All these snacks are bursting with empty calories, which provide energy but few if any worthwhile nutrients. They are high in saturated fat, sugar or salt, low in macronutrients and immensely appetizing. Try to resist the temptation as often as possible.

The human appetite seems to be influenced as much by social and psychological pressures as by internal physiological control systems. Appetite control, however, varies from person to person and remains stubbornly resistant to explanation.

It is relatively easy to study the eating habits of humans under laboratory conditions. The difficulty is that a volunteer will not necessarily mirror his or her everyday eating habits while at rest in the laboratory, sheltered from temptation. We have all seen how some people pause just long enough to grab a small energy booster, while others use mealtimes to bolster themselves against job stresses.

Eating habits and weight

Despite variations in their eating habits, most people seem to remain at approximately the same weight for considerable periods of time. A study of the population of Framingham, Massachusetts, found that, on average, people's weight varied by 4.5 to 9 kg (10 to 20 lb) over an 18-year period. The top figure of 9 kg (20 lb) may seem a lot, but it must be remembered that most of us consume about a tonne of food a year, and the energy value of each 0.4 kg (1 lb) of weight gained is only a

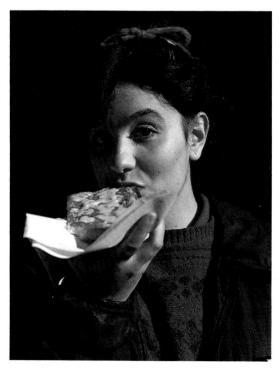

Bad habits to avoid

Don't

- Smother food with salt, sugar or relishes

- Finish up the children's leftovers.

- Serve chips with everything.

- Use food as a reward, punishment or replacement for love.

- Eat a huge meal or extra snack just before bed.

- Have second helpings to be polite.

- Snack automatically when out drinking/driving/in bed/cooking/watching a movie or TV.

- Eat when bored or depressed.

- Make a habit of eating in fast-food restaurants.

- Eat on the move.

- Cook lots of fry-ups.

- Binge and then fast.

- Eat two large meals a day.

small fraction of the energy contained in each annual tonne of food. It was also found that 5 per cent of the population controlled their weight so well that it did not vary more than 0.8 kg (2 lb).

The secret of stable weight lies in a constant food intake – at least from month to month if not from day to day. It may also be explained by the capacity to burn off excess energy, a subject at the heart of current research into obesity.

For many years, it was thought that the entire appetite control centre was seated in the hypothalamus at the base of the brain. The theory was that it contained a trigger to start eating, linked to low blood sugar levels, and a second trigger to stop eating, linked to raised blood sugar levels after eating. Unfortunately, this explanation has been revealed as too simple. The control centre within the hypothalamus is now regarded more as a sort of telephone exchange, processing and distributing information, rather than the ultimate control system (see also pp. 64-5).

One way in which we override the physical control system is to make our diet more varied. While variety ensures an adequate intake of all essential nutrients, it also leads to a pattern of behaviour in which people eat more than they need and so gain weight.

The temptation to eat
Since the early 1960s there have been continuing improvements in the range of appetizing foods available to Western societies and in culinary techniques at home. The resulting temptations, however, would be less of a problem were it not for the high levels of fat and sugar used by the convenience food and catering industries.

We are all at the mercy of seductive food advertising and high calorie menus in canteens and restaurants. Yet some succumb to overeating more easily than others. Studies in London and New York, for example, show that obesity is less common in higher socio-economic groups than in low ones. The one group under most pressure to overeat is full-time housewives. They are in constant contact with food and often feel it is better to eat excess food than to throw it away.

Eating habits are largely determined by home and family. Many parents are preoccupied with making their child 'a good eater' and use food as a reward, so while obesity is partly genetic, home environment seems to play a large part.

THE DIGESTIVE SYSTEM

The digestive system is, in simple terms, a tube 9.2 m (32 ft) long. Its function is to break down complex molecules of proteins, carbohydrates and fats into their smaller constituent molecules, to absorb those that are necessary to keep the body's biochemical systems working, and to expel the residue as faeces.

An unhealthy diet can be a factor in causing digestive problems ranging from tooth decay to gallstones. A properly functioning digestive system is also essential to well-being, since dyspepsia — indigestion — and other digestive ills can cause distress.

The digestive system is subject to stress and emotional upset (see pp. 230-3) which can lead to the formation of disabling conditions such as ulcers. The illustration and chart below show the relationship between diet and digestion.

Transit Times

A few minutes: Mouth and oesophagus

4 hours: Stomach

4½ hours: Small intestine Duodenum

about 12 hours: Large intestine

Mouth and teeth
Food is broken down by chewing and is moistened with saliva to start the digestive process, then swallowed as a bolus.

Tooth decay results from infection, which breaks down the protective enamel. The plaque-forming effect of

eating pure refined sugar often causes tooth decay.

Oesophagus
The bolus passes to the stomach via the muscular oesophagus, whose lower end is pinched shut by a valve to prevent reflux of stomach acid.

Much heartburn results from the reflux of stomach acid into the oesophagus.

Heartburn is often associated with obesity. It

requires medical treatment with antacids, but eating smaller meals can help.

Gall bladder
The gall bladder (green, left) stores bile, made by the liver, and releases it into the duodenum.

Gall stones are due to infection and the disturbance of fat metabolism.

A healthful diet, high in fibre and low in animal fats, seems to reduce the risk of gall stones.

Stomach
A muscular sac that mixes acid fluid with food which passes out in small amounts. Fatty food stays in the stomach longest.

Any upset of the stomach, from irritation, infection or too much acid can cause

pain and vomiting. The protective lining of the stomach may break down to cause an ulcer. Too much acid getting into the duodenum causes both dyspepsia and ulcers. Strong alcohol, irritant foods, such as curry, and

the effects of smoking can all cause gastritis and stomach ulcers. Duodenual ulcers are similarly related to alcohol, smoking and food and also to stress. Avoid foods and drinks that cause problems and try to stop smoking.

Duodenum
A tube 30 cm (12 in) long that receives strong alkaline juice from the pancreas and gall bladder,

which are also digestive organs. These juices act mainly to break down fats.

Small intestine
A narrow tube in which the now liquid food is mixed with various digestive juices. At its lower end,

absorption of food into the blood and lymph begin. Food is transferred, processed and stored

largely by the liver. Spasm of the small and large intestines causes severe colicky pain.

Large intestine
A wide tube in which food and fluid are absorbed. Food residue is formed into faeces.

Constipation and the formation of small, hard faeces can cause pain and discomfort.

A high-fibre diet increases faecal bulk and assists proper functioning.

Cholesterol is a fatty substance which is an essential component of the walls of body cells. To be used properly, it needs to be carried around in the bloodstream. In studies conducted in the USA, Norway, Britain and many other countries, it has been found that raised blood cholesterol levels are associated with a higher risk of having a heart attack in later years.

In trying to reduce your blood cholesterol, and thus the risk of heart disease, it is important to realize that most of the cholesterol in the blood is not eaten in the diet but is actually made by the body — mostly in the liver. Only about 15 per cent of all blood cholesterol comes from the diet, and even cutting your intake dramatically has only a minor effect on the overall level. The reason for this is that the body goes on making cholesterol, no matter how much cholesterol your diet contains. Excess dietary cholesterol is merely eliminated via the excretory system.

The best way to reduce the amount of cholesterol in your blood is to lower your intake of all kinds of fats, with particular emphasis on reducing saturated fats. High levels of dietary fat of this kind seem to encourage the liver to pour out large amounts of cholesterol, but this process can be reversed if the total level of saturated fat in your diet is reduced.

In 1976, a group of British researchers pointed out that while total cholesterol levels in heart attack surveys predicted the risk of disease, there seemed to be a proportion of the cholesterol which actually had the opposite effect and appeared to *protect* against the risk of heart attacks. The cholesterol with this protective effect is known as HDL, or high-density lipoprotein cholesterol.

In the bloodstream, fats are carried about bound to proteins. Most of the cholesterol in the blood is bound with little protein and is thus described as low-density lipoprotein, or LDL cholesterol. The remainder is bound with a lot of protein and forms HDL cholesterol. Because LDL cholesterol forms about 70 per cent of all blood cholesterol, total cholesterol remains a good predictor of the likelihood of heart disease.

It should be your aim to increase your ratio of HDL to LDL cholesterol. The best way of achieving this is through diet and, it seems, through exercise, which has some effect in increasing HDL cholesterol. Curiously, moderate amounts of alcohol may raise HDL levels. Do not forget, however, that high blood cholesterol is only one risk factor in heart disease. Smoking, high blood pressure, a positive family history and diabetes are others.

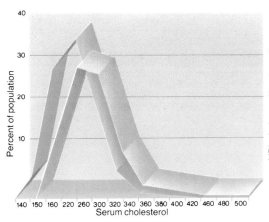

The Framingham study carried out in the USA showed that men aged 30-49 who developed coronary heart disease within 16 years (*green*) had higher levels of cholesterol in their blood than those who did not have heart attacks (*yellow*). Average cholesterol levels throughout these men were, however, extremely high. Further studies conducted in the USA and Europe have shown that reducing blood cholesterol saves lives by reducing heart disease.

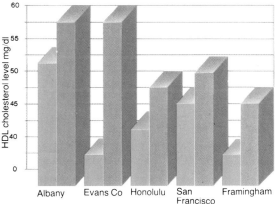

A whole range of studies of the relationship between cholesterol and coronary heart disease suggests that the higher the level of high-density lipoprotein (HDL) cholesterol, the greater the protection against such disease.The graphs show a comparison between men who developed coronary heart disease (*purple*) and those who did not (*blue*) plotted against blood HDL concentration. Figures were obtained from the areas of the USA indicated.

Metabolism is simply the sum of all the chemical activities of the body's cells. For these activities to take place, the cells must be constantly supplied with food energy. As a result of their metabolism, the cells also liberate energy, either in the form of heat or, as in muscle cells, in the form of mechanical work.

All cells, whatever their function, depend on using energy-rich molecules of adenosine triphosphate, ATP. When the high-energy bonds of ATP are split, energy is released which, in the case of muscle cells, may be used for actions as different as typewriting, walking and water-skiing.

The basic fuel

All the food you eat is broken down in the digestive system, absorbed into the bloodstream, then distributed around the body for use. Some surpluses are also stored. Glucose is the basic chemical fuel that cells are designed to use. All the carbohydrate food you eat is converted to glucose in the liver. It is then delivered back to the blood, and from there enters the cells. Here, each glucose molecule is altered chemically, then enters an extraordinary series of reactions within a kind of self-perpetuating circle, the Krebs cycle. During the course of the cycle, oxygen is used up — that is, the cycle is aerobic — and considerable energy is liberated.

One of the great strengths of this system is that other fuels can be used if glucose is in short supply. Fats, for example, can be used, and this is what happens when you lose weight on a reducing diet. When fats are burned in this way, ketones, small chemical leftovers, are produced, which the cell cannot use. If people are starving, they produce many ketones, and you can often smell them on the breath of crash dieters. They have an odour like nail polish remover, and can be a tell-tale sign that someone is trying to lose weight too quickly and may be in biochemical distress.

Alternatively, when glucose is lacking, body proteins may be used as fuel. This is a last resort, and can occur to dangerous effect in those who are starving or fasting.

Apart from chemical fuel such as glucose, the other essential for energy production is oxygen, absorbed through the lungs. Anaerobic activity — activity without oxygen — takes place when cells are being worked so hard that insufficient oxygen is reaching them. This sort of activity can last,

The Krebs cycle

In the Krebs cycle, energy from glucose and, when glucose is not available, from other carbohydrates, fats and proteins is converted into chemical form capable of rebonding phosphates and re-forming molecules of ATP or (adenosine triphosphate), (*right*). These are needed not just for running but for all other body activities. As a result of the chemical reactions of the cycle, the waste product carbon dioxide and water are formed, which are then eliminated from the body through the lungs.

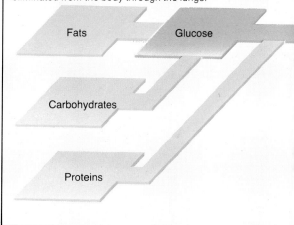

however, for only a limited period. In muscles, for example, anaerobic exercise leads to the build-up of lactic acid, which causes pain and thus 'tells' that part of the body to stop moving.

Storing food energy

As many people know to their cost, an excess intake of food energy is stored in the body as fat. Extra food not burned off in the course of daily activity is converted to fat and stored in cells under the skin and within the abdomen.

A little carbohydrate is also stored in the liver and muscles as glycogen, but in much smaller amounts than fat. A normal 70-kg (154-lb) man contains, for example, only 1 kg (2.2 lb) of glycogen but some 12 kg (26.4 lb) of fat. An obese man contains the same amount of glycogen but much more fat.

Glycogen consists of many glucose molecules joined together and is easily broken down into glucose when needed. In an attempt to boost their energy supplies, many marathon runners try glycogen loading. By reducing their carbohydrate intake for 2 or 3 days, then eating large quantities of pasta or other high-carbohydrate food the night before the race, they aim to maximize their

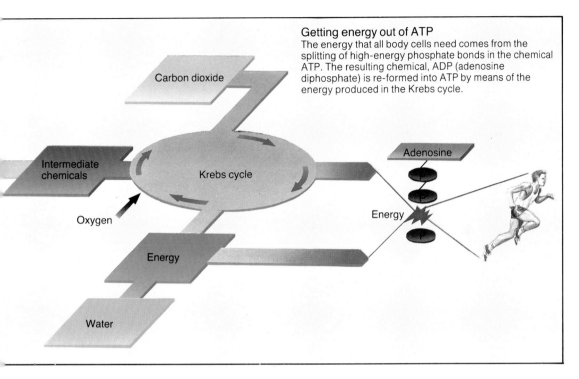

Getting energy out of ATP
The energy that all body cells need comes from the splitting of high-energy phosphate bonds in the chemical ATP. The resulting chemical, ADP (adenosine diphosphate) is re-formed into ATP by means of the energy produced in the Krebs cycle.

Carbon dioxide

Intermediate chemicals

Krebs cycle

Oxygen

Energy

Water

Adenosine

Energy

glycogen stores and help delay the onset of fatigue. There is evidence that, in fact, this technique does work.

Metabolic rate

While everyone can store extra food as fat, some people seem to do so much more readily than others. This difference depends on the overall efficiency of food-burning. Some individuals can 'waste' excess food energy by burning large amounts of glucose and fats, allowing the extra energy to escape as heat.

It has been suggested that brown fat, a special form of fat found in isolated sites around the body, may be responsible for generating this extra heat. While brown fat is undoubtedly important in baby rodents, its role in humans is still uncertain. What is certain, however, is that some people can maintain their body weight, however much they eat and drink, while others increase it by storing food as fat, despite a drastic reduction in their food intake. Most of us fall between these extremes and know from personal experience our tendency for fat storage.

The rate at which the body burns food energy is measured as the basal metabolic rate or BMR.

The BMR varies widely with age, sex and body size and shape. It tends to be lower in women than in men, for example, and decreases dramatically with age but rises with exercise. And the larger the body, the higher its BMR and the more fuel it needs to keep going. So, as a rule, the younger you are and the more exercise you take, the more food you can eat without putting on excess weight.

Somewhat in contrast to this observation is the theory that everyone has a 'set weight' which the body strives toward. According to this theory, the metabolism adjusts itself so that the set weight is maintained. Thus, if you eat more than is required to keep at the set point your metabolism speeds up, but if you eat less than is required the metabolism slows down.

It is also argued, however, that by taking aerobic exercise on a regular basis you can make a permanent, downward adjustment to your set point. The effect of exercise is to persuade the body metabolism to act according to a new set of ground rules. This may certainly help explain why the combination of attention to diet and increased exercise is the most effective means of permanent weight control.

The purpose of eating is to provide the body with the energy essential to sustain life. About 70 per cent of the energy you take in as food is used just to keep the essential processes going within the body – to keep your heart pumping, your liver and kidneys functioning and so on. Only about 30 per cent of all the food you eat is turned into 'external energy' to be used in conscious activities such as walking, jogging or working in the garden.

Although food comes in many different forms and can be cooked in a multitude of ways, it can all be considered in terms of the amount of energy it liberates when it is finally burned up by the body cells. Foods vary in their energy content, depending on how much water, carbohydrate, fat and protein they contain, but the higher the fat content of a food, the greater its calorific value. Depending upon their chemical composition, fats may be saturated or unsaturated. Saturated fat tends to increase the cholesterol level in the blood, but you should realize that there is no calorific difference between the two.

Energy and calories

The energy values of foods are commonly thought of in terms of 'calories'. In fact, what most people call a calorie is actually a kilocalorie or 1,000 calories. In scientific terms, a kilocalorie is a measure of the amount of heat needed to warm up a litre of water by one degree Centigrade. (A true calorie is thus a thousandth of this.) In many countries, including Britain, there is a move toward adopting a new unit of work energy, the kilojoule (as an approximation, 1 cal equals 4.2 kJ). But in practice it will be a long time before the word calorie is deleted or dropped from the vocabulary.

Energy expenditure

On a day-to-day basis, the body metabolism has to keep its energy intake and output in balance. If you burn more energy than you eat, you will start to use your own body constituents as fuel (notably fat from your fat cells), so you will lose weight. Similarly, if you eat more than you burn, then you will store the excess as fat and gain weight. As a rough calculation, it takes about 3,500 unburnt calories (14,700 kJ) to produce 500g (17.6 oz) of body fat.

The exact number of calories that people need to maintain their body weight at a constant level

Comparing foods according to the calories they contain reveals the high energy content of fatty and sugary foods. The following amounts of food all add up to an energy total of between 400 and 500 calories, which, for an inactive woman, is roughly a quarter of her day's recommended allowance.

Fast foods	100g (3.5 oz) hamburger, sesame seed bun and 28g (1 oz) French fries; *or* 110g (4 oz) fried cod and 90g (3 oz) fries; *or* 90g (3 oz) humous and 1 pitta bread
Meat	110g (4 oz) bacon; *or* 78g (2.75 oz) bacon and 1 egg; *or* 170g (6 oz) grilled sirloin steak; *or* 140g (5 oz) steak, 1 grilled tomato and 1 baked potato; *or* 225g (8 oz) roast chicken
Fish	900g (1.6 lb) oysters; *or* 170g (6 oz) tuna in oil; *or* 200g (7 oz) fried white fish; *or* 550g (1.2 lb) steamed white fish; *or* 350g (12 oz) smoked salmon
Dairy produce	110g (4 oz) Cheddar cheese; *or* 750 ml (26 fl oz) low-fat natural yoghurt; *or* 1,400 ml (2.5 pints) skimmed milk; *or* 700 ml (1.25 pints) whole milk
Fruit	1.4 kg (3 lb) apples; *or* 200g (7 oz) dates; *or* 770g (1.75 lb) grapes; *or* 600g (1½ lb) canned peaches in syrup; *or* 1.6 kg (3.5 lb) fresh peaches
Vegetables	225g (8 oz) avocado pear; *or* 600g (1½ lb) boiled potatoes; *or* 160g (5.5 oz) thin French fries; *or* 5 kg (11 lb) boiled cabbage; *or* 2.3 kg (5 lb) raw carrots
Snacks	110g (4 oz) chocolate cake; *or* 85g (3 oz) peanuts; *or* 90g (3.2 oz) potato crisps; *or* 3 large scoops vanilla ice-cream
Pasta and cereals	450g (1 lb) boiled spaghetti; *or* 225g (8 oz) boiled spaghetti and 55g (2 oz) Cheddar cheese; *or* 200g (7 oz) wholemeal bread; *or* 100g (3.5 oz) wholemeal toast and 25g (1 oz) butter; *or* 135g (5 oz) cornflakes
Alcohol	1,500 ml (53 fl oz) beer; *or* 1,300 ml (46 fl oz) cider; *or* 680 ml (24 fl oz) dry white wine; *or* 200 ml (7 fl oz) vodka or gin

The amount of energy you burn up in a day depends on how much exercise you take. The chart below shows the number of calories burnt per hour in a variety of activities. These figures are only a guide; some people naturally burn calories faster than others.

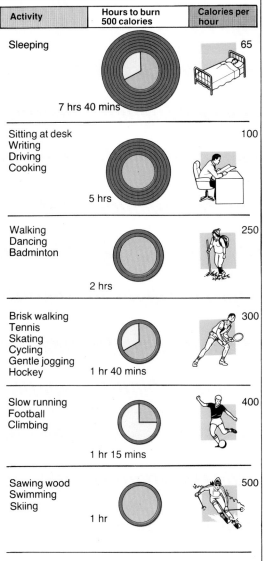

Activity	Hours to burn 500 calories	Calories per hour
Sleeping	7 hrs 40 mins	65
Sitting at desk Writing Driving Cooking	5 hrs	100
Walking Dancing Badminton	2 hrs	250
Brisk walking Tennis Skating Cycling Gentle jogging Hockey	1 hr 40 mins	300
Slow running Football Climbing	1 hr 15 mins	400
Sawing wood Swimming Skiing	1 hr	500
Running Squash Competitive swimming Water polo Weight-lifting	45 mins	650

varies according to their age, size, lifestyle, body composition and heredity. Energy needs decline with age, and it takes much more energy to maintain muscle tissue built up through exercise than it does to keep sluggish fat cells going. This, and the fact that the rate of energy-burning increases with exercise, make exercise a vital part of the body energy equation.

The figures below give recommended average daily energy allowances for men, women and children. If you are much larger or smaller than the average, or are extremely active, then you will need to increase the figures accordingly. If you have a small body and take little exercise your calorie needs will be lower than the average.

To calculate your calorie intake, and adjust it as necessary (taking account of its protein carbohydrate and fat content as well as its energy value), use the tables on pp. 54–5 and 302–4.

Men			
Age	Lifestyle	Cal/day	kJ/day
18-35	inactive	2,500	10,500
	active	3,000	12,600
	very active	3,500	14,700
36-70	inactive	2,400	10,080
	active	2,800	11,760
	very active	3,400	14,280
70+	inactive	2,200	9,240
	active	2,500	10,500

Women			
Age	Lifestyle	Cal/day	kJ/day
18-55	inactive	1,900	7,980
	active	2,150	9,030
	very active	2,500	10,500
56-70+	inactive	1,700	7,140
	active	2,000	8,400
Pregnant		2,400	10,080
Breast-feeding		2,800	11,760

Children		
Age	Cal/day	kJ/day
1	1,150	4,790
2	1,350	5,670
3-4	1,550	6,510
5-6	1,700	7,140
7-8	1,950	8,190
9-11	2,200	9,240
12-14 boys	2,650	11,130
girls	2,150	9,030
15-17 boys	2,900	12,180
girls	2,150	9,030

The concept of the healthful diet is a distillation of all the advances in nutritional thinking that have taken place since World War II. Its aim is to promote growth, body development and maintenance and vitality, and to protect against obesity and heart disease.

Specifically, the healthful diet is based on recommended daily energy allowances (see pp.66-7) and on the percentages of macronutrients within that allowance (see pp.54-5). The most significant aspect of these figures is a move away from fats and proteins and toward carbohydrates as a source of energy. In the early 1980s, for example, 40 per cent of the total calories in the average Western diet were provided by energy-dense fat. The healthful diet recommends that everyone should reduce this to 34 per cent, with a long-term aim of dropping below 30 per cent. And of this fat, only half should be saturated (hard) fat.

In practice, there is no need to eat measured quantities of food each day. Rather you should adopt a pattern of eating that will last you and your family for life. As a general rule, you should eat liberal amounts of fruit and vegetables and four or more servings a day of bread, cereals and/or grains. Meat or eggs should be eaten only once, or at most twice, a day, but fish, nuts and pulses can be eaten twice a day. You should try to restrict your servings of eggs and of high-fat milk products such as Cheddar cheese to two a day.

To give you some idea of amounts, work on the principle that a serving of cooked meat, fish or poultry amounts to about 85 g (3 oz). A serving of bread is one 35 g (1½ oz) slice, while a serving of cheese is about 55 g (2 oz).

As well as fat, the other feature of your diet crucial to health is the amount of salt you eat (see pp.74-5). High salt intake is related to raised blood pressure and heart and circulatory disease. Your daily diet should contain no more than about 8g (0.3 oz) of salt, and preferably less.

The meals illustrated on this page add up to a healthful day's eating based on a total daily intake of 2,000 calories — the average needed by a woman. The total fat content is 34 per cent. Most men would need about 500 more calories. The accent is on freshly cooked rather than processed foods.

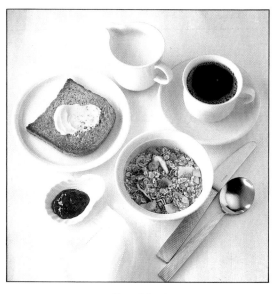

Breakfast

Unsweetened muesli; semi-skimmed milk;

wholemeal toast; polyunsaturated margarine; jam;

coffee with semi-skimmed milk.

The healthful breakfast in this example of a day's eating is based on cereals rather than on animal protein. As well as providing carbohydrate, both the cereal and the toast are excellent sources of fibre (see p.57). Other cereals are also recommended, but keep a careful watch on their sugar content.

Using both polyunsaturated margarine rather than butter and semi-skimmed rather than whole milk helps to reduce the level of saturated animal fats in the diet. Semi-skimmed milk is preferable for adding to drinks such as tea and coffee throughout the day.

Despite the absence of meat, eggs or cheese – all of which are high in animal fats – this breakfast is not lacking in protein. Weight for weight, the muesli contains about half the protein of bacon, which is perfectly adequate. If you do like a cooked breakfast, allow yourself a boiled or poached egg twice or three times a week, but restrict breakfasts such as fried bacon and eggs to a once-a-week treat.

Do not be tempted to miss breakfast. As long as its ingredients are sensibly chosen, it provides a valuable start to a day's healthful eating and will help you to resist snacking.

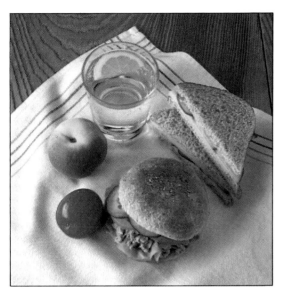

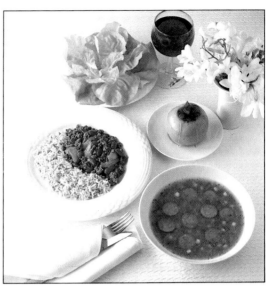

Lunch	Dinner
Wholemeal sandwich with cheese and cucumber;	*Vegetable soup (not processed); chili con carne; brown rice;*
wholemeal roll with salmon and salad;	*green salad with vinaigrette dressing;*
peach; plum; soda water.	*baked apple with dates and honey; glass of red wine.*

This lunch illustrates one of the essential aspects of the healthful diet, namely its move away from the notion that a meal is not a meal unless it contains red meat. Significantly, bread forms the staple of the meal, supplying protein and fibre as well as carbohydrate.

The animal protein in the meal comes from fish and cheese. There are great dietary advantages in using fish as a protein source rather than red meat. Not only does it contain much less saturated fat, but there is some evidence that the oils in oily fish, such as salmon, may have some protective effect on the heart and blood vessels. Cheese is a food that should be eaten in moderation, especially if it is high in fat. It is always possible to choose a low-fat cheese, such as cottage cheese, to help reduce your fat intake, but remember that all cheese is high in salt.

Salad vegetables and fresh fruit should form a substantial part of a healthy day's eating. They contribute vitamins and minerals to the diet. If you eat fruit and vegetables raw, there is no chance of losing vitamins in the cooking.

Choose a soft drink that does not contain a lot of sugar, and throughout the day be wary of the amount of salt you are consuming.

This dinner demonstrates the way in which the healthful diet uses red meat with care. As a rule, you should try to eat meat only once a day, and it is a good idea to 'stretch' it with vegetable protein, as the chili con carne illustrates. Beans are an especially rich source of vegetable protein, but the brown rice also makes a significant contribution; both ingredients contain plenty of fibre. Brown rice also demonstrates the value of 'whole' cereals: compared with polished white rice it contains significant amounts of B vitamins.

Fresh vegetables and fruit are again featured strongly in this meal, the vegetables contributing to the soup and salad, the fruit to the dessert.

Remember that clear soups are more healthful than rich, creamy ones and that salads should be sparingly dressed. It is easy to consume a whole day's allowance of fats in salad dressing alone. Similarly, the dessert is best eaten without cream and is cooked to conserve the fibre the fruit contains.

The healthful diet need not be totally abstemious, but alcohol, if you drink it at all, should only be consumed in moderation. On average, one glass of wine a day is included in the daily recommended intakes.

Eating a healthful diet should become a way of life. There are circumstances, however, in which it is difficult to choose sensibly; for example, when eating out in restaurants and when choosing between-meal snacks. Similarly, you may feel it is hard to entertain guests without offering large portions of meat and creamy sauces.

Use the guidelines beneath the illustrations to help you maintain your healthful eating pattern. The tips below will help you plan your shopping and cooking.

Food buying and preparation
● Avoid processed foods high in fat, salt and sugar. These include ready-made cakes and pastries, sausages, pies, pâtés, cooked meats, most canned foods and dried soups and quick snacks designed to be reconstituted with water.
● Buy lean meat and trim off all the visible fat before cooking.
● Buy cheese less often and choose low-fat cottage cheese or medium-fat hard cheese.
● Check all food labels carefully before you buy.
● Choose whole fruit rather than fruit juice.
● Buy 'whole' foods, such as brown rice, wholemeal flour and wholewheat pasta, rather than refined products.
● Look for fruit canned in water or natural juice.
● Choose low-calorie soft drinks.
● Buy foods canned without added salt and/or sugar.

Cooking
● Bake, boil, steam or grill food in preference to frying.
● If you do fry, stir-fry in a wok or a non-stick pan, using a little polyunsaturated vegetable oil.
● Cook casseroles a day ahead, cool and remove the fat before reheating and serving.
● Drain as much fat as possible from the pan before making gravy.
● Use salt sparingly. Try adding herbs, spices or lemon juice in place of salt.
● Use yoghurt or quark (a low-fat soft cheese) in place of cream. (Yoghurt will not curdle if you 'stabilize' it with a little plain flour.)
● Cook potatoes, apples and other fruit and vegetables in their skins.
● Mix mayonnaise with yoghurt before serving.
● Make your own salt-free stock rather than using high-salt cubes.

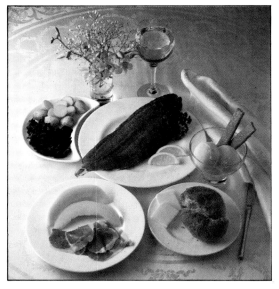

Restaurant meal
Melon with prosciutto (Parma ham); wholemeal roll with butter; grilled white fish (sole); leaf spinach; orange sorbet; wafer; glass of wine.

In restaurants, the food may be delicious, but the accent of the cooking is often on animal fat and fibre-free food. This is not a problem if you eat out only occasionally, but if your business or social life regularly involves restaurant or hotel meals, it is well worth seeking out eating places that offer more healthful food. Fortunately, the trend toward *nouvelle cuisine*, which lays less emphasis on meat and cream, is a move in the right direction.

The meal illustrated gives an idea of the sort of dishes to choose. It is essentially healthy, but rather low in fibre. Having prosciutto with your melon starter is acceptable on special occasions, but it is too salty to have a regular place in your diet. Whether you choose meat or fish as a main course, ask for it to be grilled if possible. Avoid rich, creamy sauces with all courses – this is not usually a problem since the amount of cream used in cooking is generally advertised on the menu. Similarly, request vegetables that are not buttered or fried.

For dessert, select a fruit sorbet or fresh fruit. Try to resist the temptation to smother it with cream. Restrict alcohol intake to a maximum of two glasses of wine.

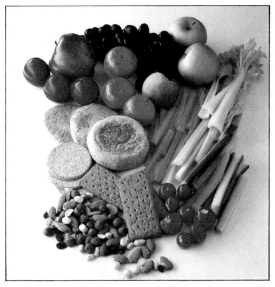

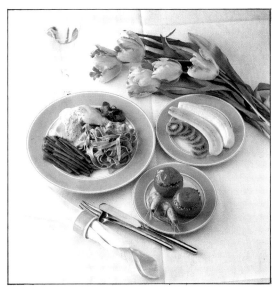

Snacks

Wholewheat or bran crackers; wholemeal rolls,

muffins or pitta bread; unsalted nuts; dried fruit;

sticks of raw vegetables; fresh fruit.

Home entertaining

Tomatoes with prawn, breadcrumb and herb stuffing;

poached chicken with watercress and yoghurt sauce,

wholewheat tagliatelle, green beans;

baked bananas with kiwi fruit; glass of wine.

Eating snacks between meals can prove to be disastrous, both to the waistline and the healthiness of your diet. With a little thought it is easy to direct your tastes — and those of children, to whom snacks are important — toward snacks that make a valuable contribution to your diet.

There is no need to feel guilty about eating the occasional chocolate bar, but remember that traditional snacks often contain hidden saturated fat, as in cookies and chocolate, or may be 'empty' calories of pure sugar. Potato crisps, pretzels and popcorn may be high in fat, salt, sugar or all three, yet provide little or no fibre.

Sensible snacks should be substantial enough to fill you up for a while, yet be free of 'danger' ingredients. This makes crackers and bread products based on wholemeal flour a good choice; but beware of spreading them with high fat or salt spreads such as butter, peanut butter or meat or yeast extract. Raw vegetables and fruit are less filling but contain fewer calories. Dried fruit is higher in calories and should be eaten in moderation, as should nuts. Try not to choose salted nuts and avoid cashews and coconut, which are high in saturated fat. Other snacks to eat only occasionally are olives, which are both fatty and salty.

At home, there is almost unlimited scope for producing enterprising and exciting food for entertaining in a healthful way. Most guests will be glad of a change from the traditional heavy cuisine, which is not only rich but can make you feel unpleasantly overfull.

The meal illustrated uses both shellfish and poultry but no red meat. The poached chicken is served without its fatty skin and with a low-fat, sharp-tasting sauce. Wholewheat tagliatelle makes an interesting change from potatoes and contains more fibre than refined white or green pasta. The baked fruit dessert has a delicate flavour that does not need enhancing with cream or ice cream.

Other good ideas for home entertaining include dishes from Chinese, Italian, Mexican and Indian cuisine, all of which can have their accent on 'filler' such as rice, pasta and pulses rather than on animal protein. It is always fun to experiment with new recipes or to adapt old favourites, using less fat, sugar and salt.

A cheeseboard was once a customary end to a meal but is really best left out if you wish to keep the food as healthful as possible.

Man is a successful omnivore, but the vegetarian way of eating has a lot to recommend it. Vegetarian diets are, in many ways, closer to the ideal of the healthful diet than traditional omnivorous ones, since as a rule they contain little saturated fat and plenty of fibre. They are also inexpensive.

Most people are vegetarians because of their religious beliefs or because they hold that animals should not be killed for food. Or they may believe that a diet provides spiritual advantages beyond the boundaries of nutrition. However, many omnivorous people are now considering the vegetarian style of eating as a serious alternative.

The degree to which vegetarians avoid animal produce varies considerably. Some vegetarians eat dairy produce and eggs or even fish; these are ovolactovegetarians. At the other end of the spectrum, vegans will avoid anything derived from the animal kingdom. Macrobiotic diets are mostly based on brown rice and vegetables.

The more strictly vegetarian you are, the less fat is likely to find its way into your diet. However, fats are a concentrated source of energy, and without them you may have to eat a lot of other food to make up your energy requirements. This can, of course, be an advantage if you are trying to lose weight.

Ovolactovegetarians avoid this problem, since they consume dairy produce, including convenient calorie sources such as cheese. This can, however, produce problems, for it is possible to err on the side of over-consumption of animal fats if you rely too heavily on cheese and eggs.

Some people worry that vegetarian diets may lead to nutritional deficiencies. In most cases there is certainly unlikely to be a shortage of proteins, but some vegans are known to suffer from the lack of vitamins D and B_{12}, so supplements are advisable. Symptoms of vitamin D deficiency include inadequate bone growth (rickets) in children and bone softening in adults. Lack of vitamin B_{12} leads to a type of anaemia known as pernicious anaemia and may damage nerve cells. Ovolactovegetarians need not worry — both these vitamins are amply supplied by dairy products.

Rather than being unhealthy, the evidence suggests that vegetarians may be healthier than meat-eaters. Their blood cholesterol levels are often significantly lower, as is their blood pressure. If this is so, then they are less prone to narrowing of the arteries and heart disease.

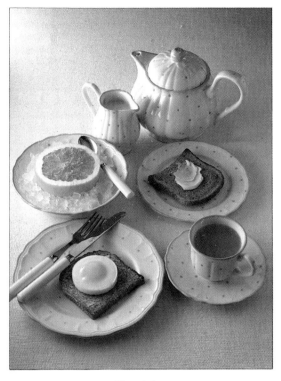

Breakfast

Grapefruit with brown sugar;

poached egg; wholemeal toast; polyunsaturated margarine;

tea with semi-skimmed milk.

Non-vegetarians can learn a lot about healthy eating from vegetarians. If you have 2 or 3 meatless days each week, you will gain many dietary advantages.

● You do not need to eat meat to be healthy. The evidence is incomplete, but it suggests that vegetarians live longer than their omnivorous contemporaries.

● Vegetarians get enough protein in their diets. Animal protein has no special virtue and carries injurious animal fat with it. However, you do need a varied vegetarian diet to avoid vitamin deficiencies and to promote growth in children.

● The non-vegetarian can use meat or fish more as a tasty garnish than as the centrepiece of a meal.

Vegetarian diets in children
Although vegetarian diets are a healthy way of eating for most adults, they present some risks to

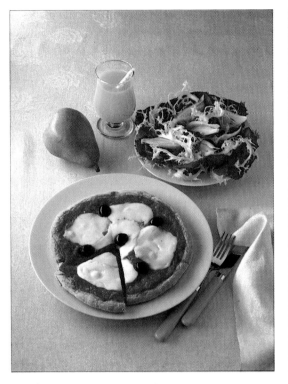

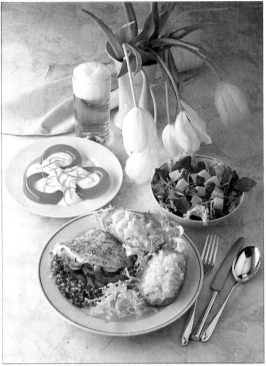

Lunch
Wholemeal pizza;
mixed salad; pear;
unsweetened orange juice.

Dinner
Buckwheat and vegetable casserole;
baked potato; tofu salad;
orange jelly with yoghurt; glass of lager.

growth and development in children.

A study of growth in a large number of vegetarian children under six years of age, carried out at Tufts University in Boston, suggested that their growth was indeed somewhat diminished. The number of children in the study was not large enough to show whether vegans fared worse than ovolactovegetarians, but there was a suggestion that this was the case.

It seems that it is the level of energy provided by a vegetarian diet that may be at fault in diminishing growth, rather than any protein deficiency. Fat provides many calories for a small weight of food consumed, and there is little fat in a vegan diet. However, a reasonable amount of additional dairy produce will provide the extra energy needed and, at the same time, avoid any risk of vitamin D and B_{12} deficiency.

The meals shown on these pages are an example of a balanced day's eating for an ovolacto-vegetarian. The total calorie content, excluding the lager, is about 2,000 calories, which is about the average needed for a woman (a man would need about 500 calories more). The fat content is 34 per cent. As in all healthy diets, there is considerable emphasis on wholefoods and on fresh fruit and vegetables.

These dishes show how vegetarian food can provide a valuable extension to the culinary repertoire of non-vegetarians in search of a healthful diet. Vegans would, however, dispense with the breakfast egg, with the cheese on the pizza and with the yoghurt on the dessert. A strict vegetarian would make the orange jelly with a vegetable setting agent, such as agar agar, not with gelatine derived from animals. The tofu, or bean curd, makes an interesting variation.

There are many other possibilities for you to choose from, including the use of nuts and pulses, both of which are excellent sources of protein.

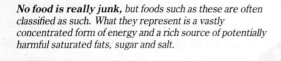

No food is really junk, but foods such as these are often classified as such. What they represent is a vastly concentrated form of energy and a rich source of potentially harmful saturated fats, sugar and salt.

The Western diet, typified by a hamburger, French fries, a thick milk shake and a slice of cream-topped cheesecake, is one of potentially dangerous excesses. High in calories, saturated fats, sugar and salt, but low in fibre, it puts its consumers at risk from the two great problems of Western health, namely obesity and heart and circulatory disease.

The superfluous energy in the Western diet comes from fats, which are undoubtedly implicated in heart disease (see p.63) and sugar. Sugar is a constituent not only of obvious foods, such as cheesecake and apple pie, but of processed relishes and ketchups and of factory-made hamburgers. In fact, sugar is present in all manner of processed foods, from curry to chicken soup and from baked beans to barbecue sauce. When buying food for home consumption, look at the label (the sugar may be described as glucose, caramel, maltose or fructose).

The problem with sugar is twofold. First, it is a concentrated energy source, and eating concealed sugar is a hindrance to those on the verge of serious obesity. Second, sugar is the single greatest cause of dental caries. If average sugar consumption in the West was cut from its present 37 kg (81 lb) a year to 20 kg (44 lb), the disease could be significantly reduced.

Even more than its sugar content, the most serious criticism of all prepared and processed food is its high salt content. The reason why salt intake is important is that high sodium consumption (salt is the chemical sodium chloride) seems intimately bound to the problem of high blood pressure. And high blood pressure is a significant contributory factor to blood vessel diseases,

This meal totals more than 1,500 calories and is around 60% fat.

A portion of French fries weighing 100 g (3¼ oz) contains about 215 calories. The smaller they are, the larger their surface area for absorbing fat.

The hamburger with the bun, cheese and relishes totals about 555 calories.

The milk shake contains about 315 calories.

The cheesecake, weighing 200 g (7 oz), contains more than 550 calories.

which can lead to heart attacks and strokes. As societies develop, so they start adding salt to their diet, and the blood pressure in developed societies tends to rise with age.

The risk of salt in the diet is in fact probably not the same for everybody. Part of the population — possibly around 20 per cent, although the exact figure is unknown — is more likely to develop blood pressure problems from salt. There is no way of telling which category you fall into, but the chances are that you are more at risk if you have a family history of high blood pressure. However, everyone living in the West would be well advised to reduce salt intake from its current daily level of some 10 to 13 g (0.35 to 0.42 oz) to 8 g (0.3 oz) or, ideally, to between 6 g (0.2 oz) and 3 g (0.1 oz). One of the disadvantages of this is that you will have to adapt yourself to a blander taste and to find other ways of making your food taste palatable. The human taste mechanism is, however, extremely adaptable and you will be surprised how quickly you become used to less salt.

It is encouraging that if you eat a healthful diet, you will naturally tend toward a lower sodium intake. Eating plenty of fresh fruit and raw vegetables will also increase the amount of potassium in your diet; and there is some medical evidence to suggest that decreasing the ratio of sodium to potassium may be just as important in preventing high blood pressure as reducing your total sodium intake alone.

Avoiding sodium

As well as salt, other chemicals added to processed foods can add unwanted sodium to the diet:

● MSG (monosodium glutamate): a flavour enhancer.

● Sodium nitrite: added to meat and fish as a curing agent and preservative.

● Baking soda (sodium bicarbonate): a raising agent.

● Sodium phosphate: a wetting agent.

Salt content rises dramatically when food is processed or cured, as the figures show. They also reveal the high salt content of cheese, butter and margarine. Apart from avoiding processed foods, the best way of cutting down on salt is to add less salt in cooking and reduce sprinkling at the table.

As well as avoiding sodium, choose foods with a low sodium/potassium ratio. These include most fresh fruit and vegetables.

Percentage contribution of foods eaten in the home to average daily intake of salt

Table salt	32
Cereal products	27
Meat, eggs, milk	19
Cheese, cream, ice-cream, fats	5
Root vegetables	2
Other vegetables	3
Fish	1
Fruit and sugar	trace
Beverages	trace
Total	100
Equivalent to 9.8 g (0.33 oz) salt	

Sodium/potassium content of some common foods

Food	Sodium mg/ 100 g (3.5 oz)	Sodium/ potassium ratio
Bread, wholemeal	560	3.5
Cheese, Cheddar	610	5.08
Butter, salted	870	58
Margarine	800	160
Bacon, unsmoked, raw	1,470	6.39
Haddock, fresh	120	0.40
Haddock, smoked	1,220	4.2
Potato, boiled	4	0.01
Potato, crisps	550	0.46
Peas, fresh	1	0.002
Peas, canned	230	1.77
Peas, frozen	2	0.02
Tomato ketchup	1,120	1.90

OBESITY AND SLIMMING/1

In the overfed Western world, many people spend their lives worrying about how to hold back the expansion of their waistlines. Being overweight is undoubtedly unhealthy: it can be a contributory factor in diabetes, heart and kidney disease and may make surgery more risky. But before rushing out to put yourself on a crash diet and making yourself miserable and guilty about failing to be slender, it is appropriate to ask, not 'Is obesity bad for you?', but 'How bad is obesity for you?' In other words, how much overweight do you have to be before the risk of ill-health is unacceptable?

The risks of obesity

In the authoritative 'Report on Obesity' published in the *Journal of the Royal College of Physicians* in London in 1983, this question was carefully considered. The conclusion was that while there is little doubt that obesity carries a mortality risk, there is no clearly defined point at which being obese suddenly increases that risk. And it seems that slight degrees of obesity carry only a slight mortality risk.

The graphs of mortality figures for men and women, *right*, show the risks of obesity. In order to surmount the problem that people come in all shapes and sizes, the graphs use the body mass index as a measure of the degree of obesity. To obtain the index, the weight of a person in kilograms is divided by the square of his or her height in metres, *below right*.

The figures in the graphs were calculated for both non-smokers and those who smoked more than 20 cigarettes a day. They are a striking version of the parable of the mote and the beam — there is no point in worrying about a minor degree of obesity if you have a separate major risk to health. At a glance, it is easy to see that a non-smoker has to reach gigantic proportions to have the same risk of death as a smoker of acceptable weight.

Suppose, for example, that you are a woman, a non-smoker with a body mass index of 29, which represents a considerable degree of overweight. Your risk of death is exactly average for the whole population. It would be smaller if you were thinner, but not a lot. It is probable, but certainly not proven, that the risk will be less if you eat a healthy diet and are physically fit, even if you remain exactly the same weight.

This said, there are certainly advantages in losing weight if you are over the acceptable figure. It is easier to be fit if you are thin and the desires to have less weight to carry about, to look good, to feel comfortable with your body and to fit into last year's clothes are more than reasonable objectives. And the less over-burdened you are with anxiety and guilt about obesity, the more likely you are to achieve those objectives.

Many people will find that they tend to lose weight as they move toward eating a healthful diet (see p.54 ff). The reduction in the intake of fats, which are a concentrated source of calories, sensible alcohol consumption (see pp.250–3) and an increase in fibre all help weight loss.

If, however, you still have surplus weight to shed, there is no other solution than to reduce the total amount of calories in your diet, by eating smaller quantities of all the foods in the healthful diet except fruit and vegetables, and thus to encourage the body to burn its fat stores as an energy source. Another important aspect of weight control is to establish an eating pattern that is right for you (see pp.60–1). Set yourself reasonable targets and do not try to lose weight too fast or cut out one group of foods altogether.

It has also been suggested that the metabolic changes that accompany crash dieting slow down the body's use of energy and thus make it doubly hard to lose weight by calorie restriction — and also doubly likely that you will regain it when you liberalize your diet a little.

Perhaps most important of all is the place of exercise in a reducing regimen. Any attempt at slimming should be accompanied by a reasonable amount of physical activity. Many people find that they are able to maintain a stable weight once they are taking regular exercise, even though it is hard to be precise about the reasons.

Tips for parents

To help prevent children from becoming obese, and to encourage the loss of 'puppy fat', make sure you provide a healthy diet for the whole family. Encourage children to exercise, and make them your allies, not your enemies, in the pursuit of a better style of eating that will promote weight loss. Do not insist that the children finish up all the food on their plates nor use food as a reward. If possible, try to ensure that children cut back on sweets, ice-cream and fatty fast foods.

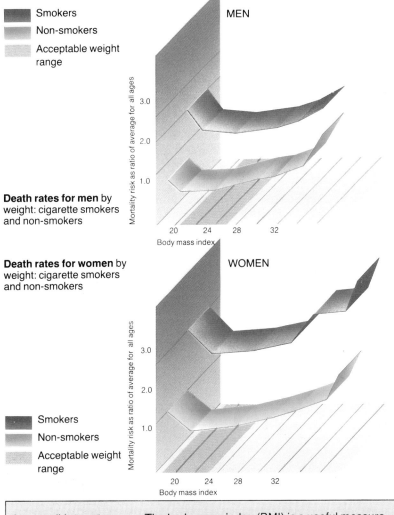

Smokers

Non-smokers

Acceptable weight range

Death rates for men by weight: cigarette smokers and non-smokers

Death rates for women by weight: cigarette smokers and non-smokers

Smokers

Non-smokers

Acceptable weight range

MEN

Mortality risk as ratio of average for all ages

3.0

2.0

1.0

20   24   28   32

Body mass index

WOMEN

Mortality risk as ratio of average for all ages

3.0

2.0

1.0

20   24   28   32

Body mass index

Tips for losing weight
● Set yourself a realistic target.

● Concentrate on eating a healthful diet.

● Don't feel guilty if you eat cakes or chocolate occasionally.

● Eat 3 small meals a day rather than 1 or 2 large ones.

● Choose low-calorie snacks.

● Cut down on alcohol.

● Eat more slowly.

● Use a smaller plate — it will look full with less food on it.

● Do not feel you have to finish all the food on your plate.

● Avoid eating large meals late at night when you cannot 'burn' off calories with exercise.

● Prepare food that looks attractive.

● Don't binge and fast alternately.

As a sensible target, you should aim to lose no more than 1 kg (2¼ lb) of weight a week. Work out your own body mass index with the help of the examples given here, then calculate a target weight within the acceptable range.

The body mass index (BMI) is a useful measure of obesity (or the lack of it). Both BMI and target weight can be easily worked out with a calculator.

$$BMI = \frac{weight\ in\ kilos}{height\ in\ metres^2}$$

Take the example of a woman who weighs 168lb and is 5ft 5in (65in) tall. To convert pounds to kilograms, multiply by 0.45, i.e.,
$$168 \times 0.45 = 75.6kg$$
To convert inches to metres, multiply by 0.025, i.e., $65 \times 0.025 = 1.62$ metres

$$Thus\ BMI = \frac{75.6}{1.62 \times 1.62} = \frac{75.6}{2.62} = 28.8$$

This BMI is well over the upper limit of the acceptable range. To calculate a target weight corresponding to a BMI of 23, which is within the acceptable range, the only sum needed is $23 \times Ht^2$, i.e., $23 \times 2.62 = 60kg$. To reconvert this to pounds, divide by 0.45, i.e., $\frac{60}{0.45} = 133lb$.
The target weight for this woman is thus 133lb, which means a weight loss of 35lb.

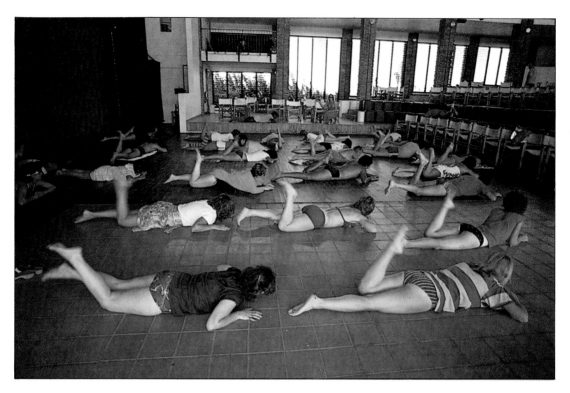

The rational way to try to lose weight is simple and straightforward – at least in theory. If you adopt a healthful diet, which is recommended by nutritional agencies on both sides of the Atlantic, then you may well lose weight. If you do not, you should attempt a modest reduction in your total calorie intake, but within the same nutritional framework, and combine this with an increase in aerobic exercise.

In this way, many people do find that they can lose weight without any other form of help. But if you are not such a person, then you may well find it helpful to join some group or organization. Those groups that are well known and also well established are most trustworthy, since they have achieved their position by some measure of success. The organizations to beware of are those that offer some new, 'effortless' cure for the problem of overweight.

Worldwide, the most famous slimming organization is Weight Watchers, which began life in the USA in the 1960s and reached Europe in the same decade. Like so many of its imitators, Weight Watchers gives participants the benefit of mutual support in a common goal. Its overall aim

is to teach members new attitudes toward eating and new eating habits so that they will not only lose weight but stay slim for life.

Although groups such as Weight Watchers help members to shed excess pounds, there is some evidence that some members regain weight once they stop attending meetings. The group experience and element of competition would seem to be what such people need for sustained weight loss and should be continued.

Health farms and spas, often nicknamed 'fat farms', work on an entirely different principle. Most offer high-quality or even luxurious accommodation, supplemented by a restricted dietary regimen and combined with exercise, massage, saunas and the like. However, the very nature of the health farm approach is one that encourages crash dieting, which is a method that is almost certainly doomed to failure.

Even if you do not wish to attend a group, you can use some of their methods at home. Make a habit of weighing yourself at the same time each week and on the same scales, so that you can gain an accurate record of your progress, and take aerobic exercise regularly (see pp. 87ff).

At a health farm or slimming spa, (right) the approach to weight loss is usually one of a low-calorie diet eaten in luxurious surroundings. The problem with health farms is that visitors stay for only a short time. This inevitably means that there is an element of crash dieting involved in the weight loss. Despite this, many people who treat themselves to a holiday at a health farm find it valuable in terms of well-being, even if they do not achieve any permanent weight loss.

Exercise groups, such as those of the slimnastics organizations (left), emphasize physical activity in helping people to slim. Participants are also given advice about controlling their calorie intake and are advised to cut down on fat consumption. Members are weighed then carry out an exercise routine, often to music.

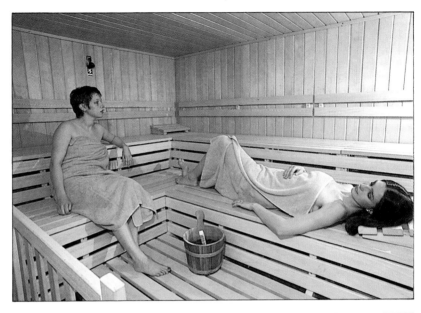

The weekly weigh-in is an essential part of the Weight Watchers approach to slimming (right). At meetings, members are encouraged to talk openly about overweight and are given help to handle the emotional problems with which overeating and overweight may be associated. Advice is given on choosing an appropriate eating programme with the aim of educating members into recognizing and accepting a lower energy input.

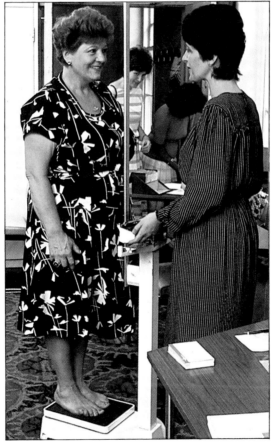

Chart your progress

Even if you do not attend a group weighing session, you can use similar methods at home to chart your progress.

● Write a list of numbers, say 1 to 20, representing your target weight loss in kilograms or pounds. Cross off each kilo or pound as you lose it.

● Make a graph of your weight against time. Fill in points on the graph each week as you weigh yourself.

SLIMMING DIETS

New slimming diets of every kind, published with monotonous regularity year after year, always seem to be a commercial success. All that is needed is a promise of 'effortless weight loss' — with this, success, at least in the overfed, overweight Western world, in which 'slim is beautiful', seems guaranteed.

The diets featured in diet books range from those that make reasonable sense from a nutritional point of view, to those that are so unsound nutritionally that severe problems can result if you remain on them for more than a week or two And compared with slimming groups and organizations, diet books have the added disadvantage that they provide no emotional support for the slimmer. This is a significant reason for the low success rate of most of them.

Another disadvantage of specific reducing diets is that, in the main, they do not encourage slimmers to adopt a pattern of eating that they can use for life. Nor can many of the suggested meals be adapted to feed all the members of a family. Such diets are largely doomed to failure, with the dieter left feeling guilty and depressed when the lost weight immediately goes back on again.

All the main trends that have emerged from the diet-book industry are illustrated on these pages; some of them have much more to recommend them than others.

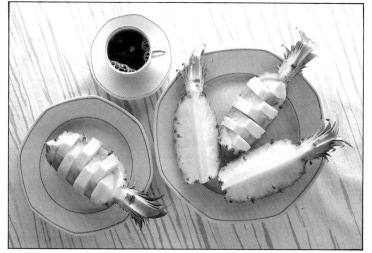

All-fruit diet

The principle underlying this diet is that fruit is largely water. You have to eat a lot of fruit to obtain calories, so that a fruit diet will result in weight loss. The same reasoning applies if you merely drink water and do not eat — the only difference is that malnutrition strikes a little sooner. ***All-fruit diets represent the extreme of nutritional danger.***

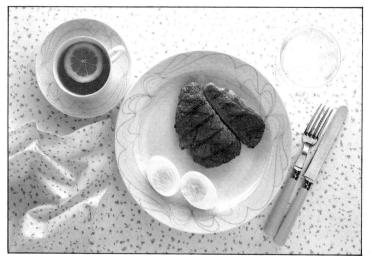

All-protein/high-protein diet

The idea behind protein-based diets is that eating large amounts of protein may speed up the body's metabolism and thus burn off some of its fat stores. And, the theory goes, the body has limited capacity to convert protein to fuel so that much of what is eaten is wasted. Such diets are expensive, hard to stick to and, in the long term, nutritionally unbalanced and thus unsound. ***Not recommended.***

Meal replacements

All types of meal replacements work on the theory that you can cut down on calories by eating (or drinking) something that will fill your stomach but which contains few calories. **Some people may lose weight using this approach, and there should be no nutritional deficiency, but it does nothing to encourage healthy eating habits when 'normal' foods are eaten.**

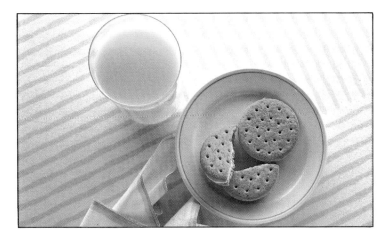

High-fibre diet

As long as they include a wide variety of foods, high-fibre diets are to be recommended. Aiming for a fibre intake of between 30 and 50 grams a day, and combining this with a reduction in fat of all sorts and unsaturated fat in particular, is the healthy way of eating. One word of warning. **Avoid any diet that suggests sticking to a single food or small group of foods, even if they are high in fibre.**

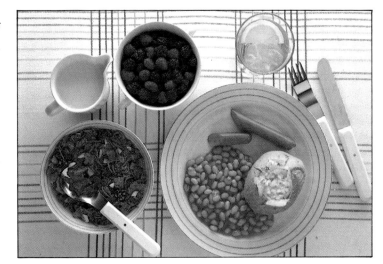

Very low calorie diets

Diets based on raw vegetables, cottage cheese and the like, with recommended daily energy intakes of less than 1,000 calories (4,200 kJ) are hard to stick to, and the evidence is that within a short time most people regain any weight they succeed in losing on such a diet. It is also difficult to eat adequate fibre in a diet with a very low calorie count. **Diets based on massive calorie reductions are locked in the vicious spiral of inevitable failure to stick to the diet, subsequent bingeing and weight gain.**

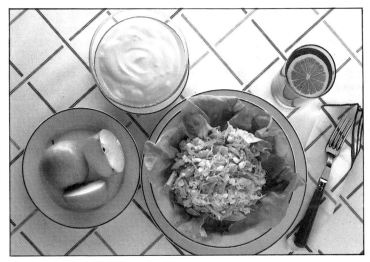

HEALTHFOODS AND WHOLEFOODS

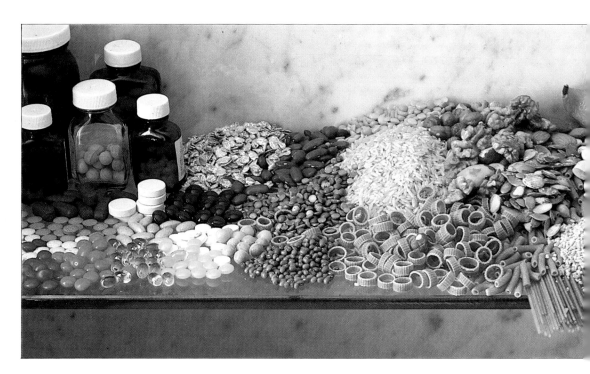

In the United States alone, the total annual sales of diet supplements exceed $700 million. These supplements consist of vitamins and minerals to add to a normal diet. The healthfood business also spills over into providing 'organic' and 'naturally grown' products unavailable through normal outlets. This vast and highly profitable industry is ostensibly scientific but, in reality, is generally the reverse.

Vitamins and minerals

Among the falsehoods that form the kernel of the healthfood industry is the notion that the normal diet is deficient in vitamins and minerals. This is not so. Another false idea is summed up in the statement: if 'vitamins and minerals are good for you; more must be better for you.' This statement is the basis of the megavitamin approach, in which people regularly take amounts of all kinds of vitamins well above the levels needed to prevent deficiency.

In large doses, vitamins and minerals are toxic. The most common forms of trouble occur with the fat-soluble vitamins A and D. Excess vitamin A causes dry skin, loss of appetite, headaches, irritability and even enlargement of the liver. It can also slow growth in children. Too much vitamin D brings about pain in the abdomen, pain in the bones and stones in the kidney due to the release of too much calcium into the blood. Even water-soluble vitamins — including vitamin C for which megadoses are often taken as a cold remedy — can be dangerous if taken in large enough amounts. Nausea and the development of kidney stones are two possible effects of vitamin C overdosing.

The diligence of the vitamin sellers is almost certainly making such diseases more common. In August 1983 the *New England Journal of Medicine* published seven cases of a new vitamin toxicity disease resulting from overdose of pyridoxine, a B vitamin which, in excess, causes nerve conduction problems. In an editorial accompanying the report, it was also pointed out that the acceptable level for impurities in vitamin manufacture is set at 2 per cent, a perfectly safe level for the minute doses needed in medical practice. But if you multiply these doses by many hundreds, you are inevitably taking in large amounts of impurities with your vitamins.

Adequate minerals are supplied by a mixed diet, with two possible exceptions. Fluorine may not be present in sufficient amounts to prevent tooth decay, and there may not be enough iron for

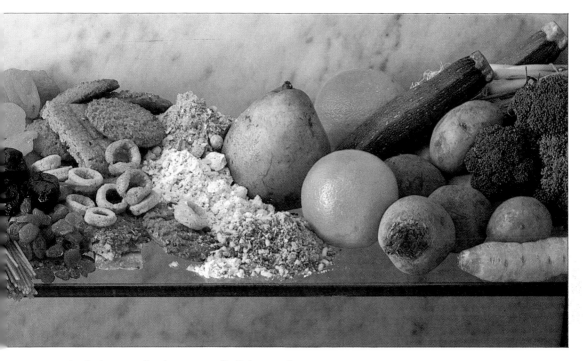

women in their reproductive years. Deficiency of iron causes anaemia, which is identified by a simple blood test. If you are not anaemic, you do not need extra iron, and excessive amounts can cause liver damage.

Perhaps the greatest absurdity of mineral supplementation is the fact that healthfood stores even offer sodium or salt pills for sale, despite the fact that salt is a major health risk for some people. These pills contain the same active ingredients as your salt-cellar.

'Natural' and 'organic' foods

Similar misconceptions underlie the 'natural' and 'organic' food markets. Most customers imagine that such foods contain lower levels of pesticides than 'normal' ones and are nutritionally superior, but, in fact, most studies fail to demonstrate this. And to a plant it makes no difference whether its nitrogen comes from organic manure or from inorganic fertilizer. Concern for the environment is well placed, but without pesticides and fertilizers, even more of the world's millions would be starving.

Food additives and preservatives are also essential to the worldwide mass marketing of food. Many additives are, in fact, naturally occur-

The shelves of the typical healthfood store are laden with goods such as those illustrated here — vitamin tablets; pulses, beans, wholewheat pasta and cereals, dried fruit and nuts; a variety of processed foods, including biscuits, canned food and dried soup mixes; and organically grown vegetables. The problem for the customer is to differentiate between which are worthwhile and which potentially harmful to health.

ring chemicals. An example is antioxidant E 330, which is citric acid, a chemical made by all body cells. Not all additives and preservatives are, however, above suspicion. Nitrites, used in meat preservation, have been investigated as a possible cause of cancer, and methods traditionally used to smoke meat and fish are also thought to be responsible for causing cancer.

Apart, perhaps, from their relatively high price, there is nothing detrimental about the wholefoods, such as pulses, nuts, cereals and grains, sold by healthfood stores. These foods are no better or worse than their supermarket equivalents. Beware, however, of 'healthy' looking and processed foods in healthfood stores. Muesli bars, nut crunches, soya mixes and the like may contain as much saturated fat, sugar or salt as a 'non-healthy' product bought from an ordinary supermarket.

ALLERGIES AND FOOD PROBLEMS

The subjects of food allergy and intolerance are among the most obscure and difficult areas of modern medicine. While many doctors are sceptical, a large industry has arisen devoted to convincing people that their multiple symptoms and general dissatisfaction with life are due to allergy to, or intolerance of, the food they eat. The truth lies somewhere between these extremes, but exactly where it is hard to say.

Allergy and intolerance

An allergy to food means that a person's immune system — the system that defends the body against infection — is mounting an attack against the food. Some people clearly suffer symptoms such as asthmatic wheezing, urticaria (raised red blotches on the skin, often called hives), swelling of the lips or symptoms like those of hay fever in response to certain foods.

In contrast, other people may experience less clear-cut symptoms, such as nausea, vomiting, abdominal pain or headache, which can be reliably shown to be brought on by a particular food and which disappear once that food is eliminated from the diet. This is food intolerance and may or may not be due to true food allergy.

In babies, food allergy may be a cause of eczema. Certainly eczema seems to run in families, and it has been shown that if babies of parents prone to eczema, asthma or hay fever are breast fed, they are less likely to experience the problem. It is also wise for parents to delay the introduction of cow's milk until the latest possible moment or to use formula feeds which are not based on cow's milk.

The other food-allergy disease from which infants may suffer is coeliac disease. In this, the intestine reacts adversely to wheat protein, and loses its capacity to absorb nutrients. Although the problem is not common, delaying the introduction of wheat-based foods until at least four months may help to reduce the symptoms, but the disease is usually one that lasts for life.

By the nature of things, the diagnosis of food intolerance is always less clear than that of food allergy, and unfortunately there is no single test to distinguish the two. Another problem in the diagnosis of food allergy and intolerance is that the emotions may also be involved. The mere thought or expectation of a food may bring on symptoms. Food intolerance or allergy may be

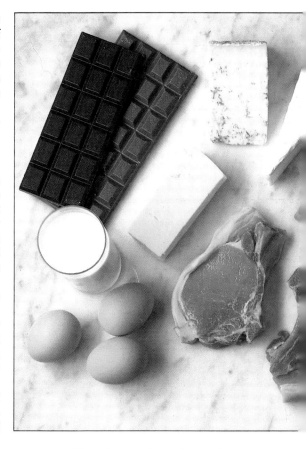

suspected if abstinence from the food leads to a disappearance of the symptoms. Experimentally, this has to be done by 'masking' the suspect food by encasing it in a gelatine capsule.

It it a widely held view that food additives and colourings are triggers of food allergy. The case for this is not clear, but they can be held responsible in some cases. In one study of migraine in children, for example, the common colorant tartrazine was shown to produce headaches in 30 out of 88 cases, and the preservative benzoate in 33 of the 88. In adults, urticaria can be set off by these and similar compounds. When children have eczema, it may well be worth avoiding food colorants to see if there is any improvement.

Elimination diets

In attempts to discover the cause of food allergies, doctors recommended full-scale elimination diets. In these, all food is cut back to a few basic staples, such as·lamb, rice and pears, for about

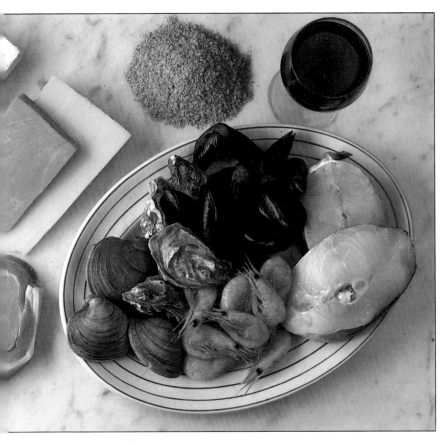

Food is often the trigger *that starts an attack of migraine. Some of the most common foods are illustrated here. Reactions to nuts, coffee, rye, maize and soya and to the additives benzoic acid and tartrazine have also been recorded as triggers in migraine studies.*

three weeks, then other foods are added gradually to see whether symptoms recur. This is a massive operation and should be undertaken only under medical supervision.

If you think you or your child may have a food problem, it is, however, worth trying a simple 'avoidance' diet. A week of avoiding a particular food is usually long enough to see if it solves a problem, but in cases of eczema you may have to persist for three weeks to be sure. Start with dairy products, eggs, nuts, fish and artificial colourings, but remember to eliminate only one food or food additive at a time.

Almost every sort of food *has been blamed, at some time, for causing problems. The chart gives the results of a study, conducted at Guy's hospital in London, of 100 adults.*

Food	Numbers affected
Milk	46
Eggs	40
Nuts	22
Fish/shellfish	22
Wheat/flour	9
Chocolate	8
Artificial colorants	7
Pork/bacon	7
Chicken	6
Tomatoes	6
Soft fruits	6
Cheese	6

Less commonly, problems occurred with yeast, bananas, beef, cucumber, onion, pineapple, sweetcorn, tea, coffee, apple, celery, cream, ginger, peas, potatoes, soya and sultanas. It was noteworthy that more than 200 instances of food problems were recorded in the 100 subjects, showing that food problems may well be multiple.

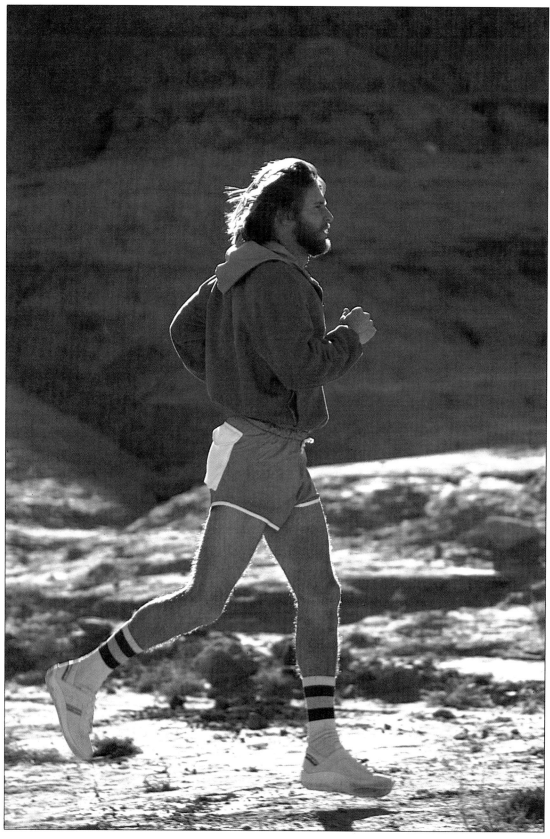

GETTING FIT, STAYING FIT

Health, vitality and long life are the goals that everyone would wish to aim for. These are not, however, achieved automatically. Because the 'civilized' habits of Western life do more to diminish health than to increase it, fitness is something that has to be worked at.

If you are resolved to take a positive attitude toward your health and well-being, and to prevent problems rather than simply treating them as and when they occur, then physical fitness must be an essential part of your life. Being fit has many advantages, from helping you to control your weight to giving you a better night's sleep. Most important of all, there is impressive and mounting evidence that people who exercise frequently and in the right way are less prone to 'killer diseases', such as heart attacks and strokes, and live longer than people whose existence is sedentary.

The key to effective exercise, that is, exercise that will make a measurable improvement in your fitness and thus decrease the risk of disease, lies in the parts of the body that carry oxygen to the exercising muscles. These, collectively known as the aerobic system, are the ones that profit from any sort of endurance activity such as running, swimming or cycling. This explains why it is endurance activity that needs to be built up and maintained if you are to help your heart and arteries to maximum effect.

There are various ways in which you can build up the efficiency of your aerobic system. This chapter gives you many examples, as well as specific programmes to follow. It should thus be possible for everyone to find all activity, or a mixture of activities, that will be both enjoyable and a help to aerobic fitness.

Although most children and young people are encouraged to take part in sport and to be fit, this kind of activity often declines sharply from early adulthood onward. It is not possible, however, to build up a store of fitness that will last you for life. You not only need to exercise regularly all your life but, if anything, you should exercise more, not less, as you get older.

Exercise, above all, makes you look and feel well. Few adults who have taken the trouble to get fit will ever allow themselves to become unfit again. You owe it to yourself to get your body fit and to maintain that fitness for as long as you possibly can.

By being fit, you will enjoy life more. This is certainly a startling claim, and one that is hard to back up with facts and figures. But if you talk to anyone who has transformed themselves from a sedentary, unfit individual to an active, fit one, you will find that — almost without exception — they go on keeping themselves fit because they feel so much better for being fit. They do not continue to exercise because of some belief that they will live longer.

If you find this sort of claim hard to believe, and if you tend to be put off by the messianic zeal of people who are newly dedicated to a fitter life, there is still some hard evidence you should consider about the benefits of aerobic fitness.

Does aerobic fitness prolong life?

The central question to be asked about the advantages of aerobic fitness is whether or not it prolongs life. And it is important not to muddle this with questions about the mechanisms that might be involved if the answer is 'yes'.

From the scientific viewpoint, the only truly satisfactory experiment to test whether fitness improves life expectancy would be to take two large, matched groups of people and allow all those people in one group to get fit. They would then have to be followed for at least 20 years, and possibly much longer, to see how they fared.

In practice, such experiments are not possible. Instead we have to rely on 'natural' experiments, which roughly parallel these ideal conditions. The first of these was conducted by Professor J. N. Morris of the University of London, and his subjects were the drivers and conductors of London's double-decker buses. It was found that the conductors suffered from less heart disease, possibly because they spent so much of their time running up and down stairs.

Similar studies were conducted in the USA by Dr Ralph Paffenbarger of Stanford University. He looked at San Francisco longshoremen (dock workers) and at graduates from Harvard. Of 3,700 longshoremen studied, Paffenbarger found

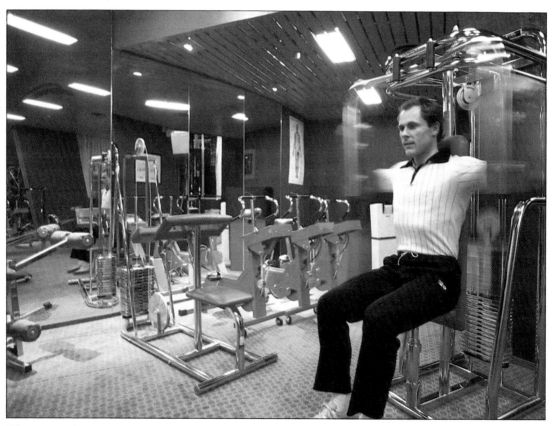

The corporate multi-gym is testament to the fact that many companies and corporations are now realizing that they have much to gain by promoting the pursuit of fitness. Not only may sickness rates be lowered, but fitter staff may well perform more efficiently and live longer.

that those with the most energetic jobs had the lowest death rates from heart attacks and strokes. It may be that the most energetic of these men were healthier to start with, and they may have been in their jobs by virtue of greater fitness; but in a natural experiment, such matters are impossible to assess or control.

When Professor Morris looked at the leisure activities of nearly 18,000 Whitehall civil servants, he too found that those who were most energetic in their leisure time fared better from the point of view of heart attacks. Those with the highest exercise level had a heart attack frequency 40 per cent lower than those with the lowest exercise level. But while this study is impressive, it still does not completely dispel the notion that people may avoid exercise because they already have some undiagnosed heart problem.

Paffenbarger's second study on 17,000 Harvard alumni shows the same order of benefit from exercise as in the civil servants. He also found that those who were college athletes — and so, presumably, 'naturally' fitter — did no better in the long run than any of the other subjects, unless they continued to exercise.

While all this evidence is not, scientifically speaking, wholly conclusive, for practical purposes it is quite good enough, and it is becoming stronger as a result of ongoing surveys. So it can be said with confidence that it is extremely unlikely that getting fit does *not* prolong life.

The body mechanisms
The way in which the body's physiology becomes changed by exercise is not entirely clear. It is, however, beyond reasonable doubt that a type of cholesterol, known as high-density cholesterol or HDL (see p. 63), increases as a result of exercise. This cholesterol is thought to help protect arterial disease and heart attacks.

Evidence from work on laboratory animals also suggests that blockage of the coronary arteries, which supply blood to the heart, can be prevented, or at least reduced or delayed, by exercise. Other factors that may contribute to cardiac risk, such as blood pressure, the levels of fats circulating in the blood, and the efficiency of the blood clotting mechanisms, may all be significantly reduced by increased activity, including the intensive energy output of some sports.

SHAPE AND PSYCHE

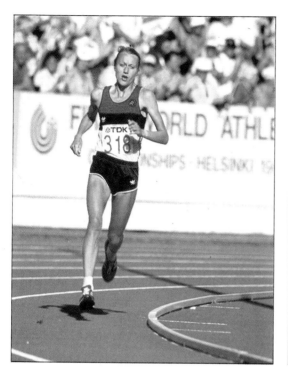

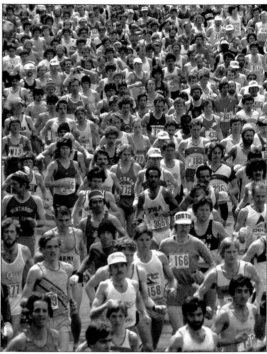

The type of aerobic exercise you choose must be the one that you enjoy most. Otherwise you will find it hard to stick to. When making their choice, however, many people feel that their bodies are the 'wrong shape' for certain types of exercise.

Overall body shape, and the physiology of the muscles (see pp. 94-5) are important considerations for those whose job it is to select and train champion athletes. However, they do not really matter for individuals attempting to find a fitness strategy that will be both effective and self-fulfilling. Mental approach is far more significant than physical make-up.

Women often feel at a particular disadvantage when it comes to exercising. Certainly the tilt of the female pelvis, which is tailored more for childbearing than athletic performance, may be a disadvantage at the highest level. More of a hindrance to most women is their high proportion of body fat (with its concentration in the breasts) at the expense of muscle. Their body fat means that women have proportionately more weight to carry, and, because of fat's insulating effects, women lose heat less readily. Exercise is, however, an excellent way of getting rid of some of this fat, once a woman has motivated herself to

start an aerobic exercise routine. Another disadvantage women have is that they sweat less than men. During exercise, this speeds up the onset of fatigue.

The men and women who find it easiest to get into a regular pattern of basic aerobic exercise, such as running or cycling, are often those who are happy with their own company. They are not necessarily lone wolves. Rather they do not need the stimulus of other people to enjoy themselves.

There is no doubt, however, that even self-sufficient people may find running boring and feel that they do not have the time to devote to

Human performance, over all distances, continues to improve. This is related to the selection of athletes, by shape and aptitude for particular events at an early age, to improved training based on a better understanding of human physiology, and to advances in running tracks and equipment.

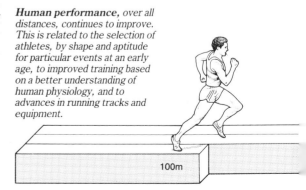

Sprinters such as the American Calvin Smith (right) are the ultimate, anaerobic, explosive athletes. Typically built, Smith is well muscled and slightly stocky. Specialists in longer distances, such as 400, 800 and 1,500 metres tend to be taller and less heavily built.

Norwegian Grete Waitz, the world-class marathon runner, (far left) is a typical example of an endurance athlete, being slightly built, with little body fat, and of medium height. Athletes who specialize in middle-distance events, such as 5,000 metres, tend to be taller than average, but are also slim.

Size and shape need be no barrier to participation, as a group of marathon runners shows (left). Among these everyday athletes are men and women of a wide range of dimensions. The message is that you can achieve a great deal in terms of aerobic exercise if that is your ambition.

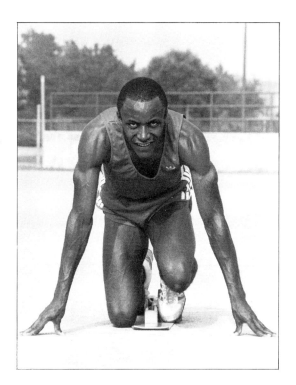

cycling or walking. For a good many of them, swimming is the answer. It has the same advantages as running, in that much aerobic training can be packed into a short time. Fortunately, non-runners often take readily to swimming.

The stimulus of competition is what many people find they need to keep them exercising; but if you play competitive sport, it is essential that you do not deceive yourself into thinking you are fit when you are not. A half-hour game of squash once a week, for example, will do little to improve your aerobic fitness. You should use aerobic training between squash sessions to help

you improve your on-court performance.

If you find it hard to motivate yourself to run, swim or cycle on your own, or even with friends, try one of the aerobics classes now widely available. The presence of others taking part, perhaps aided by the knowledge that you are paying to be there, may be all the motivation necessary for you to exercise.

At the opposite end of the spectrum, psychology is an essential ingredient of performance in competitive or championship sport. Suitability of approach to, say, long-and short-distance events can be as critical as body shape and training.

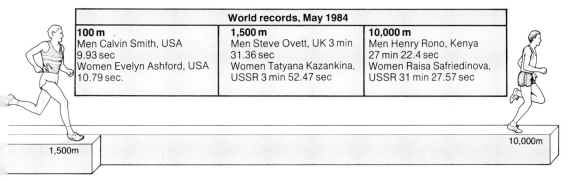

World records, May 1984		
100 m Men Calvin Smith, USA 9.93 sec Women Evelyn Ashford, USA 10.79 sec.	**1,500 m** Men Steve Ovett, UK 3 min 31.36 sec Women Tatyana Kazankina, USSR 3 min 52.47 sec	**10,000 m** Men Henry Rono, Kenya 27 min 22.4 sec Women Raisa Safriedinova, USSR 31 min 27.57 sec

1,500m

10,000m

FITNESS TESTING

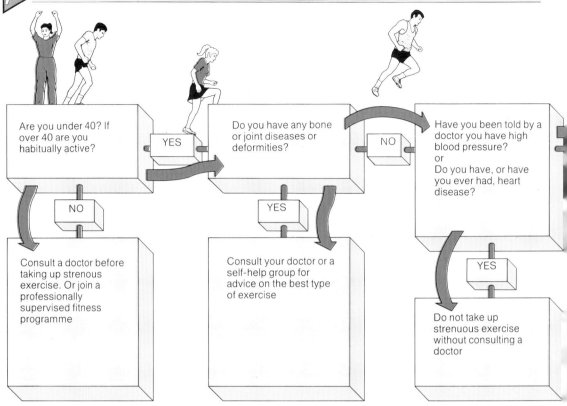

Are you under 40? If over 40 are you habitually active?

YES

NO

Do you have any bone or joint diseases or deformities?

NO

YES

Have you been told by a doctor you have high blood pressure?
or
Do you have, or have you ever had, heart disease?

YES

Consult a doctor before taking up strenous exercise. Or join a professionally supervised fitness programme

Consult your doctor or a self-help group for advice on the best type of exercise

Do not take up strenuous exercise without consulting a doctor

Fitness testing is useful on two counts. It can determine whether you are at risk — particularly of heart attack — if you take up exercise. It can also assess your levels of heart-lung, or aerobic, fitness and of muscle performance. As a result of this type of testing, your need for increased aerobic activity can be assessed.

A full fitness test includes a physical examination and measurements of height, weight and percentage of body fat. Blood and urine are also analysed to detect signs of disease. The blood analysis includes a measure of its cholesterol content, since cholesterol levels are related to the risk of heart disease (see p.63).

The electrical activity of the heart is measured as an electrocardiogram (ECG), both when you are resting and when you are exercising. This dual measurement is important in the detection of heart problems that might make exercise risky, since the signs of heart trouble do not necessarily show up on the trace taken while you are sitting or lying quietly at rest. The heart rate is also a useful guide to fitness, indicating the improvements that might be expected with increased aerobic exercise.

Blood pressure measurements, both at rest and during exercise, are taken, again with the aim of detecting cardiovascular problems that could be improved by a more judicious lifestyle. The exercise part of the fitness assessment is usually performed on some kind of treadmill or on an exercise bicycle.

As a result of the fitness test, a doctor will advise you about your fitness and the steps you should take to improve it. He may suggest that you lose weight and recommend a healthful reducing diet combined with regular aerobic exercise. Increased aerobic activity could also be indicated as a result of the heart and lung function tests. Giving up smoking and more controlled use of alcohol might also be recommended.

If it is discovered that you have heart disease, the advice you are given will depend on the extent of the problem and on your doctor's attitude toward treatment. But whatever your state of fitness, and whatever recommendations are made, you will be advised about the need for, and frequency of, follow-up fitness tests. These will assess the progress you have made in improving your fitness level.

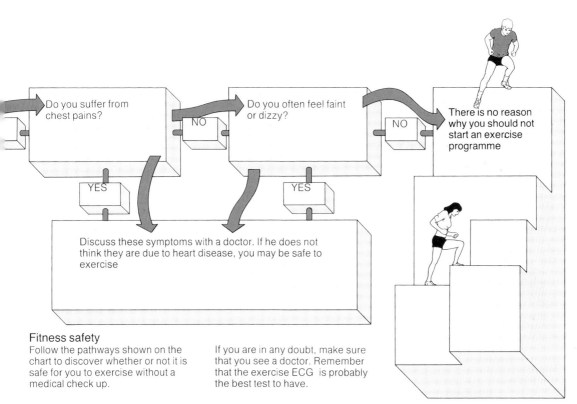

Do you suffer from chest pains?

NO

Do you often feel faint or dizzy?

NO

There is no reason why you should not start an exercise programme

YES

YES

Discuss these symptoms with a doctor. If he does not think they are due to heart disease, you may be safe to exercise

Fitness safety

Follow the pathways shown on the chart to discover whether or not it is safe for you to exercise without a medical check up.

If you are in any doubt, make sure that you see a doctor. Remember that the exercise ECG is probably the best test to have.

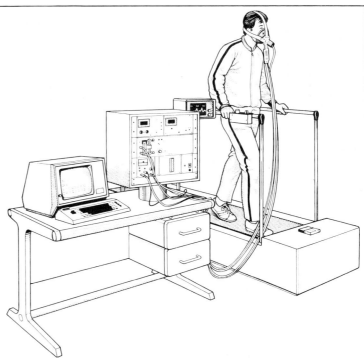

The treadmill is a piece of equipment central to fitness testing. The person being tested is 'wired up' for ECG recordings and breathes into a mouthpiece connected to a computerized air analyzer. (In non-computerized systems, air is collected in huge bags for laboratory analysis.) At the start of the test, the belt of the treadmill moves so that the person is moving at walking pace. As the test progresses, the speed can be increased so that the person breaks into a run, or the treadmill may be made to rise into an incline. In both instances this means that the person's aerobic system is having to work harder.

The test continues until the doctor supervising it considers (from the subject's age, his degree of distress and from the readings on the recording apparatus) that it is no longer safe to continue. Analysis of the results are followed up with advice about future activity.

WARM UP AND COOL DOWN

Warming up and cooling down should be an integral part of any type of aerobic exercise, for it is dangerous and inefficient to leap immediately from cold to maximum activity. A few minutes' slow swimming, jogging or cycling before you start to work a little harder is usually quite satisfactory. As with all exercises, stop at once if you experience any pain.

It is especially important to warm up before a race or competition, for cold muscles are much more likely to be injured, and the extra stimulus of competition tempts many people to drive too hard before the full blood flow through their muscles is established, so precipitating problems. Remember that the fitter you are, the longer it takes for the muscles to warm up for full exertion, since they have a greater capacity. It is important, however, to recognize that these exercises are an adjunct to aerobics and should not exhaust you before you begin to cover any ground.

Runners benefit particularly from warm-up exercises, since running incorporates only a limited range of movements. Use the toe touch, arm rotation, waist stretch and wall stretch for warming up. These exercises are designed to put the big muscle groups through a variety of motions. Gradually increase the duration of each exercise so that you give each muscle a stretch lasting for 30 seconds or more.

In many ways, the period after exercise is even more important because the body can suffer from shock if you stop exercising suddenly. If you sit down and rest immediately after aerobic exercise, the muscles tend to shorten, with subsequent loss of flexibility and stiffness. First reduce the exercise you are doing to a slow pace, then use the exercises suggested here — squats, hamstring stretch, knee hugs and book or kerb drop. These are designed to give the important muscle groups a mild stretch before you shower and rest. As with the warm-up exercises, gradually increase the duration of each.

For runners, the wall stretch and book or kerb drop exercises, which prevent shortening of the achilles tendon, are particularly important.

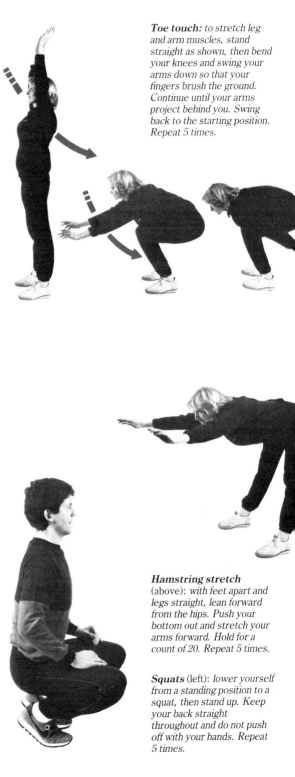

Toe touch: *to stretch leg and arm muscles, stand straight as shown, then bend your knees and swing your arms down so that your fingers brush the ground. Continue until your arms project behind you. Swing back to the starting position. Repeat 5 times.*

Hamstring stretch (above): *with feet apart and legs straight, lean forward from the hips. Push your bottom out and stretch your arms forward. Hold for a count of 20. Repeat 5 times.*

Squats (left): *lower yourself from a standing position to a squat, then stand up. Keep your back straight throughout and do not push off with your hands. Repeat 5 times.*

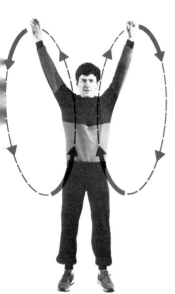

Wall stretch (right): *stand 1 m (3 ft) from a wall, tree or post and reach out to touch or grasp it. With back straight, lean in close until your forearms touch the support, then push away. Repeat 5 times.*

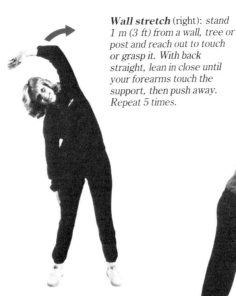

Arm rotation (above): *rotate your arms backward in large circles 5 times, then forward 5 times.*

Waist stretch (above): *stand with feet apart, then bend to the right as shown. Repeat 5 times on each side of the body.*

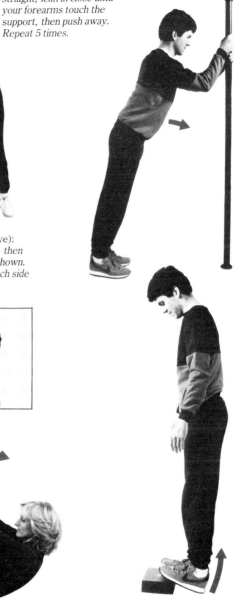

Knee hugs: *from a standing position (above left), pull up and hug each knee alternately, pulling it toward your chest. Repeat 5 times. Alternatively, perform these knee hugs in a lying position (top).*

As a variation, follow each knee hug with a leg stretch (above). Raise the leg to a straight position as shown, and pull it toward you with both hands. Do 5 repeats for each leg.

Book or kerb drop: *stand with your heels on the ground and your toes on a book or the kerb. Rise up on to your toes, then lower your heels again. Repeat 5 times.*

FLEXIBILITY

Those who concentrate on cardio-respiratory fitness often neglect the importance of flexibility in a general training programme.

A supple body may be of no direct benefit to your heart and lungs, but it allows the body to exercise aerobically with greater ease. The joints have a natural tendency to lose mobility from adolescence onward and, without the benefit of regular exercise, normal forms of exercise become increasingly hard to perform. By putting all the main joints in your body through their full range of movements every day, you can help to maintain their function and possibly even prevent arthritic problems later in life.

The exercises on this page provide a basic flexibility package which will keep you in trim if used two or three times a week. They are a good way of backing up your aerobic training, and an essential aid to maintaining flexibility if you are a runner. You can use them either immediately after a day's exercise or on their own after the warm-up exercises on pp. 100-101. Build up the number of repeats from the basic number given with each exercise. Remember that the trunk and limbs should feel pleasantly warm with circulating blood before the body's main groups of muscles are put through their paces.

Warmth increases the benefits of flexibility exercises, so choose a warm room or wear warm clothing outside. Try not to rush, but maintain a comfortably even pace, increasing the number of repetitions as you improve. The neck rolling exercise needs to be performed slowly to loosen the neck. The squat thrust, however, can have an aerobic effect if you increase the speed.

As you follow the exercises and feel the relevant muscles under tension, it is important to respond to your body's own signals. The muscles should feel extended, but not pulled, for if you overstretch shortened muscles too suddenly, you may tear the body of the muscle. The aim is to allow a gradual and comfortable lengthening of the muscle fibres.

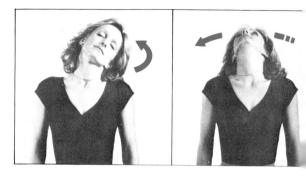

Head roll (above): *drop your head forward, then slowly roll it clockwise 5 times, and counter-clockwise 5 times. Work up to 10 repeats.*

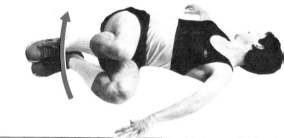

Double knee roll (above): *lie on your back, with knees bent and arms by your sides. Roll your head to one side, your knees to the other. Hold for a count of 5, then roll over to the other side. Repeat 5 times.*

Sleeves up (left): *grasp your forearms as shown, then push your hands towar your elbows. Repeat 5 times.*

Hurdle stretch (right): *sit in a hurdle position as shown. Pull your left foot back with your left hand, your right foot back with your right hand. Repeat 5 times for each side.*

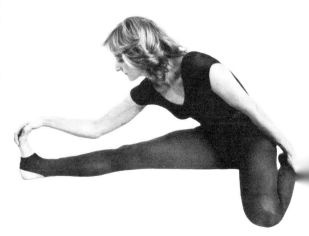

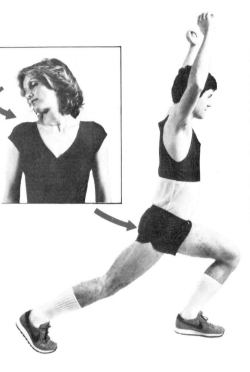

Lunge stretch (left): *stand with feet apart, then take a step forward with one leg and, at the same time, shoot your arms above your head. Repeat 5 times for each side of the body.*

Knee diamonds (right): *stand with feet together. Using a chair for support, slowly bend from the knees to create a diamond shape as shown. Return slowly to the starting position. Repeat 5 times.*

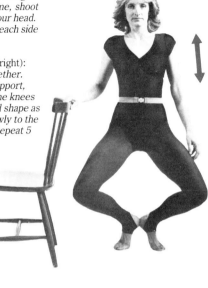

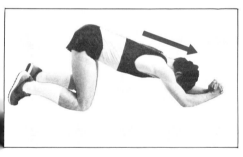

Pectoral stretch (left): *kneel down, then slide forward until your elbows, then your upper arms, touch the floor as shown. Repeat 5 times.*

Thigh shift (right): *flex your left knee sideways as shown. With hands on hips, bounce up and down 5 times. Repeat with the right leg.*

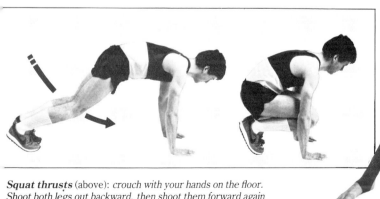

Squat thrusts (above): *crouch with your hands on the floor. Shoot both legs out backward, then shoot them forward again as shown. Repeat 5 times.*

EXERCISING THE BACK

More muscular pain and injury occur in the back than in any other part of the body, but exercises can protect your back by improving its flexibility and strength.

In order to maintain an upright posture, the muscles of the back are constantly in action. It is wise to do exercises for your back, however, especially if you have a sedentary lifestyle. Back exercises also aid lifting and twisting movements which tend to put a strain on the back. In addition to the exercises shown here, you may wish to do some strength training (see pp. 128-9).

It is most useful to exercise for correct posture and to build up the muscles of the abdominal wall, for, if these are strengthened, they automatically correct any postural faults.

The exercises on this page are designed for those people who have never had any serious back trouble and wish to prevent trouble arising. If you have suffered problems, however, these exercises may also be used, but only after consultation with your doctor or physiotherapist.

The backswing device has become very popular over the last few years to relieve bad backs

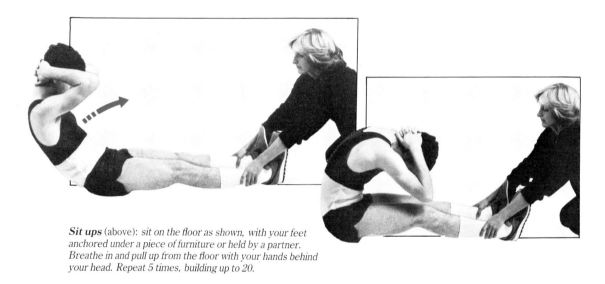

Sit ups (above): *sit on the floor as shown, with your feet anchored under a piece of furniture or held by a partner. Breathe in and pull up from the floor with your hands behind your head. Repeat 5 times, building up to 20.*

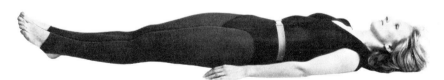

Head and shoulders up: *lie flat on your back as shown. Pull your head and shoulders up, tightening your abdominal muscles. Repeat 5 times, building up to 30 repeats.*

although its use is controversial. By hanging upside down, its proponents argue, all the strain is taken off the back, thus allowing it to resume its correct shape. It may well relieve recurrent back pain, but consult your doctor or osteopath if you are under treatment and stop immediately if the pain gets worse (see p. 155).

Back weakness and poor posture need to be put right gradually. If you rush at it, you may simply end up exchanging one set of bad habits for another, so take each sequence of exercises and improvements slowly and gently.

Cat back (below): *kneel with your weight evenly distributed between hands and knees. Breathe in; then, keeping your head up, curve your back down into a U shape. Then reverse the curve, and push your back up. Repeat 5 times, building up to 20.*

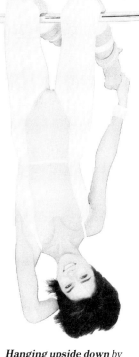

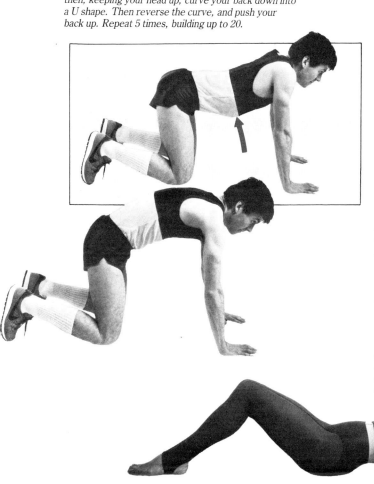

Hanging upside down *by your knees, or with your feet in specially designed gravity boots, is beneficial to the back. The weight of the body acts to pull the bones of the spine apart into the correct alignment. Use this exercise to prevent back problems and, if your doctor so advises, to help treat back pain.*

Pelvic tilt (below): *lie flat on your back, with knees bent and arms by your sides. Tilt your pelvis upward, tightening your buttock and stomach muscles so that you make an arch behind your buttocks. Repeat 5 times, building up to 20.*

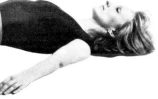

Aerobic exercise is one of the keys to improving and maintaining fitness and well-being (see pp. 88-95). To find out your current fitness level, test yourself by completing the quiz and tests on pp. 12-14, then use the guidelines on this and the following pages to help you set up and maintain your own exercise programme.

There are only a few means of aerobic conditioning available to everyone. The 'big three' are running, swimming and cycling, which are all excellent forms of aerobic training. Walking is a good starter for runners, and if your current fitness level is low, you would not be able to start on the running programme without completing a walking programme first. Other aerobic programmes you can try in this section, and use as alternatives on selected days if you wish, include stair climbing, aerobic dancing, and skipping and using a rowing machine.

About the programmes
The programmes for running, swimming and cycling give distances and times for beginners, intermediate and advanced performers, and for men and women. The walking programme opposite takes you from beginner stage to a level which is equivalent to about week 4 of the running schedules.

The swimming programme is structured rather differently, since not everyone has the same natural ability at swimming. The beginners' programme is for those who have never felt they were good swimmers. Readers who are starting a training programme, but who have been reasonable or even good swimmers in the past, should start on the intermediate programme.

The cycling and running programmes are designed to be interchangeable, and this should present no problems. You can also interchange them with aerobic dancing, skipping and using a rowing machine. If you wish to interchange any programme with swimming, however, it is wise, because of the different skills involved, to advance in both programmes concurrently.

Using the programmes
Before you start to use the programmes, have any necessary medical checks (see pp. 98-9), take note of your resting pulse rate (see pp. 12-13) and warm up (see pp. 100-1). If you are not used to exercise, be sure to start with the beginners' programme of your chosen exercise.

The times in each programme are guides to use once or twice a week. The important element in these schedules is a steady increase in distance covered and thus of energy expended. Time is, of course, a guide to energy expenditure in programmes such as rowing. It is speed that is the optional extra.

Because beginners are injury-prone, do not start off too fast. You cannot get fit in a week, but you can get a long way toward it in a month. If you feel stiff the day after exercise, change activities or simply do some warm-up exercises so that you allow your body a chance to recover.

Exercise at a time of the day that is most convenient, but preferably not until 2 or 3 hours after a meal. Never exercise if you feel ill or have a cold or a temperature. Do not start training again until you are free of symptoms, and keep your distance down to half your normal level for a week. For every day's exercise you miss, backtrack at least 2 days on the programme. If you wish to exercise more, than five times a week, be sure to make your extra sessions slow. Although you should feel physically stretched by the programmes, you should not exercise to exhaustion point. Keep a check on your pulse (pp. 12-13) and do not exceed the safe maximum. If you feel dizzy, or in pain, **stop at once**.

Anyone below 35 should be able to work through the programmes with no trouble. If you are over 50, progress at about half the recommended rate, spending 2 weeks at each stage instead of one. If you are aged 35 to 50, attempt the first half of the beginners' programme on a weekly basis, then cut back to a fortnightly progression.

Once you have completed the beginners' running and cycling schedules, 20 to 30 minutes at these levels three times a week is enough to maintain fitness. For swimming, aim to complete a 1,000-metre swim three times a week. For walking, allow 60 to 75 minutes a session.

Natural ability does impose some restrictions on achievement beyond the beginner stage. Once you feel you have reached your own limit, it will be more useful to stick at this stage and to measure your improving fitness by the decrease in your resting pulse rate and by an increase in the time in which you reach your safe maximum pulse rate.

Walking

The walking programme below is a 16-week programme well within the capabilities of anyone who can walk 1.6 km (1 ml). This makes it suitable for people of all ages and for everyone but the severely unfit. Start off walking at your own pace. For the first 8 weeks, targets are offered in terms of either time or distance, but you will find that your pace increases naturally as you progress. Check by week 5 or 6 that you can walk 3.2 km (2 ml) in 30 minutes – nearly everyone will be able to achieve this. If you cannot, stick at the 3.2 km (2 ml) level and increase your pace before continuing the programme.

To maintain an adequate level of fitness after completing this programme, you will need to walk a minimum of 8 km (5 mls) three times a week. Take all possible opportunities to walk during your daily routine rather than using motorized transport.

Stair-climbing

This is an excellent form of aerobic exercise. The programme below is a brisk one, but is ideal for all but the over-60s. Increase your time and/or rate each week. The set rate of climbing includes the time taken for descents. Thus if you have 15 steps in your flight of stairs, you will need to go up and down 4 times a minute to achieve the rate of 60 steps a minute.

Steps/min	Time spent climbing/ min
40	2
40	4
50	4
50	5
60	6
60	7
60	8
60	9
60	10
70	10
70	11
70	12

Walking programme

Week	Distance/ km/(mls)		Time/ min	Repeats/ week
1	1·6 (1)	or	15	5
2	2 (1¼)	or	20	5
3	2·4 (1½)	or	23	5
4	2·8 (1¾)	or	26	5
5	3·2 (2)	or	30	5
6	3·2 (2)	or	30	3
	4 (2½)	in any time		2
7	4 (2½)	or	30	3
	4·8 (3)	in any time		2
8	3·2 (2)	or	30	4
	any distance	in	60	1
9	3·2 (2)	in	28	4
	any distance	in	60	1
10	3·2 (2)	in	27½	4
	any distance	in	60	1
11	4 (2½)	in	35	4
	any distance	in	60	1
12	4 (2½)	in	34	4
	6·4 (4)	in	58	1
13	4·8 (3)	in	42	4
	6·5 (4)	in	58	1
14	3·2 (2)	in	27	3
	6·4 (4)	in	56	2
15	3·2 (2)	in	26½	3
	8 (5)	in	75	2
16	3·2 (2)	in	26	3
	8 (5)	in	70	2

Racewalking

This is a form of high-speed walking that is becoming increasingly popular as a means of achieving aerobic fitness. The speed of this type of walking is such that many people would find it more comfortable to run, but it imposes a discipline on body performance that you may find stimulating. The amount of energy used in racewalking is probably greater than that consumed in running, and more groups of muscles are exercised, so that mile for mile (at the speeds given below), It has a better training effect.

As a guide, use the walking programme, but aim to walk each 1·6 km, (1 ml) in 9 to 10 minutes.

Running—also known as jogging when performed at a slow pace—is the most popular and accessible of all the aerobic sports. Use the running programme below according to the guidelines given on p. 106. It is designed to produce an acceptable level of fitness by the beginning of the intermediate stage and a run of 5 km ($3\frac{1}{10}$mls) three times a week will maintain fitness.

At the advanced stage, the men's programme should eventually enable you to complete a full marathon in less than $3\frac{1}{2}$ hours. The women's advanced programme should lead to a marathon time of $3\frac{3}{4}$ to 4 hours.

Once you begin running, you should quickly fall into a style that suits you, but remember to run with a heel-first action, making a clawing action as

| Men's running programme | | | | | | | | | | | |
| Beginners | | | | Intermediate | | | | Advanced | | | |
Week	Distance/ km (mls)	Repeats/ week	Time/ min	Week	Distance/ km (mls)	Repeats/ week	Time/ min	Week	Distance/ km (mls)	Repeats/ week	Time/ min
1	1.6(1)	5	—	1	3.2(2)	3	17	1	4.8(3)	2	$24\frac{1}{2}$
					4.8(3)	2	—		12.8(8)	3	70
2	1.6(1)	5	12	2	4(2½)	4	22	2	6.4(4)	2	33
					any distance	1	45		12.8(8)	3	—
3	1.6(1)	3	11	3	3.2(2)	4	—	3	6.4(4)	3	32
	2.4(1½)	2	20		6.4(4)	1	35		12.8(8)	2	68
4	1.6(1)	3	$10\frac{1}{2}$	4	4.8(3)	4	26	4	11.2(7)	4	58
	2.4(1½)	2	18		any distance	1	55		16(10)	1	—
5	1.6(1)	3	10	5	4(2½)	4	—	5	6.4(4)	2	31
	2.4(1½)	2	16		8(5)	1	44		11.2(7)	3	—
6	1.6(1)	3	$9\frac{1}{2}$	6	4.8(3)	4	$25\frac{1}{2}$	6	6.4(4)	1	30
	3.2(2)	2	$22\frac{1}{2}$		any distance	1	65		9.6(6)	4	49
									16(10)	1	—
7	2.4(1½)	3	15	7	4(2½)	4	$21\frac{1}{2}$	7	4.8(3)	1	23
	3.2(2)	2	22		11.2(7)	1	63		11.2(7)	4	58
8	2.4(1½)	3	14	8	6.4(4)	4	$34\frac{1}{2}$	8	8(5)	3	—
	3.2(2)	2	20		any distance	1	75		12.8(8)	2	66
									16(10)	1	—
9	2.4(1½)	3	14	9	4(2½)	4	21	9	4.8(3)	1	22
	4(2½)	2	26		8(5)	1	44		12.8(8)	4	64
10	2.4(1½)	3	13	10	6.4(4)	3	34	10	9.6(6)	2	47
	4(2½)	2	24		any distance	2	60		12.8(8)	3	—
									16(10)	1	80
11	2.4(1½)	3	$12\frac{1}{2}$	11	4.8(3)	3	25	11	4.8(3)	1	$21\frac{1}{2}$
	4.8(3)	2	30		8(5)	2	—		11.2(7)	3	55
									19.2(12)	1	—
12	3.2(2)	3	$17\frac{1}{2}$	12	6.4(4)	3	34	12	6.4(4)	3	29
	4.8(3)	2	27		12.8(8)	2	—		12.8(8)	3	62
									24(15)	1	—

the rest of your foot hits the ground and pushing off from the ball of your foot at each stride. Hold your arms loosely at your sides and curl your fingers a little to aid relaxed running. Adopt an erect action, with relaxed neck and shoulders, rather than one in which the buttocks protrude. Start with small strides and alter them until you find the natural, most comfortable stride length.

Try to breathe rhythmically and deeply.

Test whether you are running within your capabilities by keeping a check on your pulse (see pp. 12-13) and by making sure you are breathing easily. A good test is to see whether you can chat to a fellow runner as you exercise.

Wear proper shoes for running (see pp. 156) and absorbent clothes suited to the weather.

Women's running programme											
Beginners				Intermediate				Advanced			
Week	Distance/ km (mls)	Repeats/ week	Time/ min	Week	Distance/ km (mls)	Repeats/ week	Time/ min	Week	Distance/ km (mls)	Repeats/ week	Time/ min
1	1.6(1) 2.4(1½) (walk/jog)	3 2	— —	1	3.2(2) 4.8(3)	3 2	17½ —	1	4.8(3) 6.4(4)	3 2	27 —
2	1.6(1) 3.2(2) (walk/jog)	3 2	13 —	2	3.2(2) 6.4(4)	4 1	17½ —	2	6.4(4)	5	36
3	1.6(1)	5	12½	3	4(2½) 6.4(4)	4 1	23 —	3	4.8(3) 9.6(6)	3 2	26 54 ·
4	1.6(1)	5	12	4	4(2½) any distance	4 1	34 40	4	6.4(4) 12.8(8)	4 1	35 —
5	1.6(1) 2.4(1½)	3 2	11½ —	5	3.4(2) 6.4(4)	3 2	17 —	5	4.8(3) 8(5)	4 2	25 45
6	1.6(1) 2.4(1½)	3 2	11 18	6	4(2½) any distance	4 1	22 50	6	6.4(4) 16(10)	4 1	35 —
7	1.6(1) 2.4(1½)	2 3	10½ 17½	7	3.2(2) 8(5)	3 2	— 45	7	6.4(4) 12.8(8)	4 1	34 —
8	2.4(1½)	5	16½	8	4(2½) any distance	4 1	21½ 60	8	8(5) 12.8(8)	3 2	45 —
9	2.4(1½) 3.2(2)	3 2	16 22	9	3.2(2) 6.4(4)	3 2	17 36	9	4.8(3) 12.8(8)	3 2	24 72
10	2.4(1½) 3.2(2)	3 2	14 21	10	4(2½) any distance	4 1	21 65	10	4.8(3) 8(5) 19.2(12)	1 4 1	23 44 —
11	2.4(1½) 3.2(2)	2 3	13½ 20	11	4.8(3) 8(5)	3 2	28 44	11	4.8(3) 9.6(6) 19.2(12)	4 1 1	22½ — 108
12	3.2(2) 4(2½)	3 2	18 24	12	4.8(3) 11.2(7)	4 1	27 63	12	4.8(3) 12.8(8) 24(15)	3 2 1	22 70 —

To undertake the cycling programmes on these pages, it is not necessary to possess a smart, 10-speed bicycle. Cycling is a most efficient form of transport. It demands less energy to move a moderate weight over a given distance than any other method. With a good bicycle, almost all your effort is used against air resistance or drag, *not* in forward propulsion.

This drag increases according to the square of the relative wind speed, so that an increase in wind or bicycle speed will create extra resistance; to reduce this effect, racing cyclists adopt a crouching position. The gradient also affects the level of effort that is required; even the mildest of gradients can double the amount of work.

Since the terrain and the relative wind speed make such a difference to cycling energy levels, the times and distances in this programme are inevitably a less accurate guide than they are in the running and swimming programmes. The basic rule for beginners is to go by time rather than distance and to keep up a reasonable level of effort. You should be cycling hard enough to sweat a little, but easily enough to continue a conversation. Keep a check on your pulse (pp. 12–13) and do not exceed the safe maximum.

Most modern cycles have gears, and beginners are inclined to start in too high a gear. Try to increase your pedalling speed as much as possible in the early stages. As you progress, vary the terrain to include some work on hills.

When you reach the intermediate programme, add 2 intervals of 1 minute each during 20 to 30 minutes of each cycling session. During each interval, cycle as fast as you can (within the bounds of safety). Warm up thoroughly before each interval and recover slowly after each one. In the advanced programme, gradually increase the time and frequency of the intervals. As a guide, aim for 4 intervals of 2 minutes each at the beginning of the advanced programme and build up to 5 intervals of $2\frac{1}{2}$ minutes each.

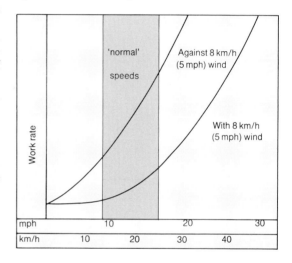

Each small increase in wind resistance imposes a huge strain on the cyclist. The graph (above) shows the levels of energy needed to cycle when faced with a 8 km/h (5 mph) wind. The cyclist must work 9 times as hard cycling into this light wind at 8 km/h (5 mph) as when cycling with a wind of the same speed.

Exercise cycles
If you really want to exercise at home, an exercise cycle can give a high level of aerobic training. Choose a good one with a chain drive and flywheel. It must be stable with a reasonable range of saddle and handlebar adjustments. It is also essential to have an adjustable tension mechanism, which varies the stiffness of the pedals and indicates your progress on a graduated scale. This 'gearing' mechanism should be adjustable while you are in motion to avoid the need for stopping to increase the level of work. Remember to warm up gently before gradually increasing the tension during your session.

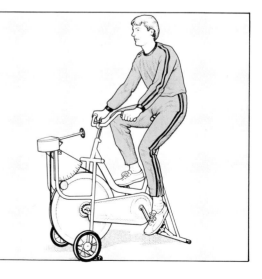

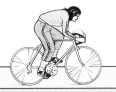 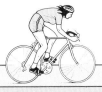

Cycling programme: Beginners

Week	Distance/ km (mls)	Time/ min	Repeats/ week
1	any distance	10	5
2	3.2 (2) / any distance	12 / 15	3 / 2
3	3.2 (2) / 4.8 (3)	11 / 18	3 / 2
4	4.8 (3) / any distance	17 / 25	3 / 2
5	3.2 (2) / 8 (5)	10 / 30	3 / 2
6	4.8 (3) / any distance	16 / 35	3 / 2
7	4.8 (3) / 9.6 (6)	15 / 38	3 / 2
8	4.8 (3) / any distance	14 / 40	3 / 2
9	4.8 (3) / 11.2 (7)	13 / 42	3 / 2
10	6.4 (4) / any distance	18 / 45	3 / 2
11	6.4 (4) / 12.8 (8)	17 / 45	3 / 2
12	8 (5) / 16 (10)	22 / 60	4 / 1

Cycling programme: Intermediate

Week	Distance/ km (mls)	Time/ min	Repeats/ week
1	8 (5) / 16 (10)	20 / 55	3 / 2
2	6.4 / 12.8	16 / 40	3 / 2
3	8 (5) / 16 (10)	20 / 50	3 / 2
4	9.6 (6) / 19.2 (12)	24 / —	3 / 2
5	6.4 (4) / 16 (10)	15 / 48	3 / 2
6	11.2 (7) / 19.2 (12)	28 / 58	3 / 2
7	8 (5) / 16 (10)	18 / 45	3 / 2
8	11.2 (7) / 24 (15)	26 / —	4 / 1
9	6.4 (4) / 19.2 (12)	14 / 53	3 / 2
10	9.6 (6) / 32 (20)	22 / —	4 / 1
11	8 (5) / 16 (10)	17 / 42	3 / 2
12	4.8 (3) / 8 (5) / 48 (30)	10 / 17 / —	2 / 2 / 1

Cycling programme: Advanced

Week	Distance/ km (mls)	Time/ min	Repeats/ week
1	9.6 (6) / 19.2 (12)	21 / 50	3 / 2
2	11.2 (7) / 19.2 (12)	25 / —	3 / 2
3	12.8 (8) / 32 (20)	30 / —	3 / 2
4	8 (5) / 16 (10)	17 / 40	2 / 3
5	6.4 (4) / 24 (15) / 48 (30)	13 / 58 / —	2 / 2 / 1
6	9.6 (6) / 24 (15)	19 / —	3 / 2
7	11.2 (7) / 24 (15) / 48 (30)	22 / 54 / 115	2 / 2 / 1
8	12.8 (8) / 24 (15)	26 / —	4 / 1
9	12.8 (4) / 24 (15) / 48 (30)	25 / 52 / —	2 / 2 / 1
10	16 (10) / 32 (20) / 48 (30)	32 / 70 / 110	2 / 2 / 1
11	12.8 (8) / 32 (20)	24 / 67	2 / 1
12	16 (10) / 32 (20) / 48 (30)	30 / 65 / 105	2 / 2 / 1

GETTING FIT/SWIMMING

Swimming is an excellent way of getting plenty of aerobic exercise in a short space of time. And being able to swim well has the added advantage that it might help to save your own or someone else's life. Because the work you are performing when you swim is against water resistance rather than against gravity, the risk of injury to body muscles and joints is low.

If you look at a group of people in a pool, you will notice how markedly they differ in their swimming capability. The programmes on these pages are designed to take account of this enormous variation in natural swimming ability. Use the programmes according to the general guidelines given on pp. 106-7.

If you are already a competent swimmer, and especially if you can swim front crawl continuously for 100 metres or more, start off with the intermediate programme. The same applies if you are adept at back crawl, which is almost as fast as front crawl when swum well and has a breathing technique that is much easier to master. Its chief disadvantage is the degree to which it reduces your visibility of other swimmers.

As you progress through the programme, you should aim to include more and more lengths of

Men's swimming programme

	Beginners				Intermediate				Advanced		
Week	Distance/ m (yds)	Repeats/ week	Time/ min	Week	Distance/ m (yds)	Repeats/ week	Time/ min	Week	Distance/ m(yds) mixed strokes	Repeats/ week	Time/ min
1	50	3	—	1	200	5	5	1	500	2	13
									500	3	11
2	50	2	—	2	200	3	5	2	500	2	12
	100	2	—		300	2	8		500	3	10
3	100	2	—	3	300	5	7½	3	500	2	12
	150	3	—						800	3	17
4	150	2	—	4	300	3	7	4	800	2	20
	200	3	—		500	2	13		800	3	16½
5	250	3	—	5	400	5	10	5	800	2	20
	300	2	13						800	2	16
									1200(1100)	1	—
6	300	5	12	6	500	5	12	6	800	2	19
									1000	2	21
									1200(1100)	1	—
7	300	3	11	7	500	3	10	7	1000	2	24
	400	2	—		700	2	16		1200(1100)	2	25
									1500(1400)	1	—
8	400	5	15	8	600	5	12	8	1000	2	24
									1500(1400)	3	31
9	400	3	14	9	600	3	11½	9	1000	2	23
	500	2	—		800	2	17		1500(1400)	3	30
10	500	5	19	10	700	5	14	10	1000	2	23
									1600(1450)	3	32
11	500	3	16	11	800	5	16½	11	1000	2	22
	600	2	—						1800(1600)	3	36
12	600	5	22	12	800	3	16	12	1000	2	21
					1000	2	22		2000(1800)	3	40

front or back crawl. You will probably need to do this to achieve the times set in the schedules, but the programmes do not specify 'mixed strokes' until you arrive at the advanced section. In this section you should spend an equal amount of time on your chosen strokes — ideally front crawl, back crawl, breast-stroke and butterfly if you can manage it. Whatever stage you are at, keep a check on your pulse rate (see pp. 12–14) and do not exceed the safe maximum.

The programmes are given in terms of metres for the short distances, at which the difference between metres and yards is not significant.

However, both metres and yards are given for the longer distances. Ask the pool attendant the length of the pool or pace it out at approximately one large stride per metre. Count the lengths as you swim and do not cheat.

To avoid the crush at public pools, try swimming early in the morning or late in the evening. You could also consider joining a club, which would offer coaching as well as reserved pool times. Protect your eyes from chlorinated or salt water with goggles and wear a swimsuit that will not cut into you and that will not slip off when you swim or dive.

Women's swimming programme

	Beginners				Intermediate				Advanced		
Week	Distance/ m (yds)	Repeats/ week	Time/ min	Week	Distance/ m (yds)	Repeats/ week	Time/ min	Week	Distance/ m (yds) mixed strokes	Repeats/ week	Time/ min
1	50	3	—	1	200	5	5	1	500	2	14
									500	3	11
2	50	2	—	2	200	3	5	2	500	2	13
	100	2	—		300	2	8		500	3	10
3	100	2	—	3	300	5	$7\frac{1}{2}$	3	500	2	13
	150	3	—						800	3	18
4	150	2	—	4	300	3	7	4	800	2	21
	200	3	—		500	2	13		800	3	17
5	250	3	—	5	400	5	10	5	800	2	21
	300	2	14						800	2	16
									1200(1100)	1	—
6	300	5	13	6	500	12	20	6	800	2	20
									1000	2	21
									1200(1100)	1	—
7	300	3	12	7	500	3	11	7	1000	2	26
	400	2	—		700	2	16		1200(1100)	2	25
									1500(1400)	1	—
8	400	5	16	8	600	5	$13\frac{1}{2}$	8	1000	2	26
									1500(1400)	3	32
9	400	3	15	9	600	3	13	9	1000	2	25
	500	2	—		800	2	19		1500(1400)	3	30
10	500	5	20	10	700	5	15	10	1000	2	25
									1600(1450)	3	32
11	500	3	18	11	800	5	$17\frac{1}{2}$	11	1000	2	24
	600	2	—						1800(1600)	3	36
12	600	5	24	12	800	3	17	12	1000	2	23
					1000	2	24		2000(1800)	3	40

GETTING FIT INDOORS

Rowing machine: Beginners			Rowing machine: Advanced		
Week	Repeats/week	Time/min	Week	Repeats/week	Time/min
1	3	15	1	1	20
				3	22
2	1	15	2	3	22
	2	16		1	23
3	3	16	3	1	22
				4	23
4	1	16	4	3	23
	2	17		2	24
5	3	18	5	2	24
				3	25
6	1	17	6	4	25
	1	18		1	26
	1	19			
7	3	19	7	3	26
				2	27
8	2	18	8	5	27
	2	19			
9	3	19	9	2	27
	1	20		3	28
10	1	19	10	4	28
	2	20		1	29
	1	21			
11	2	21	11	3	29
	2	22		2	30
12	4	22	12	5	30

Plenty of opportunities exist for indoor aerobic training. Aerobic dance, a highly effective and, for many, the most enjoyable form of exercise, has the added advantage of improving strength and flexibility. Having learned the basics at formal classes, you can use these schedules to build up your fitness levels in your own home. If you find any exercise painful, stop immediately.

Skipping was first popularized by boxers and has now been recognized by other sports people as a most convenient form of aerobic training. It needs no equipment beyond an ordinary skipping rope and can be done almost anywhere. Start off with a basic rocking skip, with the same foot leading, then with alternate feet leading before progressing to double jumps, one foot hops and other variations.

Although a rowing machine cannot duplicate the sensation of actual rowing, it provides an acceptable substitute and puts the same range of muscles through their paces. The rowing programme aims to build up your work level gently.

As with all aerobic exercise programmes, follow the general guidelines on pp. 106-7. Keep a check on your pulse and do not exceed the safe maximum (see pp. 12–13). These programmes can be interchanged with the beginners' and intermediate running and cycling programmes.

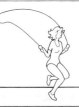

Skipping programme: Beginners			Skipping programme: Advanced		
Week	Repeats/week	Time/min	Week	Repeats/week	Time/min
1	3	5	1	5	10
2	3	$5\frac{1}{2}$	2	5	$11\frac{1}{2}$
3	4	$5\frac{1}{2}$	3	5	12
4	4	6	4	5	13
5	4	$6\frac{1}{2}$	5	5	14
6	4	7	6	5	15
7	3	7	7	6	15
	1	6			
8	4	8	8	6	16
9	4	9	9	6	17
10	4	10	10	6	18
11	5	11	11	6	19
12	5	12	12	6	20

Aerobic dance: Beginners			Aerobic dance: Advanced		
Week	Repeats/week	Time/min	Week	Repeats/week	Time/min
1	3	3	1	4	15
2	3	4	2	2	15
				2	18
3	3	5	3	4	18
4	3	6	4	4	19
5	4	6	5	4	20
6	4	7	6	4	20
7	4	8	7	2	20
				2	22
8	4	9	8	4	22
9	4	10	9	3	22
				2	25
10	4	12	10	5	26
11	4	14	11	5	28
12	4	15	12	5	30

Tips for keeping it going

● Enter, and train for, a fun run, or a race such as a half- or full marathon.

● Train with a friend.

● Add plenty of variety to your training routine.

● Train with someone better than yourself to provide extra stimulus.

● Enter and train for a sponsored event, such as a run, swim or cycle.

● Find and use a fitness trail.

● Try some interval training in each session.

● Join a club or group.

When you start out on a fitness programme, you will probably be spurred on by enthusiasm. There may well come a moment, however, when that first enthusiasm begins to wane. This is a danger point, since small improvements in aerobic fitness can easily disappear. Thus, while you can make definite steps forward in, say, a fortnight of fitness training, the same backward steps occur in a fortnight of inactivity.

With longer periods of initial training (beyond eight weeks), the overall effect on aerobic fitness is little affected by short lay-offs. If you stop exercising completely after this period, there is a rapid loss of 20-30 per cent of endurance from your peak level, followed by a slow decline. As far as muscular strength is concerned, there is no marked early loss, and the fall off rate is slow. These figures should not, however, be used as an excuse for laziness because of the benefits to health of regular exercise.

One of the essentials to strive for in keeping an exercise programme going is a 'happy medium'. Do not forget that the idea of fitness training is to improve your maximum oxygen uptake and to use as high a percentage as possible of this maximum oxygen uptake during regular exercise. You can do more than three sessions a week but the main reason for exceeding this minimum is sheer enjoyment. Exercise should be fun, and the fitter you get, the more fun it becomes.

There are many ways in which you can add extra stimulus to your training schedules. As a guide, use some of the tips suggested or seek out a fitness trail such as the one shown opposite. Alternatively, try to inject some interval training into your regular sessions.

Interval training

Interval training can make an exercise programme more fun and can help build up your speed.

The basic type of interval training is to exercise at maximum capacity for short bursts and to intersperse these with periods of rest or low-level activity. To produce the maximum effect on your 'sprint' or fast-twitch muscle fibres, these bursts of speed need last for only 40 seconds. As you progress, you can build them up to 2 to 5 minutes, while keeping going slowly between each. This will then build up speed in the context of endurance.

As you get fitter, you can cut down the time spent on rest or low-level activity between bursts.

Runners may find it helpful to mix their interval training with flexibility exercises (see pp. 102-3).

The idea of fitness training *is to get you up to your own maximum capacity for oxygen uptake, to keep you there, and to be able to utilize a large percentage of this maximum capacity. The graph of improvement in oxygen uptake, or VO₂ (max), shows that once you have reached a certain point, improvement levels off. Your aim should be to stay on this plateau, not to slip back.*

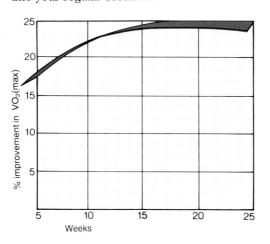

% improvement in $VO_2(max)$

Weeks

Many parks and open spaces now have fitness trails or *parcours* built into them. These trails not only provide some extra interest and incentive to keep you going, but also provide a valuable additional range of exercises.

The idea of the fitness trail is that you start off on a marked run with exercise stations placed every 100 metres or so. The exercises are designed to help build up strength and improve flexibility and balance, as well as

to improve your level of aerobic fitness.

A well-planned fitness trail will begin with simple warm-up exercises, progress to a range of strenuous activities, such as those shown below, then end with groups of exercises that help you to cool down. The instructions at each station should suggest the number of repeats to be done by participants at different levels of fitness. Stop at once if you are in pain or feel ill.

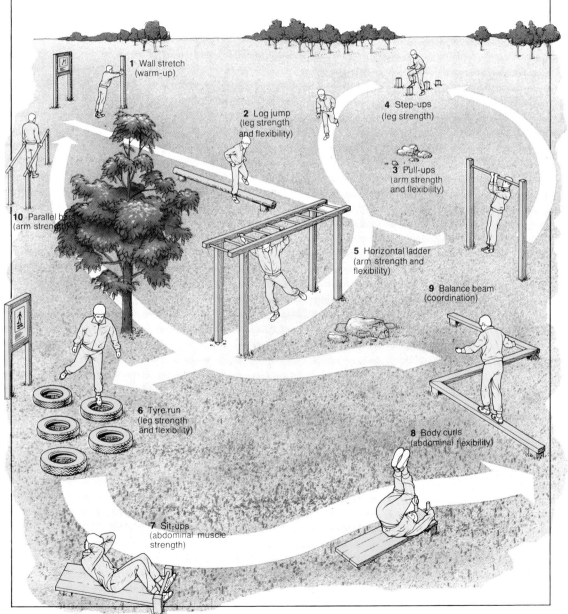

1 Wall stretch (warm-up)

2 Log jump (leg strength and flexibility)

3 Pull-ups (arm strength and flexibility)

4 Step-ups (leg strength)

5 Horizontal ladder (arm strength and flexibility)

6 Tyre run (leg strength and flexibility)

7 Sit-ups (abdominal muscle strength)

8 Body curls (abdominal flexibility)

9 Balance beam (coordination)

10 Parallel bars (arm strength)

FAMILY FITNESS

The pursuit of fitness should be a family affair, not something confined to just one or two family members. If everyone in the family is keen on getting and staying fit, this will avoid the inevitable friction that arises over conflicts of interest.

Getting children fit

One good way of enabling all the members of a family to get fit is to take out family membership of a sports club with a wide variety of facilities. Such clubs also offer coaching facilities, which can be useful for both adults and children alike.

If such a strategy is beyond your means, or not available in your area, you still have plenty of scope. Activities such as swimming, cycling and walking, or the use of a fitness trail are easy to organize on a family basis. Or the family might pursue their chosen exercise in pairs, depending on ability and inclination. Children from the age of ten and above can start on the beginners part of the fitness programmes (see pp. 106-15).

It was once thought that children gained sufficient aerobic exercise through play. For many children, however, this is not true. Parents may thus need to foster a pattern of regular aerobic exercise from early on in life.

As well as helping to keep children fit, sport is an ideal way to encourage the development of physical skills. This is an area in which parents can and should become involved, even if they are unable to supply the specialist coaching needed for certain sports. All children should be taught to swim and to ride a bicycle by the age of about seven, but the earlier the better. By encouraging the development of hand-eye coordination, which is central to all kinds of ball games, you can ensure that your children do not get left out of such sports or become labelled as 'useless'.

If children are left behind by their peers in the development of their physical skills, they will lose the drive to catch up and will convince themselves that they are no good at sport. This commits them to a downward spiral in the teens and twenties, leaving them dangerously unfit in their thirties and beyond. For this reason alone, the fostering of any kind of sporting activity must be a goal worth pursuing.

Risks of sport in children

As children have become caught up in the fitness boom, so younger and younger children have begun to take part in endurance events. There is considerable concern in medical circles and among sports administrators about the safety of such activity. Is it safe, for example, for 11 and 12-year-olds to run marathons?

The plain truth is that we do not know the answer to that question at present. Time alone will tell. There are certainly theoretical reasons for believing it may be dangerous. The growth of

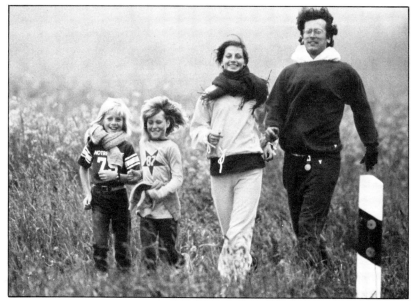

Children adopt the habits of their parents, whether these are good or bad. This makes it important to introduce children to the value of physical fitness and regular aerobic exercise at an early age. Children should be encouraged to try a wide selection of sports and activities rather than concentrating on just one or two. This will promote the development of strength and flexibility, and of hand-eye and eye-foot coordination as well as muscular endurance.

Tips for encouraging children

● Allow children to join in with your own fitness training. Even the smallest children can be taken for a warm-up, even if it is only a few hundred metres, before you start off on a run.

● Remember that any kind of teaching that makes children physically aware is excellent. Dancing and music and movement classes should be encouraged for both boys and girls.

● Do not try to coach an average performer to be a champion. If your child is a champion in the making, this will soon be obvious.

● Play ball games with children from the earliest possible age to help develop hand-eye and eye-foot coordination.

● Encourage children to try a wide variety of sports. They will eventually settle on the ones they most enjoy and in which they have most ability.

● Join in with your children whenever possible. Let them see that you enjoy exercise and let them feel that 'exercise is something we all do in our family.'

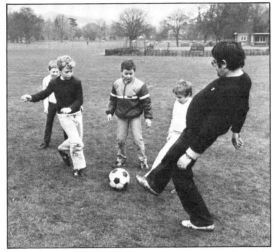

Coordination *between foot and eye is not fully developed until at least the age of 12, but from the age of 5 or 6, if not sooner, parents can help children to develop such ball skills. When practising with children, make the sessions structured so that they work on a variety of skills.*

Training with a partner

Sharing a fitness routine can be fun, but there are some problems when you train with a partner.

As a rule the maximum aerobic capacity in men tends to be greater than in women. This means that men need to train at greater intensity, for example at a greater running or cycling speed, to improve their aerobic capacity. Thus it is generally inadvisable for a man and a woman to train together exclusively.

If necessary, work out some training strategies to accommodate the needs of both partners. The female partner can, for example, start out first on a course that takes her past home at half or three-quarters of the distance her male partner will cover. Or the man may do some basic training with his partner then add speed work or interval training (see pp. 116-17) to his schedule.

bone takes place at the ends of the long bones, such as the femur in the leg, in areas known as growth plates. It is possible that much road-running may damage these. However, it is also claimed — with justification — that contact sports, such as rugby and American football, are even more likely to cause severe injury.

The body's full capacity to lose heat through sweating does not develop until the early teens. It has thus been suggested that young children risk heat exhaustion if they run in long races. Again there is a cogent counter argument: children's bodies have a relatively large surface area, which means that they lose heat more easily and so do not need to sweat so efficiently.

Although there is an element of physical risk in allowing children to take part in endurance races, such as marathons, there may be as much psychological risk in pushing children too hard in sport. Children should obviously be encouraged to use all their talents to the full, but enjoyment remains an essential element of sport. The keys to enjoyment are variety and a reasonable degree of skill. Other than in exceptional circumstances, there is no justification for trying to develop young children into champions in a single discipline. For every first-class performer you train, there will be 10 or 20 who will class themselves as 'failures' by the age of 16.

Aerobic exercise is undoubtedly the way to improve your physical fitness. It can, however, become addictive. This addiction is useful in the sense that it keeps people exercising and thus maintains fitness. On the other hand, it can make people obsessional about their sport, to the detriment of the rest of their lives.

In one Canadian survey it was shown that runners have a higher divorce rate than non-runners. And in an article published in the *New England Journal of Medicine*, in 1983, three doctors from the University of Arizona put forward a well-argued case that obsessional running in men in their thirties and forties is the male counterpart to anorexia nervosa or obsessional starvation.

In physical terms, obsessional participation can endanger your health (and possibly your life) if it means that you run when you are ill or in extreme weather conditions.

The reason why exercise has such powerful psychological effects seems to lie in a group of chemical compounds called endorphins. The compounds, which bear a close chemical relationship to the powerful, and potentially addictive painkiller morphine, were first discovered in medical research into the cause of narcotic addiction. They are found in the highest concentrations within the brain and nervous system, and here there are special receptors, which ensure that they key into and react on certain nerve cells.

Exercise, it seems, increases the levels of endorphins in the brain. This explains why hard endurance training, which might appear both painful and exhausting, is in fact enjoyable. The phenomenon of 'runner's high', in which athletes feel euphoric and capable of effortless exertion, almost certainly depends upon endorphin release.

Endorphins have physiological as well as psychological effects. They interact closely with the pituitary gland, for example, and can interfere with its function of controlling hormonal output in various parts of the body. This helps to explain why high levels of training can lead, in women, to menstrual irregularity or even a complete cessation of periods.

Competition

At all levels of sport, and at all ages, competition is an important element. This is because it provides goals for people to aim at and gives training a valuable purpose. At the same time, people may

Mishaps are an occupational hazard in many kinds of competitive sport, but are unlikely to deter the keen participant. What is important is to keep the prospect of severe injury or illness in perspective. Obsession can place your health and happiness at risk.

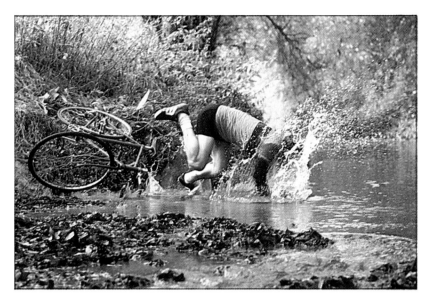

use their will to win as a way of preserving their own personal identity.

Competition, in the sense of beating the person next to you, is important for children, adolescents and young people. Learning to lose is also important to psychological maturity — nobody can win all the time. As an adult, however, it is important to keep the element of success in perspective. The need to win should, thus, diminish with increasing maturity so that, in the words of one expert in this field, 'the end point of sporting competition should be to wean the individual off the need for it.'

One of the great advantages of the 'running boom' has been that it is now possible to train for, and participate in, events in which there is no need to beat the person next to you. In such events, it is more likely that you will team up with someone in a joint attempt to complete the course in a reasonable time so that, in fact, you are competing against no one but yourself. In events such as the New York and London marathons, the proportion of entrants with serious thoughts of winning is a mere tenth of one per cent of the total field. Remember that the desire to win at all costs can do more than make you disappointed. It can increase the possibility of your suffering from those stress-related illnesses, such as heart attacks, that exercise should reduce.

In hot weather, dehydration and heat exhaustion are the major risks to exercisers. Remember that high humidity, because it prevents evaporation of sweat from the skin and thus lowers the effectiveness of the body's cooling mechanism, is as dangerous as a high air temperature.

If you wish to exercise in hot conditions, choose the coolest part of the day, such as the early morning or late evening. If you are running or cycling, search out as much shade as you can. Remember that it takes time for the body to acclimatize to hot conditions (see pp. 58–9). Keep a steady, slow pace and take plenty of breaks for rest and drinks, Wear light, reflective clothing, protect your head with a hat and, if you can, keep your body wet. After you have finished exercising, drink plenty of water in order to replace the lost fluids.

In cold weather, remember that the wind can provide an additional, unwelcome chilling factor, as can being wet through to the skin. As a general guide, it is safe to exercise in temperatures down to $-32°C$ ($-25°F$), as long as you are properly protected. Wear plenty of separate layers of light clothing, and keep your head covered (20 per cent of body heat is lost from the head). Protect any exposed areas of the skin with Vaseline. If it is raining, sleeting or snowing, make sure that your outermost layer of clothing is waterproof but allows for the escape of water vapour. Warm up indoors before you begin. When you have completed your period of exercise, change out of any wet clothes immediately.

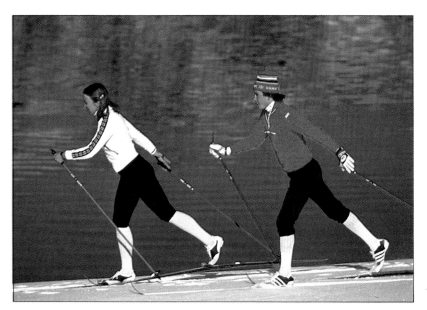

Nordic, or cross-country, skiing is a near-ideal form of aerobic training. A wider range of muscles is used than in cycling or running, and there are added advantages in terms of flexibility. Even a beginner can soon learn to move easily and to expend large amounts of energy.

Running, swimming and cycling, and other everyday aerobic activities such as dancing, are available to almost everyone, everywhere, which is why they form the core of an aerobic fitness programme. There are, however, many other pursuits which are equally good for training the aerobic system. The problem is that they are not all universally available.

Winter sports
Worldwide, downhill skiing is the most popular winter sport. As you master the extensive skills required to become a proficient downhill skier, you undoubtedly begin to improve your aerobic performance. Many occasional skiiers never reach this stage, so, even if you are already competent, you will find that aerobic training will help you to get more out of skiing.

In contrast, Nordic skiing is one of the best forms of aerobic training. With it comes the pleasure of moving through varied terrain. Skating is also good aerobic exercise.

Water sports
Rowing and canoeing rank high among the effective forms of aerobic exercise. Both require a reasonably high degree of skill before they begin to become enjoyable. Rowing is essentially a team sport, which demands a heavy work-load from the back, and considerable skill is needed to protect the back from injury. It is thus unwise to take up rowing much over the age of 30.

Dinghy sailing can be an aerobic sport as long as the wind is strong enough for you to reach high levels of energy expenditure. Ideally, you should sail more than once or twice a week. Windsurfing or board sailing is, however, more advantageous aerobically and demands even more balance and flexibility. The greatest disadvantage of windsurfing is that you have to be skilled to stay on the board at all, and the learning process demands much trial and error.

Orienteering
Although orienteering does not need snow or water, it does need an organization. Fortunately, however, there are now orienteering clubs that hold regular meetings in many countries. An orienteering course contains a number of checkpoints. These are marked on a map, which you carry. You do not have to reach the checkpoints in any specified order, and skills of map- and compass-reading are as important as speed over the ground.

Orienteering is not expensive and, at meetings, courses are offered of varying difficulty so that all family members can join in. Overall, it is excellent aerobic training, with enough mental stimulus to satisfy both the inexperienced and the most seasoned of performers.

Canoeing (below) is an easier sport to take up than rowing, since the initial degree of skill required is less, but it rates just as highly as a form of aerobic exercise. Both canoeing and rowing have the disadvantage that they tend to exercise the upper body more than the legs.

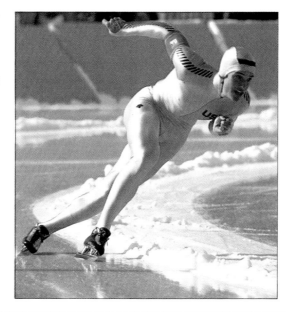

Speed skating, for those who have access to it, is an excellent form of aerobic exercise and is exhilarating into the bargain. To gain aerobic advantage, it is not strictly necessary to adopt the typical technique of world-class performers.

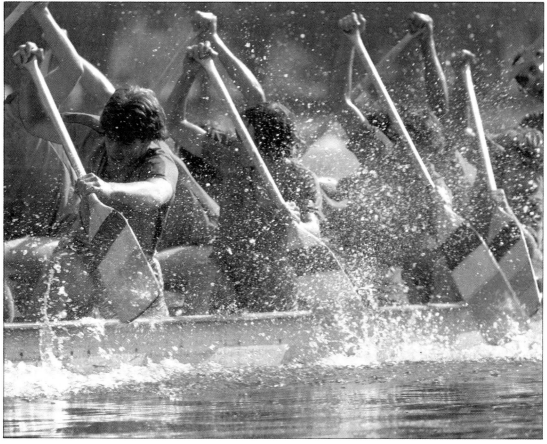

123

ANAEROBIC SPORTS

Many of the sports traditionally regarded as mainstays of a get-fit routine depend, in fact, on a succession of short-lived, largely anaerobic efforts, rather than on continuous aerobic exercise as experienced in sports such as running or swimming. The world-famous tennis star Bjorn Borg described his fitness as the ability to run 'thousands of ten-yard races'. This statement neatly sums up the overall physical requirements of many racket games, including squash, racketball, badminton and tennis itself.

The fact that these games depend more upon anaerobic than aerobic effort certainly does not mean that they are bad for you. It is desirable and healthy for people to play squash, tennis or some other racket sport once or twice a week, and the many devotees of these sports find them absorbing and energetic. Racket sports fail only in that they do not, in themselves, comprise a complete exercise programme. If, however, you combine your tennis, squash or other chosen sport with some aerobic training, you will not only get fitter but will improve your performance on court. And as you become fit enough to play longer and harder, the game itself will come to provide more and more in the way of aerobic training.

Team sports
Another popular way of exercising in social surroundings is by playing team sports. Such sports vary widely, however, in the extent to which they provide aerobic training. American football is little more than a series of sprints, while games such as basketball, netball and volleyball are essentially larger-scale versions of the racket games and work on the 'thousands of ten-yard races' principle. With sports such as ice and field hockey, soccer and rugby, much depends on the players and their place on the field. Rugby forwards, for example, tend to get much more aerobic exercise than the backs.

The quality of exercise you get from a team game depends also on the way it is played. If the teams are ill matched and the play is one-sided, you may find that you are either lingering far from the play with little to do, or exercising enormously energetically in frantic defence. And there are some team games, such as cricket and baseball, in which some of the players may do little more than stand on the field during the course of the average game.

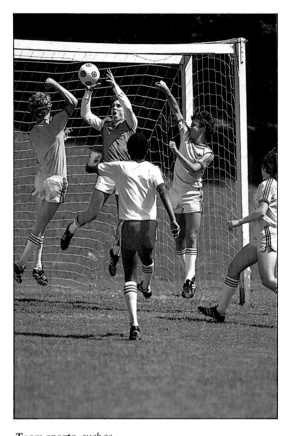

Team sports, such as soccer, provide, for many people, the stimulus they need to get fit. In soccer, players move over reasonable distances for most of the game, so there is a definite aerobic training effect, although its extent will depend on the amount an individual exerts himself.

Whatever your chosen individual or team sport, it is well worth training for that sport's specific demands as well as for all-round aerobic fitness, since the more skilful you are, the more enjoyable will be your participation. All participants in ball games benefit from improved co-ordination and ball control, which can only be gained through practice. Improved strength and flexibility of particular body areas will also be helpful. Better mobility of back, waist and hips are, for example, helpful in tennis and squash, while jumping skill is needed for sports such as soccer and volleyball, as are balance and agility.

Ice hockey is an exciting sport for spectators and participants alike. As long as players achieve periods of continuous activity, the sport can have an aerobic training effect. However, as with other team sports, additional aerobic training will improve performance considerably.

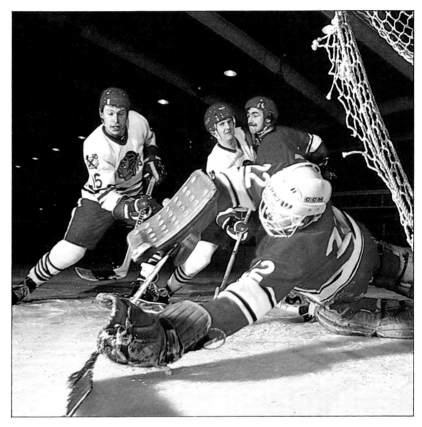

Squash is one of the world's most popular court games. It is excellent for developing muscle strength and flexibility, and provides the vigorous arm exercise that many sports lack. But because squash, except at the highest level, depends on a series of sprints rather than on continuous lower-level muscle activity, it is more anaerobic than aerobic. To improve aerobic fitness, squash is thus best combined with an activity such as running.

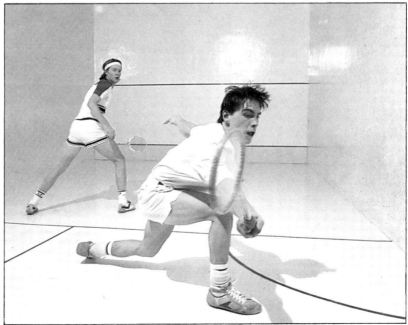

RELAXATION SPORTS AND ACTIVITIES

Most of us feel that if we are doing something that takes us out into the open air, or away into the countryside, then we are doing something that is essentially healthy. The desire to get away from the pressures of life at the week-end, and to recharge the batteries for the week ahead, is widespread. This can do wonders for your state of mind, but does not necessarily do anything to improve or maintain physical fitness.

In assessing the value to aerobic fitness of relaxation sports, the most important consideration is the amount of walking or other muscular activity involved. A round of golf, for example, involves a walk of about 8 km (5 mls); hilly terrain will add to the training effect.

The various forms of hunting, shooting and fishing that take people out into the country on their feet for reasonable distances also have their aerobic benefit, by virtue of the time spent in walking. If, however, your form of participation involves little more than getting your gear from the car and walking a few yards with it, you may be doing wonders for your relaxation but little indeed for your fitness.

In sport, as elsewhere in life, mechanization has taken over. Thus there are many forms of motor sports, and although they are a form of relaxation, few involve much in the way of physical exertion. The chief exceptions are cross-country motor cycle events and water-skiing.

Leisure activities, such as darts, billiards and pool, rate high in relaxation but low on fitness. If played in an atmosphere laden with cigarette smoke, and accompanied by the consumption of large quantities of alcohol, they may well do much more harm than good in physical terms.

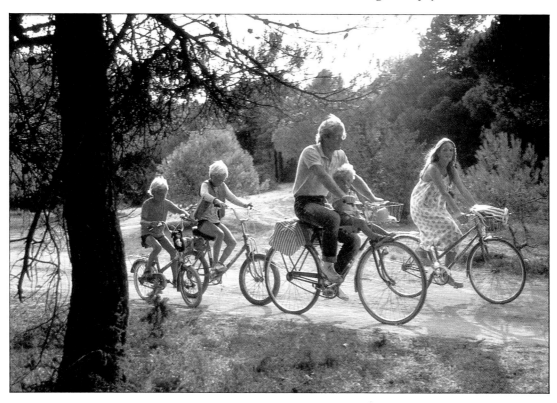

A family cycle ride, taken at a leisurely pace, is invigorating and enjoyable, but will do little to improve adult aerobic fitness levels. Children will benefit more, since they have to pedal harder to keep up with the pace of the adults.

Golf is played and followed by millions of people all over the world. It contributes a little to aerobic fitness because it involves walking a few miles each round. But this aerobic effect is reduced to insignificant proportions if you walk slowly and have a caddy to carry your clubs, and is lost altogether if you ride around the course in a motorized buggy.

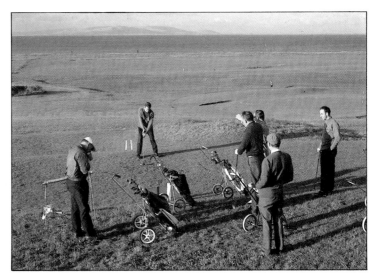

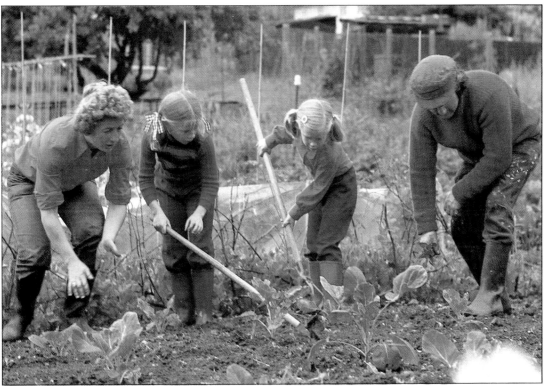

The home and the garden *offer plenty of opportunities for aerobic training. Activities such as sawing wood or digging the soil use plenty of energy and oxygen, particularly if they are performed at a steady pace rather than in short, sharp bursts.*

127

Strength training is not essential to fitness, but being strong will undoubtedly help you to build up your endurance and aid your aerobic training. There are also a number of good reasons why you might want to build up your muscle strength, as well as improving your aerobic endurance. What is important is to go about strength training in the correct way. If you do not, you may do yourself considerable harm.

Muscle strength can have a striking effect on your appearance. Your posture is better if you are strong. This not only looks more attractive than a weak, slumped posture but does much to protect your back from common ailments. Since, volume for volume, muscle weighs heavier than fat, you may gain some weight as your proportion of body muscle increases.

In many sports, both aerobic and anaerobic, strength is a positive advantage to performance. In rowing, windsurfing and swimming, strength of the upper body muscles is essential to success. In football and ice hockey, for example, leg strength is critical. Strength of both upper and lower body are helpful to squash and to the martial arts such as judo and karate.

Another bonus of strength training is that if you are relatively strong for your size, you will be more likely to stay active longer. This will, in turn, keep you aerobically fit for longer and, hopefully, help prolong your life. If you simply wish to impove your strength for its own sake, remember that strength training will not, in itself, make you fit.

How to train for strength
The simplest, and probably the safest way to train for increased strength is to use your own body weight. Press ups and pull ups are good for improving the strength of both your arms and your shoulders. Runners, and people who play sports such as football, which concentrates on lower body activity, may find such exercise particularly worthwhile, since running is good for strengthening the legs and back but does little for the upper part of the body. Before you begin, do some warm-up exercises (see pp. 100-1).

Even if they have done no strength training, most men are able to do a few press-ups. If this is so, then training is simply a matter of building up the number. Lie face-down on the floor, with your legs together and your hands flat on the floor beneath your shoulders. Straighten your arms, pushing your body off the floor and keeping it straight. Then lower your body back into the starting position. Once you can repeat this 20 or more times with ease, raise your feet on a box or low stool. This increases the work that your arms have to do.

Many women find press-ups difficult. If this is so, keep your knees on the ground and simply use the upper part of your body for the press-up, keeping your back in line with your thighs.

Pull-ups are the reverse of press-ups. In these you use your arms to pull yourself up high enough to chin a bar. (This usually needs to be done in a gym, but you can buy bars for use at home.) If you cannot manage more than two or three repeats, then modify the exercise by lying under a lower bar, placed at the level of your chest. Keeping your heels on the floor and your body straight, grasp the bar and pull yourself up.

To strengthen the abdominal muscles, the easiest exercises to do are sit-ups (see p. 104-5). These have the added advantage of helping to prevent back trouble.

Training with equipment
The best and safest sort of strength-training equipment is that in which the weights are fixed, rather than free, and are moved by pulleys of various kinds. The introduction and development of such equipment has done much to reduce the many injuries that people used to suffer when using free weights for strength-training.

The most sophisticated equipment available puts each muscle group in the body through its complete range of movement without risk of injury. If you use free weights or even a fixed pulley to put muscles through their entire movement range, the muscles are subjected to considerable strain at the extremes of their range, since they are working at a mechanical disadvantage. Variable resistance equipment, however, such as that made by Nautilus in the USA, Sports and Fitness in Germany and Daltons in the UK, automatically alters the load on the muscles as the operator carries out a range of movements. Thus the load is least when the muscles are at the greatest mechanical disadvantage.

Variable resistance equipment, which any good gym should be able to provide, has the added advantage that the exercising muscle can be put under adequate, but not excessive, tension during its relaxation phase. This prevents muscle-shortening and the consequent diminishing of flexibility that accompanies it.

If you are considering using a gym for strength-training, choose one that not only has a full range of variable resistance equipment but which provides close supervision, particularly for beginners. Look, too, for other facilities, such as the opportunity to use equipment that will measure your aerobic fitness (see pp. 98–9).

The bench press machine (below) *is designed for strengthening the muscles of the arms and shoulders. The person exercising grasps the handles of the machine and attempts to push them upward as far as possible. One of the reasons why such a machine is safer than lifting free weights in this position is that it is impossible for the person exercising to be 'trapped' by the weight of the machine.*

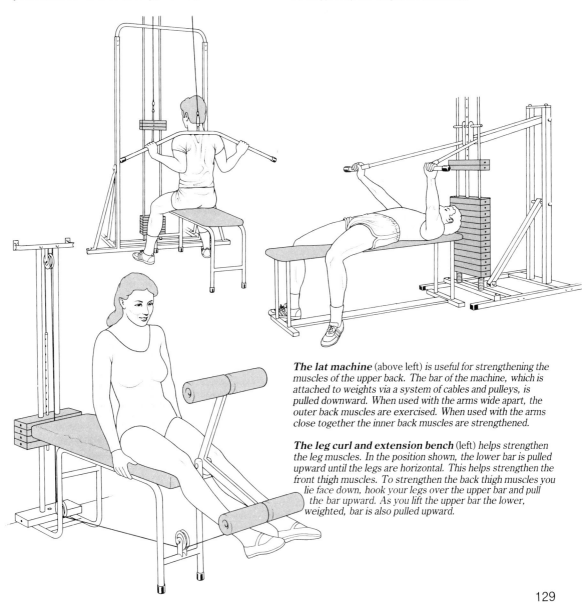

The lat machine (above left) *is useful for strengthening the muscles of the upper back. The bar of the machine, which is attached to weights via a system of cables and pulleys, is pulled downward. When used with the arms wide apart, the outer back muscles are exercised. When used with the arms close together the inner back muscles are strengthened.*

The leg curl and extension bench (left) *helps strengthen the leg muscles. In the position shown, the lower bar is pulled upward until the legs are horizontal. This helps strengthen the front thigh muscles. To strengthen the back thigh muscles you lie face down, hook your legs over the upper bar and pull the bar upward. As you lift the upper bar the lower, weighted, bar is also pulled upward.*

Fitness has become big business. There are scores of different devices on the market which are sold with the promise that, used in your own home, they will act as mainstays in your quest for increased fitness. The destiny of most such equipment is to gather dust in a garage, attic, or basement. The best of home equipment, including exercise bicycles and rowing machines, can be incorporated into an aerobic fitness schedule (see pp. 110–11 and 114–15). An assessment of the usefulness of the most popular of the remainder is given on these pages.

Massagers
These consist of a belt, which is slung round the hips or thighs, or of pads, which are strapped to various parts of the body. These machines represent the fanatical fringe of the fitness and slimmers' markets. The marketers of massage machines promise inches off the parts of the body that bulge too much, an assurance based on the unlikely assumption that if you shake up the underlying fat a little it will go away. Often this fat is called 'cellulite', which is no more than an invention of the slimming industry. Massage machines are not recommended.

Mini trampolines
These trampolines are designed to make it easier and more fun to jog indoors, on the spot. They do produce a sensation reasonably akin to real running, but unless you are housebound or live in an area where the weather is not conducive to outdoor exercise, they are probably not worthwhile. However, they can do no harm and are a less expensive alternative to a treadmill.

Treadmills
The treadmill—a moving belt on which the participant walks or jogs—is an essential part of the sports physiologist's equipment and has been successfully adapted for home use. Treadmills are obtainable powered and unpowered, and obviously unpowered ones are a lot less expensive. Many models incorporate equipment for measuring the way in which your pulse rate changes as you exercise. If you can afford one, and have the space to accommodate it, a treadmill will allow you to run effectively indoors. Treadmills work, but add nothing to ordinary running, which is free of charge.

Hand and ankle weights
Various sorts of weights are available to carry in your hands or fix around your ankles, so increasing the work that you must perform against gravity as you exercise indoors or out. They aim to increase both strength and aerobic fitness, objectives which can also be achieved by an aerobic exercise routine combined with strength training in a gym. These weights can turn an enjoyable exercise session into one of drudgery so should be used judiciously.

Chinning bars
These are bars which you fix between the posts of a door and use for strength training. Useful and inexpensive, they allow you to exercise the set of muscles opposite to the ones you exercise by doing press-ups. They rely on the sensible principle of using your own body weight for strength training and are perfectly safe, as long as you can find a secure position in which to fix them.

Bullworkers
These are sprung devices, held in the hands, which are used isometrically (see p. 90) to build up many groups of muscles, especially those in the arms. In their role as muscle strengtheners bullworkers are effective, but they are not recommended because isometric exercise is less beneficial to the heart than aerobic exercise and may raise the blood pressure.

Chest expanders/grip developers
Spring chest expanders have been popular exercise devices since the last century and are an inexpensive, effective and safe way of building up the strength of the arm muscles in an isokinetic way (see p. 90). However, press-ups and pull-ups using your own body weight are better and more effective. Grip developers are sprung isometric devices held in the hand. Like other such equipment, they can, however, raise the blood pressure, so are not recommended.

Free weights
Until the late 1970s, any sort of strength training involving the use of more than your own body weight meant the lifting of free weights. Today, however, weight-lifting devices have been incorporated into many sorts of multi-gym equipment such as the leg and arm press. Free weights

remain a favourite among body builders and competitive weight-lifters, but they can easily cause injuries. For this reason, it is not safe to use them unless you are under expert supervision.

Home multi-gyms

These pieces of equipment, incorporating devices such as the weight bench; leg raise/dip bar; lat bar; weight pulley; leg pulley and neck developer aim to provide isokinetic strength training to all the muscle groups in the body. Because the equipment is subject to a great deal of strain, it must be manufactured to high standards and will, therefore, be expensive. Remember, however, that to be effective, it must provide a wide range of activities for the various muscle groups.

A treadmill offers a means of running indoors or in your garden. It is particularly useful for exercising in spells of bad weather.

The simplest sit-up bench (below) is equipped with a strap beneath which the feet are restrained. The angle of the bench may be altered to increase the degree of difficulty of the exercise. As with other such equipment, it is wise to consult your doctor before you begin an exercise schedule. Stop if you are in any pain.

The mini trampoline (left) can be used for jogging by both children and adults.

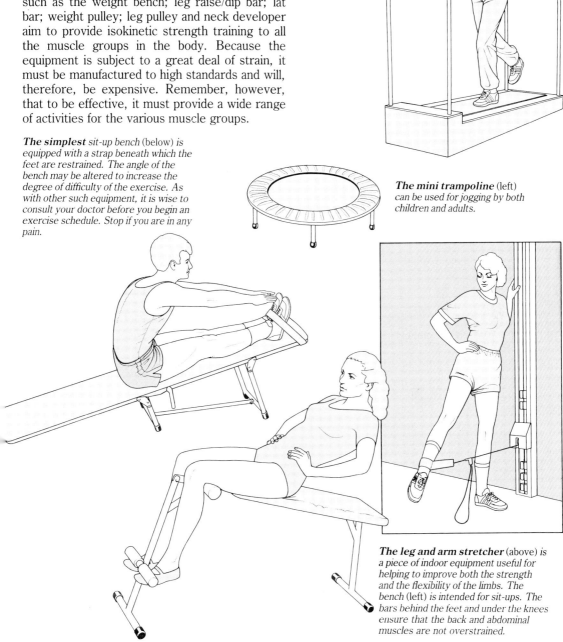

The leg and arm stretcher (above) is a piece of indoor equipment useful for helping to improve both the strength and the flexibility of the limbs. The bench (left) is intended for sit-ups. The bars behind the feet and under the knees ensure that the back and abdominal muscles are not overstrained.

EXERCISE AND SPORTS ROUND UP

The choice of sports and relaxation activities available today is huge. Everyone can find something to increase their level of activity and so become fitter.

The table below lists all the important types of active leisure pursuits, including aspects of normal daily life, and rates each according to a number of important criteria. Starred activities are those that rate highest overall.

Aerobic fitness is the most important element, since it produces the greatest long-term benefits. In this column, the lower scores may be the most revealing, for if you think that playing golf every week-end is contributing significantly to your fitness, then the score of four will help to revise your ideas. However, it is still better than playing snooker and scores high on sociability. Activities that score in the middle

	Aerobic fitness	Muscular strength	Coordination	Flexibility
Archery	2	5	5	5
Badminton	6	6	8	6
Baseball	4	5	6	6
Basketball	8	6	7	6
Billiards/Snooker/Darts	1	2	5	2
Bowls	2	3	5	2
Boxing	10	10	8	6
*Canoeing	7	9	6	7
Cricket	4	5	8	5
*Cycling	10	9	6	3
*Dancing	7	8	9	10
Fencing	5	9	9	9
Fishing	1	1	3	1
Football (American)	5	10	6	3
*Football (soccer)	6	9	8	6
Golf	4	3	7	5
Gymnastics	2	9	10	10
*Hockey (field)	6	6	6	6
*Hockey (ice)	8	6	10	9
Judo/Karate	3	6	9	9
Lacrosse	8	9	8	8
Mountaineering	7	10	8	5
*Orienteering	6	7	7	2
Riding (horse)	2	7	7	2
Rowing	10	10	6	2
Rugby	6	9	6	2
*Running	10	9	3	3
Sailing	2	6	6	2
Skating (ice)	5	5	10	8
Skating (roller)	5	5	9	8
*Skiing (cross-country)	10	9	8	7
Skiing (downhill)	5	8	9	8
Skipping	9	4	6	3
Squash	6	7	9	7
*Swimming	10	10	9	9
Table Tennis	5	3	8	5
Tennis	6	8	8	6
Volleyball	7	9	9	7
*Walking (Brisk)	6	3	2	2
Water Skiing	3	9	8	2
Weight-lifting	2	10	8	5
*Climbing Stairs	8	5	7	6
DIY (Painting)	3	3	2	5
Gardening	6	6	6	6
Housework	3	5	2	5

range of aerobic fitness are still valuable, particularly if you are also involved in other sports. More restful sports, such as fishing, can help to combat stress.

Other physical criteria, such as flexibility and coordination, are particularly important in children and adolescents, since they will help a young person develop into a fit adult. The relative safety of the various sports will also influence your choice and the encouragement you give to children. A small risk is involved in any activity, but while walking is not intrinsically dangerous, boxers have to accept that some damage is inevitable.

Other important practical considerations, such as the social side of sport, and the extent to which the whole family can participate are also given ratings for quick reference.

Relaxation	Accessibility	Economy	Safety	Sociability	Family involvement
6	2	4	9	5	4
4	5	6	4	7	5
3	4	5	8	6	4
3	5	8	7	5	1
9	6	5	9	9	3
6	6	7	9	8	2
1	5	8	1	4	1
3	2	3	4	6	2
6	5	3	5	9	6
9	9	4	4	4	9
10	8	6	6	10	2
6	3	4	3	6	4
10	8	6	10	4	7
2	2	5	1	3	2
5	5	6	3	7	3
6	6	8	2	7	6
8	3	7	2	3	1
5	3	7	6	7	3
8	3	4	3	4	8
6	5	7	2	6	8
6	2	7	6	6	1
4	2	3	1	6	3
6	6	7	6	5	3
8	4	2	3	6	8
6	2	3	6	8	1
4	2	6	2	9	2
8	10	7	5	5	4
9	1	1	3	8	8
8	2	3	2	5	9
9	7	7	3	3	9
6	2	2	4	2	5
8	2	1	2	9	9
9	9	10	8	1	8
3	5	6	4	5	5
9	6	7	8	2	10
6	5	7	7	6	8
6	7	5	6	7	7
5	6	8	7	5	2
9	10	10	10	6	9
5	2	2	2	4	4
2	7	7	5	3	2
2	10	10	9	1	0
7	10	7	8	2	6
9	7	8	9	1	7
3	10	10	10	1	10

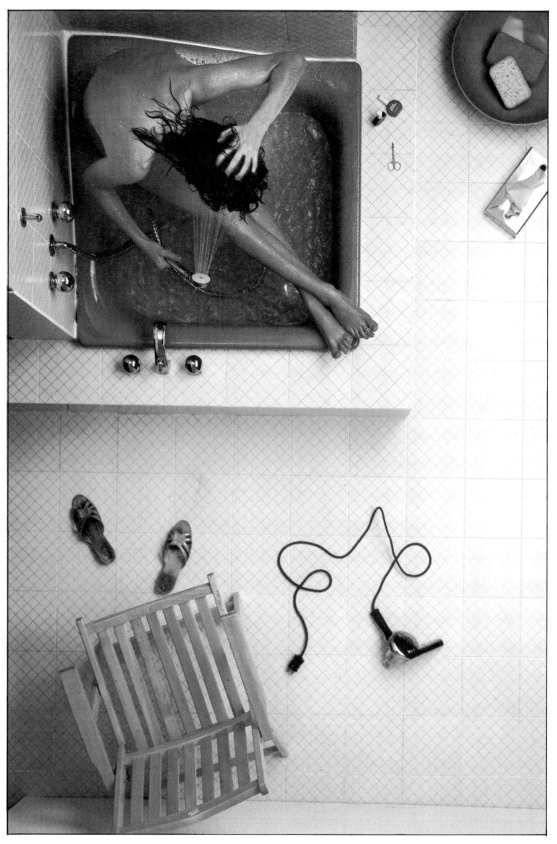

HEAD TO TOE

A body finely tuned and in good working order from top to toe promotes and reflects a sense of well-being. A feeling of vibrant health, energy and confidence is positively encouraged if you treat your body with the respect it deserves.

None of us is entirely content with our physical make-up. With self-control, some aspects, such as excess weight, can be regulated. We must, however, learn to live with those elements that cannot be changed, such as height, skin colour or hair texture — and even turn them to our advantage — instead of wasting precious time worrying about them. The secret is to capitalize on good points and to effect any possible improvements.

Understanding a little of how your body works and knowing how best to care for each part on a day-to-day basis are two of the keys to fitness and well-being. This chapter takes you on a trip around your body, selecting the most important areas of self-care and indicating when professional help may be needed.

To see ourselves as others see us is not as easy as it seems. How often have you been surprised by a chance remark about you? Many people, for example, have considered opinions about their weight — some normal-sized people think they are overweight, while others who are considered obese believe they are normal. And how many of us feel uncomfortable in the company of strangers? Yet by learning the body language of the confident, we can all begin to cope with such situations more easily. Small children reach out and touch one another to make friends, but this instinctive behaviour is so often suppressed as we grow up that it needs to be relearned later.

This chapter shows you how to know your body better and to use it wisely.

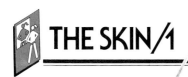

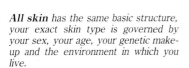

Hair
Melanin
Epidermis
Melanocyte
Basal cell layer
Sebaceous gland
Dermis
Hair follicle
Collagen fibres
Muscle
Sweat gland
Fat

All skin has the same basic structure, your exact skin type is governed by your sex, your age, your genetic make-up and the environment in which you live.

The skin is the largest of all the body organs and the one of which we are most aware. Waterproof and self-repairing, it is a reflector of health and well-being.

Most important among the skin's many functions is to act as an impervious body-covering, to control body temperature and to eliminate some wastes via the sweat glands. The nerves in the skin endow the body with its senses of touch, pressure and pain. In sunlight, the skin also makes vitamin D, essential for healthy bones. In addition, our skins reflect our emotions: fear makes the skin pale, cold and clammy, while the blush is an unmistakable sign of embarassment.

The way the skin works

The skin is structured in layers. There is an outer horny layer of dead cells, then the living, growing epidermis. Below this is the dermis and beneath it, at the bottom, is a layer of fat of varying thickness. Skin growth is from inside out. At the junction between epidermis and dermis is a basal layer of cells, which divide, grow, mature and gradually die off, moving all the time toward the surface. At the surface, all that remains of these cells is a layer of tough material, keratin, which is thickest in body areas subject to most wear and tear, such as the palms of the hands and the soles of the feet. Keratin prevents water loss and is impervious to many harmful chemicals and to bacteria.

Within the basal cell layer, melanin, the pigment that gives skin its colour and acts as a natural sunscreen, is produced by melanocytes. Everyone has the same number of melanocytes. What varies is their melanin-producing ability — the more melanin, the darker the skin.

Hair is made in the dermis, and hairs, which are made of keratin, grow outward in follicles through the epidermis, Hairs are lubricated by oily, water-repellant sebum made in sebaceous glands. These glands are particularly active and prone to infections such as acne in the teenage years (the more active they are, the greasier the skin), but they become less productive in middle age, making the skin dry. Sweat is made in sweat glands in the dermis and also exudes on to the skin surface.

Elastic tissues in the skin, its collagen fibres, give the skin its resilience. However, these tissues lose their stretchiness with age, and it is this that leads to wrinkling which is irreversible, although its effects can be removed by cosmetic

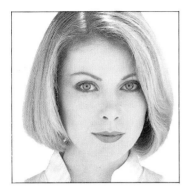

Dry skin
Fair skins are sometimes dry in childhood, but dryness is more often a problem in mature skin.

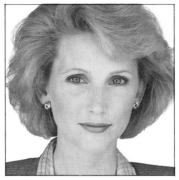

Balanced Skin
A balanced skin, with a peach-bloom appearance is rare. More common is a combination skin, a mixture of dry and oily.

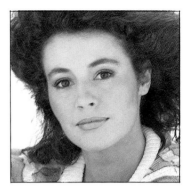

Oily skin
Most teenagers have an oily skin due to overproduction of sebum. Darker skins are often more oily than fair ones.

Do you have dry skin?
- Does your skin feel tight?
- Is it fine textured?
- Does it flake, chap and peel easily?

Do you have balanced skin?
- Is your skin even in texture?
- Are the pores visible but not obvious?
- Is your skin soft, not flaky to the touch?

Do you have oily skin?
- Are the pores of your skin clearly visible?
- Do you often get spots, blackheads or whiteheads?
- Does your skin shine?

---

surgery. Beneath the dermis, the fatty layer acts as insulator and cushion. In areas such as the face, muscles under the fat layer enable the skin to move.

Caring for the skin

Body skin takes good care of itself. Surprisingly, dirt does not interfere with the skin's proper functioning — it does not, for instance, prevent sweat being released, nor does it block the hair follicles. And any proteins, vitamins or other 'nutrients' applied directly to the skin are not absorbed by it beyond the outermost layer.

Bathing, showering and washing with soap to get rid of dirt and grease and body odour undoubtedly make the skin look and feel good. Soap can, however, lead to the development of allergic reactions, causing itching, soreness and possibly a red rash. Stop using any product that causes such a problem immediately. Instead, choose a product labelled 'hypoallergenic'.

Soap dries out the skin, stripping it of its protective sebum and making it taut. You may thus feel more comfortable if you apply a moisturiser to relubricate the skin with a light coating of an oil and water emulsion.

The skin of the face is the most vulnerable and fragile of all body skin. It should be treated with respect and with products suited to its degree of dryness or oiliness. The area around the eyes is especially likely to be damaged by aggressive application or removal of make-up. In the elderly, the whole skin area is delicate and should be treated with care – a weekly, rather than a daily, bath may be advisable.

Make-up and its use

The use of facial make-up is as old as civilization itself, but today such a vast and bewildering array of colours, creams, lotions and powders exists that it is difficult to make a choice. Have fun experimenting with colour and texture, but do not pay a lot for packaging unless the product is one you will use over and over again. Start with a clean skin and the application of a little moisturiser if the skin is not oily. Aim for an illusion of a clear, unblemished skin. As with soap, choose hypoallergenic products if you do develop any allergic reactions to make-up.

Removing make-up at night is a necessary chore. Whether you use soap or cleanser, treat your face gently. Astringents help remove excess oil from greasy skins. Use moisturiser all over your face and neck unless your skin is very oily.

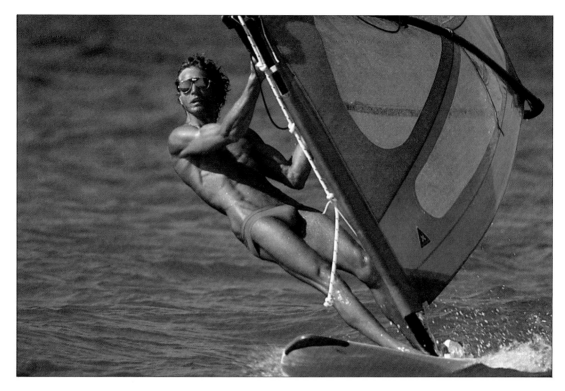

The skin is the body's automatic heat regulator. In response to increased temperatures, whether these are generated internally through exercise or externally by the sun, the many thousands of sweat glands situated in the skin all over the body respond to messages from the 'thermostat' seated deep in the brain, in the hypothalamus. The sweat released on to the skin surface cools the body as it evaporates.

Stressful and emotional situations also trigger the sweat glands into action, particularly those glands that develop during adolescence in the groin and underarms. This sweat, however, contains pheromones, odours that are thought to be involved in sexual arousal. If they are allowed to become stale, they are quickly broken down by bacteria and develop a pungent smell.

To prevent body odour developing, have a bath or shower and change underwear, socks or tights every day. Underarm deodorants help to kill the bacteria that may collect there and contain certain metal salts that close up the sweat glands. Vaginal deodorants, however, are not advisable. Any offensive vaginal secretions demand medical attention and treatment.

Cotton is the best fabric for sports gear worn next to the skin, since it allows sweat and water vapour to evaporate quickly. Choose non-constricting, stretchy clothes, watch for seams and fasteners that may rub, and wear appropriate layers to be discarded as necessary.

Sun and the skin

Sunshine gives us all a sense of well-being. We feel more relaxed and, with the acquisition of a glowing, golden tan, more beautiful. Over-exposure, however, can be dangerous. In the short term, excess water and salt loss can lead to overheating and dehydration. In the long term, it can cause skin damage and even cancer. Children are particularly susceptible to sunstroke, since, if unrestrained, they will spend considerable time running around in the sun, and particularly near water, which intensifies the effect of the sun's rays by reflection. They should always be adequately covered, particularly on their heads, and their time in the sun carefully monitored.

Tanning is the skin's defence against the sun's harmful, ultraviolet rays. Melanin, the dark pigment made by the skin, acts as a screen to

Watersports such as windsurfing can be risky unless the skin is adequately protected with an appropriate sunscreen. Even when you have developed a deep tan you should continue the applications for safety's sake. In cold conditions, the skin needs protection to prevent loss of body heat and to minimize chapping.

prevent burning. When the skin gets hot, it turns red and the blood vessels dilate. Increasing the blood supply to the surface of the skin helps to cool it down. If the skin becomes too hot, however, it will burn. A clear fluid oozes into the skin and blisters bubble up, the outer layer stretches, hardens and peels, leaving a raw layer beneath.

Repeated over-exposure produces a wrinkled leathery look to the skin and can be harmful. Fair-complexioned people produce insufficient melanin to protect the skin from the cancer-inducing rays in hot climates. The nearer to the Equator fair-skinned people live, the greater the risk of skin cancer developing.

The ageing skin

As well as becoming thinner and less elastic with age, and thus less smooth and supple, the skin commonly develops patches of peculiar pigmentation. These may be brown and like rather large freckles, or they may be reddish or purplish in colour and caused by the rupture of small blood vessels in the skin. Such marks are a normal part of the body's gradual ageing process and should not be a cause for concern.

Safety in the sun for yourself and your children

Start slowly, building up from a few minutes for baby skins, a little longer for adults, depending on skin colour. Avoid the midday sun, between 11 am and 2 pm. Radiation is at its most intense at this time.

When you cover up, wear a hat with a shady brim. A lot of heat falls on the head, and infants with little or no hair are unprotected. A hat also prevents you screwing up your eyes against strong sunlight. Adults should wear sunglasses or goggles if necessary.

Be particularly vigilant about protection during water and winter sports because the sun's rays are intensified when reflected off snow and water.

Always use a sunscreen, re-applying after bathing.

Don't wear perfume when sunbathing. Some scents can cause unpleasant reactions in sunlight. Some drugs can also cause sensitivity to sunlight.

Drink plenty and add a little extra salt to your food.

Sunscreens

Choose a preparation with good sunscreening properties, such as one containing para-aminobenzoic acid or benzophenone. Apply liberally, especially on your face, neck, shoulders and shins. Use the notes below to determine which protection factor you need. Note that each increase in protection factor allows you to double your sunbathing time. Once you have a tan, it is safe to reduce the protection factor by 2 points and stay 1 or 2 hours longer in the sun.

● If your skin always burns, do not risk more than 10 minutes without a sunscreen. Use a protection factor of 12 to 15 and try to limit sunbathing to 2 hours a day.

● If your skin usually burns, do not stay unprotected for more than 20 minutes. Use a factor of 8 to 10 and stay in the sun for a maximum of 2 hours a day.

● If you burn then tan, choose a protection factor of 6 to 8 and do not expose yourself to strong sun for more than 30 minutes a day without a sunscreen.

● If you tan without burning, 2 hours of sun a day, with a protection factor of 4, is a good start. The safe limit for sunbathing without lotion is 40 minutes.

● Use sunlamps with caution, particularly those emitting shorter-wave ultraviolet rays. Never look directly at the light.

A shining head of hair makes you look good and feel good, and it usually reflects a good state of health. Its colour and texture are genetically determined but may change during life. Many blonde babies, for example, have darker hair as adults, while in later life, loss of pigment turns hair grey, and reduced oil production makes it drier and less smooth.

Hair is composed of the dead material keratin. Deep within each hair follicle the root sprouts a strand of hair. The cells divide rapidly, so that head hair grows about 1 cm ($\frac{1}{2}$ inch) a month, or even faster in warm weather. Each strand is composed of an inner shaft, containing the pigment that gives hair its colour, and an outer cuticle. The cuticle is lubricated by sebum released by the skin's sebaceous glands (see p. 136), and this gives it a sheen.

There are four different types of hair: scalp hair; underarm, pubic, chest and facial hair; eyebrows and lashes; and the fine down of insulating body hair. The structure of the hair root, which is genetically determined, dictates whether a hair strand grows straight or curly.

A full head of hair consists of 100,000 to 120,000 hairs, but everyone loses between 50 and 100 hairs a day. A hair grows for between 2 and 6 years, although some people's hair may grow long enough to sit on. When the strand reaches full length, it rests for a few months before a new hair pushes it out. Fortunately, however, the growing and resting cycles are not synchronized in adjacent follicles. If a follicle dies, it cannot produce hair, and balding results.

Hair care

Like the skin, the hair can maintain itself in a healthy condition with little or no help. For reasons of comfort and cleanliness, however, the hair should be brushed and/or combed daily, and shampooed and trimmed regularly.

Although the hair is composed of dead material, it is possible to damage your hair if you ill-treat it (see panel, right). It is also important to remember the substances put on the hair may be absorbed into the skin. The substance that is most suspect in this context is the chemical dye 2, 4-diminotoluene, which has been found to cause cancer in some animals. For this reason, you should avoid using a hair dye containing this substance. For preference, choose vegetable dyes, which are safer.

Is your hair oily or dry?			
Shampoo your hair as you would normally. After two days check on its condition.			
Appearance	Type	Care guidelines	Special treatments
Strands separate and stick to your head	Oily	1 Shampoo as often as necessary, even if that means every day. 2 Use a mild shampoo. 3 Use very little shampoo. 4 Put a conditioner on the ends unless the hair is very greasy. 5 Don't use too hot a hairdryer. 6 Don't brush or comb more than necessary.	To help reduce sebum production, use 1 litre (2¼ pints) of water with the strained juice of 1 lemon added for the final rinse after shampooing.
Tangles easily, brittle	Dry	1 Shampoo your hair every 4-6 days. 2 Use a mild shampoo. 3 Use a cream conditioner after every shampoo, combing it thoroughly through the hair and leaving it on for a few minutes before rinsing. 4 Never brush your hair when wet, always comb gently. 5 Protect your hair from the sun, either with a hat or scarf.	Massage 2 tablespoons of warm olive or almond oil into your hair. Wrap your head in a warm, damp towel or a plastic turban and keep it on for at least 30 minutes. Do this every 3-4 weeks.
Oily roots/dry ends (most common type)	Combination	Adapt the guidelines above for your own hair type.	

When caring for your hair

Do:
● Choose brushes or combs with widely spaced and smooth-tipped bristles and teeth, to avoid the risk of splitting hairs or scratching the scalp.

● Wash combs and brushes in shampoo or soap every time you wash your hair.

● Always rinse your hair thoroughly.

● Use a conditioner to smooth the outer surface of the hair, which is roughened by washing.

● Apply extra conditioner when using a heated dryer, rollers or tongs.

● Always try a temporary rinse first, before you risk using permanent colour.

● Go to a professional colorist for a permanent dye.

● To disguise greying, try a semi-permanent colorant, which lasts for 6 to 8 shampoos.

Washing, brushing and drying

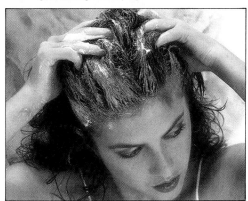

Massage shampoo into your scalp as you wash your hair, but rub gently if your hair is greasy to prevent excess sebum production.

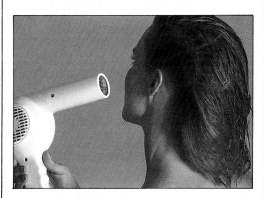

When blow-drying, take care not to burn your scalp or the skin of your neck. Remove metal necklaces which conduct heat rapidly.

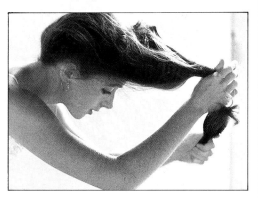

Brush your hair gently to avoid splitting the strands or pulling them out. Too much brushing and combing can exaggerate greasiness.

Don't:
● Overbrush your hair, it may increase the greasiness of oily hair and break the ends of dry hair.

● Tangle the hair while washing it.

● Give dry hair two applications of shampoo.

● Rub too vigorously when drying, it may break and tangle the hair.

● Hold the hairdryer closer than 6 in (16 cm) from the hair, and don't scald the scalp.

● Have a permanent bleach if all you really need is 'highlights'.

● Apply a permanent colour until you have tested the solution on your skin for 36 hours to check for any adverse reactions.

Did you know?
● Brushing your hair 100 times a day to make the hair shine does no good and may even damage the hair.

● Daily shampooing, although not strictly necessary, can do no harm as long as you use a mild shampoo.

● Static electricity is reduced by a conditioner.

● The hair is heavy when wet and up to 20 per cent less elastic when dry.

● A perm can give more body to lank hair, but the chemicals can make it drier and more brittle.

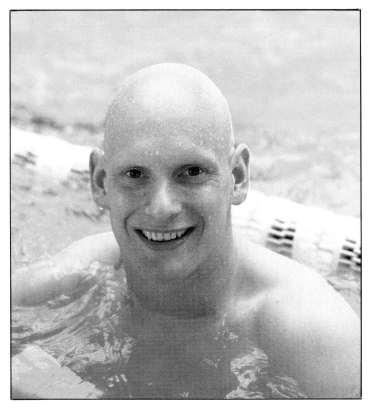

Baldness is often regarded as a threat to looks and esteem, and for many men is a severe impairment to well-being. Swimmer and Olympic medallist Duncan Goodhew turned baldness to his advantage. Having lost all his head hair, he discovered that his lack of hair improved his performance in the water by reducing water resistance. Many men swimmers now deliberately shave their heads to produce the same effect.

Human hair helps to protect the head from the sun and prevents heat loss from the body, but otherwise it performs a largely cosmetic function. Most people take hair for granted, but a lack or excess of it can give rise to acute anxieties and loss of self-confidence.

Hair problems

Pattern baldness, in which hair is lost successively from various parts of the scalp, is an hereditary male adjunct to ageing that affects around 40 per cent of all men. Women do not normally develop pattern baldness but may experience generalized thinning of head hair from middle age onward.

All men lose some head hair after puberty, when the increased androgens (male hormones) cause the hairline to recede slightly over the forehead and temples. Those with an inherited disposition to baldness also lose hair over the crown area. Men are 10 times more likely to be severely bald than women, but the total number of people severely distressed is about the same for each sex, because women find the experience of losing their hair more traumatic.

Diffuse hair loss in women may occur after childbirth, if the contraceptive pill is being taken, or after acute physical or mental stress, such as fever or bereavement. However, this reaction, which may also occur in men, is temporary, and hair should start to regrow within a few months. Excessive hair loss, however, may be caused by a hormone imbalance or lack of iron and can be medically treated.

Psychological stress may also trigger the occurrence of patches of baldness in children and young adults. Occasionally the patches coalesce into total loss of head or even body hair, but the hair that has been shed usually regrows within a period of some 6 to 9 months.

Dandruff affects over 60 per cent of the population. It is usually a mild form of eczema in which scales of dead skin flake from the scalp, but it is sometimes caused by psoriasis, a condition in which the skin cells multiply abnormally fast, forming larger, thicker, oilier flakes. The best treatment for dandruff is to wash hair regularly

Tips for men: Shaving

If your shaving method produces a skin rash, try another and consult your doctor if it persists.

● For a wet shave, use a really clean and sharp blade, work with, not against, the grain of the hair, and shave the chin and upper lip first.

● Electric shaving works best when the hairs are stiff and dry and may be better for soft skins.

Moustaches and beards

Allow up to 6 weeks for the hair to grow.
● Wash regularly with soap and water, and trim. Shape to suit your face. A drooping moustache disguises chubby cheeks or a square jaw. A beard may overemphasize a narrow forehead or hollow cheeks.

Thinning hair

There is no known prevention or natural cure for baldness. A drug, minoxidil, has sometimes helped to halt its progress.

Wigs and toupés can improve self-confidence.

Hair weaving connects new to natural hair and is an improvement on the toupé, but it also needs frequent adjustment.

Hair transplants are rarely satisfactory, since they depend on the continuing growth of transplanted hair follicles and may be of hair destined, itself, to be permanently lost.

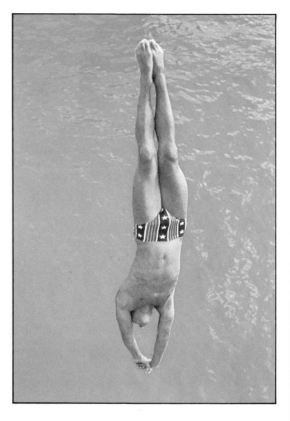

Body hair distribution in adult men varies widely. Some men have little or no hair on their chest or back while others are profusely endowed with hair. The difference is largely determined by heredity.

with a shampoo containing a selenium compound or tar extracts. If the problem is severe or persistent, you should consult your doctor.

Nits are sticky, white lice eggs found on the shaft of the hair. The minute lice that hatch cause intense itching and can be treated with a prescribed shampoo.

Fragile, brittle hair is often the price paid for frequent perming, bleaching, and using hair driers and heated curlers. The best treatment is to give your hair a rest from such processes.

Unwanted hair

Excessive hair growth in women is caused by the over-production of androgens or the skin's over-sensitivity to natural levels of androgens. Most women are able to control extra hair with a combination of shaving, bleaching, electrolysis, depilatory creams or waxes.

Tips for women: Removing unwanted hair.

Shaving:
Quick and easy. Shave legs, underarms, bikini line, but never arms, upper lips or hairs on breasts. The hairs do *not* grow back thicker and darker; this is a myth.

Depilatory creams:
Chemicals dissolve hair, leaving a smoother, more enduring result. Test on a small area of the skin before first use of any product, in case you are allergic.

Waxing:
Although painful, waxing lasts longer and leaves the skin soft and smooth. Best undertaken by a professional, but home kits are effective.

Abrasive pads:
Hairs do not regrow bristly. May destroy some hair follicles.

Plucking:
Most effective on chin and eyebrows. Never pluck hairs from a mole.

Bleaching:
Best for disguising facial hair. Always test on a patch of skin before use and rinse off.

Permanent hair removal:
Electrolysis causes a chemical reaction, and shortwave diathermy uses heat. Both *must* be performed by a trained operator, and home kits should be avoided. Although skin is left red and sore, it is an excellent way to remove facial hair.

Eyelid: protective flap.

Conjunctiva: the thin covering of the inner surfaces of the eyelids and exposed cornea.

Iris: the coloured muscle that alters the amount of light entering the eye.

Pupil: a hole whose size changes with the action of the iris in response to the amount of light.

Lens: a flexible transparent structure used for focusing.

Sclera: the 'white' of the eye.

Retina: has light-sensitive cells. Nerves transfer information to the optic nerve.

Optic nerve: carries information about an image on the retina to the brain.

Blind spot: the place where the optic nerve leaves the eye; contains no light-sensitive cells.

Choroid

Ciliary muscle: alters the shape of the lens for focusing.

Eyes are the most highly developed of our special sense organs. They feed in most of the information about our surroundings, reveal many of our inner feelings, communicate significant information to others and reflect well-being. However, the eyes need care, attention and protection, particularly when the strength of the sun or the hazards of an occupation or sport demand it. Above all, they should be regularly checked for any faults in vision, especially in children.

The bones of the skull naturally protect the eyes, and the eyelids and lashes help to prevent grit entering the eye. Above the outer corner of each upper eyelid lies the lacrimal gland. When you blink, tears, which are salty and antibacterial, sweep across the eye to keep it clean, lubricated and free from infection. When more tears are produced through crying, they drain into a channel that leads to the nose.

The eye is spherical and is operated by three pairs of muscles working in unison. The part you see through is the black pupil, which is altered in size by the muscles of the iris to control the amount of light falling on the retina at the back of the eye. Here the light-sensitive cells on the retina convey information to the optic nerve; this passes to the brain which interprets the signals as vision. A transparent, elastic lens attached to the ciliary body lies behind the iris and pupil. By causing the lens to thicken or become narrower, the muscles in the ciliary body enable the eye to focus on objects at various distances.

Eye tests

Good eyesight can only be maintained by having regular eye checks. Most people go through life without any disease of the eye itself, but most need glasses at some time. Early detection of any problem may make the difference between good eyesight and complete loss of vision.

A typical eye examination usually includes recording how much a person can see without spectacles, then improving the sight if necessary by selecting suitable lenses. The way in which the two eyes work together (binocular vision) is first assessed, followed by a careful examination of the inside and outside of the eye. Pressure measurements of the inside of the eye are performed on all patients over the age of 45 and on younger people if a near-relative has the condition glaucoma, in which there is a dangerous build-up of pressure in the eye. Width, or field, of vision is checked, then colour vision. One male in eight suffers from colour blindness — difficulty in distinguishing between certain colours, usually red and green — an important consideration for those involved in occupations requiring accurate colour judgement.

An optometrist classifies normal sight as 6/6 (or 20/20), which means you can read letters of a fixed size on a chart at a distance of 6 metres (20 ft). A measure of 6/10 (or 20/32) for example, means that you can only read at 6 metres (20ft) a line that someone with normal vision can read at 10 metres (32 ft).

The eye (left) *works like a pin-hole camera. The object observed is focused on the light-sensitive retina, just as light-sensitive film is used in a camera.*

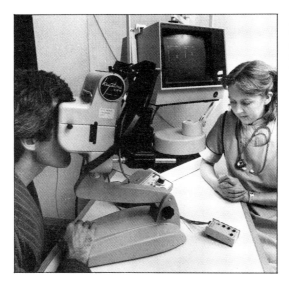

Even if your vision is not defective, regular eye tests are vital. Some serious eye disorders are symptomless in their early stages, but can be treated and cured if detected in good time. An eye test every 2 years is ideal, but any sudden changes in your vision should be reported to your doctor or an eye specialist immediately.

Eyestrain

Tired, sore eyes usually result from making the muscles around the eyes work too hard. Glare from the sun, snow or a television set, for example, can make the eyes feel sore because of the strain of keeping the eyelids protectively screwed up. Poor lighting may also overstress the eye muscles, so adequate light is important and is best directed from behind, over a shoulder for close work. No permanent damage can be done to the eye itself from prolonged study or close work, or from incorrect glasses or too much television viewing.

If your eyes feel tired or sore, bathe them in warm water, with a little salt added if you wish. There is no harm in using one of the proprietary eye washes if you find them useful.

Eye problems

Several types of eye problems are common and include the following:

Short sight (myopia) causes distant objects to appear blurred because the light entering the eye focuses in front of the retina, instead of precisely on it. This is corrected by concave lenses, which may need to be quite thick. Contact lenses (see p. 146) may be preferable to spectacles, since they give a wider field of vision.

Long sight (hypermetropia) makes close-up vision fuzzy, while distant objects are more clearly focused, because light rays focus behind the retina. This condition is corrected with a convex lens, which must be used for close work and sometimes constantly. Since focusing power diminishes with age, most middle aged people require glasses for reading.

Astigmatism (distorted vision) is the result of an uneven cornea or lens. Slight abnormalities will go unnoticed, but more severe cases need to be corrected by lenses worn most of the time.

A squint (lazy eye) arises when muscles are not holding one eye in place, so it deviates, either constantly or occasionally, in relation to its partner. Squints must be corrected or the lazy eye will deteriorate and blindness in that eye may result. Correction is usually made by covering the strong eye with a patch to make the lazy eye work, but an operation may be necessary to improve the muscle balance.

Cataract is a condition in which the lens inside the eye becomes cloudy, so light reaching the retina is gradually reduced. More than 90 per cent of people over the age of 65 has some sign of this disorder. An operation may become necessary to remove the diseased lens, but surgery is successful in 95 out of 100 cases.

Other common eye problems include styes, which are caused by an infection of the eyelash follicles, and conjunctivitis (pink eye), an inflammation of the delicate lining of the eyelid, caused either by bacteria or viruses. These infections are highly contagious, and anyone inflicted with one of them should isolate their personal towels and face cloths.

THE EYES/2

Spectacles
Use the following tips for choosing various types of spectacles.
- ●Look for lightweight plastic frames that return to shape, even when sat upon.

Sunglasses
- ●Choose high-quality lenses.

- ●Polaroid types reduce glare but will make a car windscreen appear blotchy.

- ●Photo-sensitive lenses adjust to the light intensity but can be dangerous when you move from bright sunlight into a dark tunnel.

Mirrored lenses protect the eyes from reflected glare, as when skiing and sailing.

Sports glasses give good protection during active sports.

Protective goggles are essential for much industrial work, to guard against flying metal and reflected infra-red and ultraviolet light.

Contact lenses (see chart, right) have cosmetic appeal and provide better all-round vision than glasses. Although initial discomfort can occur, a few people are unable to wear them. A specialist must be consulted for fitting, and you should have a professional check-up once a year. This is important to prevent or correct any problems.

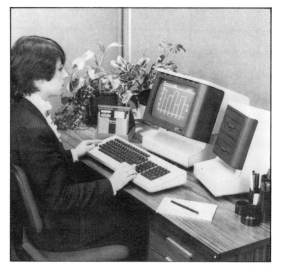

Working at a computer screen can cause the eyes to feel tired. This is because the muscles concerned with focusing are subjected to a heavy work load. Ideally, you should work at a screen for 20-minute stretches with a 5-minute break between each, and change to a different task altogether after 2 or 3 hours. If you have problems with tired, red or itchy eyes, or with headaches, you should have your eyes tested. You may be suffering from a visual defect of which you are unaware.

Type	Description	Advantages	Drawbacks
Hard	Rigid plastic, fitting over part of cornea.	Good, clear vision. Last a long time. Can be repolished to remove scratches. Easy to handle and clean. Least expensive to buy and maintain.	May be uncomfortable at first. Can distort the cornea if ill-fitting. May be unsuitable for extremely sensitive eyes. May have adverse long-term effects.
Soft	Look like drops of water. Made of a hydrophilic plastic polymer.	More comfortable initially than hard lenses and better for occasional use. Particularly good in dusty environments.	May react adversely to high temperatures and pressures. High maintenance costs. Last less long than hard lenses.
'Gas permeable' hard lenses	Rigid plastic that allows the passage of air.	Crisper vision than soft lenses. Allow more oxygen to reach the cornea than hard lenses do.	Often need soaking in special solution to remove accumulated proteins.
Extended-wear lenses	May be worn for 1 week to 3 months without being removed.	Useful for babies, small children and the elderly.	Can be harmful to the eyes if not used with careful, *regular* professional supervision. Vision less good than with hard or soft lenses.
Coloured lens filters	May be worn if one or both eyes are damaged or by actors to change eye colour.	Useful for medical camouflage of eye damage. Do not affect vision.	

The ear has three parts: *the inner ear, which controls hearing and balance, deep within the skull; the middle ear, associated with hearing; and the outer ear, extending from the eardrum outward, which concentrates sound.*

The bones of the middle ear adapt vibrations from the drum and transmit them to the inner ear.

The semicircular canals control our sense of balance.

The pinna helps to channel sound received from air waves.

The auditory nerve carries signals to the brain.

The auditory canal funnels sound toward the eardrum.

The cochlea generates signals concerned with hearing and balance.

The eardrum is a membrane that vibrates in response to sound.

The Eustachian tube links the middle ear to the back of the throat.

The human sense of hearing is developed long before birth. Recordings of sounds within the womb are well known to be soothing to a new-born baby, who soon comes to recognize his own mother's voice. However, the brain's ability to translate nerve impulses into meaningful sounds, such as the rattling of a spoon against a cup or the complexities of a conversation, takes months and even years to develop fully. A child, therefore, needs to be brought up in a world of sounds, especially words, to develop his hearing and language facilities fully. Of course, the hearing must be normal for this to be achieved.

The ears are also organs of balance. Impulses generated in the cochlea of the middle ear are sent to the brain and inform it of the body's orientation in space. This combination of functions explains why ear infections may be accompanied by dizziness. As with hearing, the sense of balance becomes less acute with age.

Care of the ears

The ears are normally efficient, self-cleaning organs and do not benefit from interference. The wax in the outer ear, which contains a bactericide, helps to trap dirt and potential irritants as they enter. Body warmth melts the wax, which travels outward with the help of movement of the hairs in the outer ear. The wax should never be poked with any type of cotton bud, hairpin, fingernail or other instrument, since this can easily damage the eardrum and cause deafness.

The most that should be done is to wipe the *outer* ear with the corner of a towel, or with a cotton bud or tissue.

If you suspect that a blockage of wax is affecting your hearing, arrange to see your doctor, who may syringe your ears with warm water. You may need to soften the wax with warm olive oil for a few days before syringing. Always protect your ears and those of your children from severe cold and do not overlook the ears when applying a sunscreen.

Air travel

Spare a little thought for the ears when you travel by air. The pressure in the middle ear is the same as atmospheric pressure because an open, air-filled channel, the Eustachian tube, links the middle ear with the back of the throat. The canal may collapse, however, with sudden changes in altitude, resulting in an alteration in pressure between the middle ear and the outside.

To keep the canal open during take-off and landing, try swallowing, sucking sweets or drinking. Alternatively, hold your nose and blow; you will feel a 'pop' as the pressure equalizes. If possible, avoid flying when you have a cold or throat infection, since bacteria in the throat are more likely to enter the middle ear under these high pressure conditions. A decongestant spray, used before a flight, should help to prevent pain. However, if pain or giddiness persist, you should consult a doctor.

The sense of hearing is essential to normal development. A deaf child cannot communicate his handicap to parents or teachers because he does not understand it. So any child with learning problems should have an ear test immediately. If an infant does not startle at a loud noise, a mother may suspect deafness, particularly if she contracted German measles (rubella) in the early months of her pregnancy.

With advancing years, the sense of hearing begins to deteriorate, albeit slowly. For this reason, it is sensible to have your hearing checked regularly after the age of about 50. However, if you suspect at any age that your sense of hearing is less than perfect, it is well worth having it tested by a specialist.

Hearing tests

Accurate hearing tests cannot be conducted until a child is $2\frac{1}{2}$ to 3 years old. Rudimentary testing, however, can be done at any age. Between 6 and 9 months, the normal baby begins to localize sounds and will turn his head to look for the source of a sound. From 18 months onward, the first formal hearing test can be given, since the child is old enough to respond in a meaningful way to various spoken words, commands and test sounds.

The most common cause of deafness in young children is infection of the middle ear, which is caused by bacteria passing into the ear from the throat. The Eustachian tube (canal) becomes blocked, and, as a natural response to infection, fluid collects in the middle ear, thus impairing its efficiency. If it persists, despite antibiotic treatment, a small hole can be made in the eardrum, the sticky fluid sucked out and a tiny ventilation tube or 'grommet' inserted into the middle ear for a period of 3 to 9 months. Children with grommets can swim if they wear a cap that covers their ears and as long as they do not put their heads under water.

Occasionally, a middle ear infection may cause the eardrum to burst, and a sticky discharge to trickle out from the ear. The severe pain of infection is relieved by the perforation of the ear drum, but although the drum usually heals within a few weeks, the ear should be kept under observation and the efficiency of hearing subsequently checked.

The prospects for improving loss of hearing

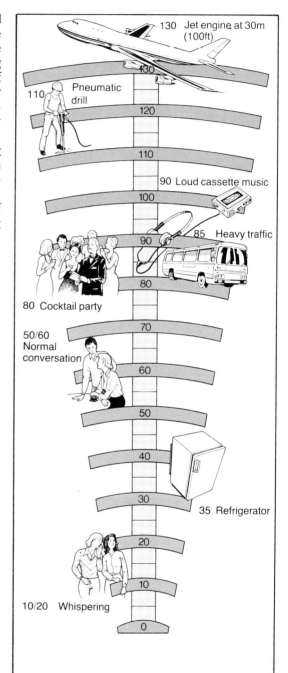

Noise levels above the value of 90 decibels can cause permanent damage to the ears and thus to the sense of hearing. The diagram shows the decibel rating of some common sources of noise, whose potential danger to your hearing can be evaluated.

Ear piercing

As long as it is carried out under sterile conditions ear piercing is safe. If conditions are unhygienic infections such as hepatitis and blood poisoning could result.

Stud or ring 'sleepers' should be made of gold, since this is least likely to cause an allergic reaction. Keep the holes clean and dry by washing night and morning with soap and water, then pat dry with cotton wool. Turn the sleepers several times a day to keep the holes open.

Conspicuous ears

Cosmetic surgery can be undertaken if ears are large, mis-shapen or protruding, although it is often possible to conceal them with the hair.

depend on its cause, and on the part of the ear that is affected. (The anatomy of the ear is illustrated on p. 147.) If a wax or dirt blockage, poor vibration of the middle ear bones or a permanently ruptured eardrum is causing poor sound conduction, the condition may be helped by medical treatment or a hearing aid. If, however, the cochlear apparatus, nerve cells and pathways involved in hearing are damaged, the problem is not easily treated, although hearing can sometimes be restored with a hearing aid. Hearing tends to deteriorate appreciably with age, but in recent years many younger people have become deaf, partly due to the increased noise levels in the everyday environment.

Hearing and noise

Noise-induced hearing loss which affects the cochlea is irreversible. The louder the noise, the shorter the exposure time needed to produce hearing loss. Noise arising from heavy machinery, pop concerts, hi-fi and from the personal earphone stereo systems that have been introduced, can all cause deafness.

Noise is measured in decibels. Sounds of about 10 decibels and below are inaudible to the human ear. Exposure to noise levels of more than 90 decibels can, however, result in permanent damage to the ears, so pop music in discotheques, with sound levels well over 100 decibels, can prove harmful. After 100 minutes of subjection to such extreme noise levels, hearing may not be restored to normal for 36 hours. If the exposure is repeated, however, hearing capacity will be diminished as a result of permanent damage to nerve cells.

A persistent ringing or buzzing in the ears usually indicates temporary damage. The most common result of damage is a reduced ability to follow discussions when several different conversations are going on at once. Firearms, fireworks, noise at work, particularly from heavy machinery, and noise at home, especially from do-it-yourself tools, garden appliances and motorbikes can also adversely affect hearing. If you work in an environment which you think may be damaging your concentration or your hearing, do what you can to effect a change. Ear plugs or muffs should be worn to prevent occupational deafness, and in many countries compensation can be claimed for industrial injury to hearing.

Ear tests: checklist

● Every newborn baby is given a general examination, but hearing problems may not emerge until later.

● At 3 months, check your baby's hearing by clapping loudly while he is crying; he should stop for a moment.

● At 6 to 9 months, a normal baby turns to face in the direction of an unusual sound.

● At 18 months, the first formal hearing test should be given.

● Always request an ear test if you suspect impaired hearing, especially after an infection.

● Consult a doctor if you experience pain, dizziness or 'gluey' ears.

● An ear test is usually given as part of a general health screen.

● In later life, if loss of hearing becomes tiresome, a hearing aid may be helpful.

TEETH AND GUMS

Teeth are an integral part of our self-image, our speech, our digestion and our appreciation of food. Yet looking after the teeth can be such a chore that they are all too often neglected. Decay (caries) in the teeth, and receeding, bleeding gums, with accompanying pain and bad breath are not inevitable. They can be prevented by understanding dental disease and by taking a little extra time and effort to clean the teeth and gums thoroughly twice a day throughout life.

Diet and teeth

A healthy diet with as little sugar as possible is the basic rule for prevention of dental problems. Eskimos rarely suffered from tooth decay until they adopted a high-sugar Western-style diet. Likewise, during World War II, when sugar was scarce, there was much less tooth decay in Europe than there is today. Having a sweet tooth is a reversible habit, but it is better to prevent children from developing one in the first instance. Remember that soft drinks contain a lot of sugar, so offer children water to quench their thirst and give them raw vegetables, bread, fruit or nuts as snacks rather than sweets or biscuits.

The total amount of sugar consumed is, however, less important than the number of times that sugar enters the mouth. Sugar eaten at mealtimes is thus less damaging than sugar eaten between meals. This is because, in the early stages of dental caries, it is possible for the saliva to repair the small amount of damage caused by the interaction of sugar and bacteria in the mouth. If the teeth are constantly bathed in a sugar solution, this repair process cannot occur and, slowly but surely, the damage continues.

The effects of fluoride

An important part in the prevention of dental decay, both during the development of the teeth and after they have erupted, is played by the mineral fluorine. The most effective way of supplying people with flourine salts — flouride — is by introducing them into public water supplies. Some towns in the USA have fluorinated their water for more than 30 years, to good effect. And where flouride exists naturally in the water supply, lifelong residents are found to be resistant to tooth decay.

No harm has ever been demonstrated from drinking water fluorinated at the level of one part fluoride to every million parts of water (1ppm: 1 mg/litre). Where fluoride levels reach 3ppm or more, however, white or brown marks may appear on the teeth (the same effect can occur when children are given certain antibiotics). If the dose is adjusted to the levels of fluoride in the water supply, it is advisable to give children up to 13 years of age fluoride tablets or drops. Fluoride toothpastes, mouth rinses and paint applied by a dentist are all helpful.

Sticky dental plaque is the primary cause of both tooth decay and gum disease. Made up of millions of bacteria, it accumulates between the teeth and around the gum margins and feels rough to the tongue. When sugar is present, the bacteria produce acid, which dissolves a hole in the protective enamel surface; other bacteria then cause caries or tooth decay.

A recently developed vaccine against these bacteria has been shown, in animals, to reduce caries by 75 per cent. Clinical trials are being conducted in the USA and in Britain and may provide a breakthrough in preventing caries.

More teeth are lost through gum disorders than tooth decay. Again, plaque is the cause. It collects around the gum margin, inflames the gum and eventually loosens the connection between gum and tooth until a pocket forms and the tooth loosens. Regular and careful brushing, flossing and massaging are the best forms of prevention, although dentists can help with regular scaling and polishing of the teeth.

Modern dentistry

The use of anaesthetic injections, high-speed drills and comfortable surroundings have made a visit to the dentist less daunting — an important factor, since this prevents unnecessary delay in filling cavities.

Today, a natural-coloured filling material is available for treating front teeth; and fissure sealants, plastic coatings for crevices in the back teeth, are used to prevent dental decay in children. Badly damaged teeth can be capped or crowned, and a fixed bridge can be made to hold new replacement teeth. Tooth-straightening (orthodontics) is best done between the ages of 12 and 16. It usually takes 2 years to complete, and invisible plastic braces help to make the treatment acceptable to young people at an acutely self-conscious age.

Dental Care

To prevent gum disease and tooth decay developing, ensure that you have the necessary equipment, (right). Chew a disclosing tablet and spread the liquid around the teeth with the tongue, then rinse. Use a dental mirror to see where the plaque is concentrated – indicated by an intense red colour. To remove plaque, floss regularly and clean the teeth daily with fluoride toothpaste, using both a standard and a single tuft or interspace brush.

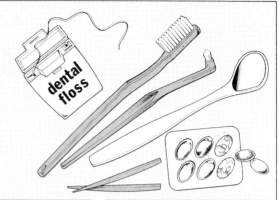

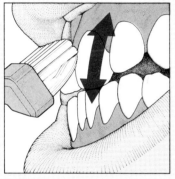

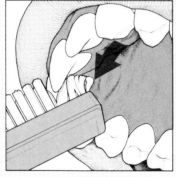

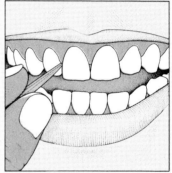

Brushing:

Use a small, soft or medium toothbrush and fluoride toothpaste. Keep the bristles at 45° to the teeth and brush up and down on all sides of each tooth.

Concentrate on a few teeth at a time and establish a routine to ensure all teeth are brushed. Begin with the inside surfaces, move to the chewing surfaces, then brush the outside of the teeth.

Massaging:

To massage the gums and remove plaque, use wooden interspace sticks. Gently scrape between the teeth and at the gum margin, but never force a stick between closely set teeth.

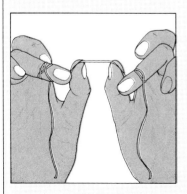

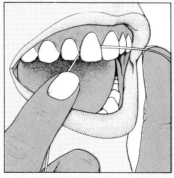

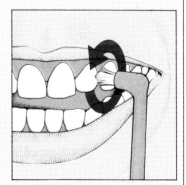

Flossing:

Cut off a piece of dental floss or tape 45cm (18in) long. Wind it around the index fingers of both hands, leaving 10cm (4in) between the two hands.

Gently push the floss between the teeth, rubbing it against the inner surfaces of each tooth, particularly at the back. Do not press too hard on the gums; if necessary ease the floss backward and forward.

Single-tuft brushes help to massage the gums and clean the more inaccessible gaps between teeth. Use a circular motion and pay particular attention to the molars.

Do you bite or pick your nails?

These are common habits, so do not feel too guilty, but make a tremendous effort to stop. It will do wonders for your confidence and will prevent repeated nail infections.

Use these tips to help you or your children stop biting their nails:

● Be determined to stop.

● Take a pride in your hands; use hand cream regularly.

● Use scissors or an emery board on rough nails *before* your teeth get there.

● Start by allowing one nail at a time to grow, then limit your biting to one nail until you have stopped.

● Ask your friends and family to remind you if they see you lapse.

● Try the bitter-tasting nail coatings, available from pharmacists, or a clear nail polish.

● Try bribery — treat yourself if you stop for a month.

● Pinpoint and try to reduce the cause of stress.

● Keep any new nails smoothly filed to avoid the risk of losing them again.

● Try hypnotism or acupuncture.

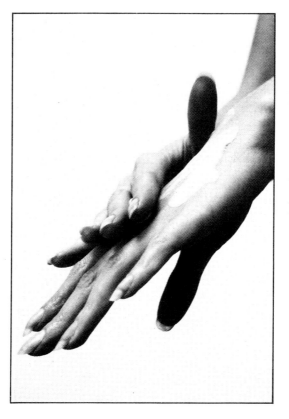

When washing your hands, always rinse and dry them thoroughly. Wear special gloves for dirty work. Rubber gloves may produce red, itchy, cracked skin, so plastic gloves are often preferred. If waterproof gloves are kept on for more than 15 minutes, the hands may sweat: you may prefer to wear cotton gloves inside them. Gardening and other similar protective gloves are also advisable, as are barrier creams. If possible, apply hand cream often, and in all circumstances, especially over the knuckles and around the nails.

Hands are great reflectors of well-being. They reveal the kind of work we do, our age, our degree of nervousness or self-esteem, and may show the first sign of any illness. Yet our hands come in for a lot of rough treatment. They suffer the extremes of weather and temperature; they are immersed in water and garden soil and subjected to irritants such as detergents. Skin problems on the hands are rarely contagious.

Hands are great communicators. They emphasize our words and silently express our feelings through gesture and touch. The new world that is opened up through the fingertips in touching or being touched, is an indefinable part of well-being. Everyone, but particularly those who live alone, feels more relaxed with a pet to stroke.

Nail care

Each fingernail grows about 1 cm ($\frac{1}{2}$ inch) every three months, and each toenail at about a third of that rate. Growth rate varies with the individual, however, but it is a myth that if the nail is persistently bitten, it grows twice as fast.

The nail

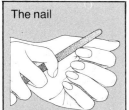

The nail is a plate of keratin — dead cells that grow from a root, where the cells divide rapidly. Blood vessels in the soft tissue beneath the nail nourish the nail bed, which is visible as a white crescent. Nails also grow from the nail bed.

Nail care

● **Keep the nails short** to stop them splitting and always use an emery board in preference to a steel nail file.

● **File from the sides** toward the centre and avoid cutting or filing down the sides, since this will weaken the growth. If the skin is pierced, a painful infection may develop.

● **Most nail problems** are caused by abuse rather than dietary deficiencies. The best prevention and cure is to file them correctly, to avoid any obvious irritants or submersion in water, and to wear protective gloves or hand creams whenever necessary. Swollen fingers may be a symptom of heart disease, which needs medical attention. If you suffer from stiff fingers, exercise them as much as possible.

Although they are made up of the tough, dead material, keratin, fingernails enhance the appreciation of fine touch, adding valuable dexterity to the fingers by enabling the hand to pick up tiny objects. Nail-biters are reminded every day of the inconvenience and 'clumsiness' arising from the loss of this ability.

The condition of nails is a signal of general health, both psychological and physical. A severe or traumatic illness may cause nail growth to slow down temporarily, until a transverse furrow develops, which indicates the approximate date of the onset of the illness. Lack of iron can make the nails depressed and spoon-shaped but, contrary to popular belief, brittleness is not caused by vitamin or mineral deficiencies, and eating extra protein, gelatine or cheese is of no use whatsoever in solving the problem.

The best cure is to keep the nails short and apply cream at night. Small white spots or flecks on the nails are probably caused by minor injuries to the nail bed rather than by any problems with calcium, and usually grow out with the nail.

All manual work damages the nails, so if necessary keep the nails short and trim them regularly. Split edges of nails and brittleness are common among people who work with their hands in water and detergents or use harsh, acetone nail varnish removers. If the hands are to be immersed in water for more than a short while, waterproof gloves should be worn. Nail polish applied underneath and on top of the nail provides an additional shield, it also prevents flaking.

Discoloration of the nails is caused by, for example, smoking, ill-health and some nail varnishes. It can only be removed by allowing the nails to grow out in the natural way.

Exercises for hands and wrists

To keep hands and wrists supple, exercise them regularly, for example while sitting watching television. Place the heel of each hand on your upper leg or the arm of a chair. Stretch your fingers and thumb out as far as they will go, then relax them. Repeat this 10 to 15 times.

To exercise the wrists, hold your arms out in front of you with your elbows straight. Point your fingers alternately toward the ceiling and the floor. Repeat this about 10 times. With your arms still outstretched, rotate your hands from the wrist, making 5 to 10 circles with each.

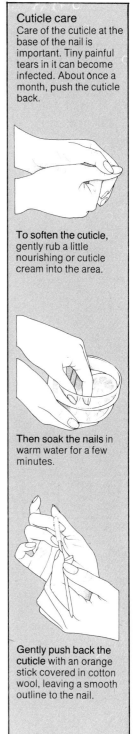

Cuticle care
Care of the cuticle at the base of the nail is important. Tiny painful tears in it can become infected. About once a month, push the cuticle back.

To soften the cuticle, gently rub a little nourishing or cuticle cream into the area.

Then soak the nails in warm water for a few minutes.

Gently push back the cuticle with an orange stick covered in cotton wool, leaving a smooth outline to the nail.

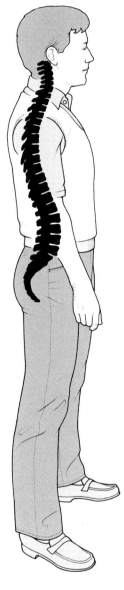

The back is the pivot of all human movement and bears the brunt of any postural problems. Man's flexible spine was originally designed for walking on all fours, and our upright posture imposes great strain on the spinal column, since it has to support the weight of the entire upper part of the body. If the muscles that link the vertebrae of the spine and transmit this weight to the pelvis and legs are weak, the spine becomes unstable and back pain inevitably follows. The abdominal muscles also lend great support, so if these are weak too, the back is more susceptible to strain.

Millions of working days are lost every year because of back pain, which is now the most common reason for adults consulting their family doctor in both the USA and Britain. The most widespread cause is simple muscle weakness, particularly in the abdomen.

The anatomy of the spine

Between the base of the skull and the pelvis lie 24 vertebrae, separated by elastic discs, which allow flexible movement and absorb shock; tough ligaments hold the discs and vertebrae in correct alignment. Twelve pairs of ribs are attached to the spine and curve around to the front, where the upper ribs join the breast bone, forming a protective cage for the lungs and heart.

The spinal cord lies within the vertebral column, just as the thread of a necklace lies inside each bead. The spinal cord is made up of a vast number of individual nerves, connecting the brain with the rest of the body. Each shock-absorbing disc in the spine is a rigid ring surrounding a compressible, pulpy centre. If subjected to a heavy load while the vertebrae are misaligned, a disc may slip out of place or extrude its soft

Are you insulting your back?
● Are you overweight? This puts extra strain on the spine.

● Do you slouch and hunch your shoulders?

● Are your stomach muscles flabby?

● Do you wear high heels? These push the body's centre of gravity forward.

● Do you carry a baby or parcels on one hip? This causes a sideways tilt to the spine.

● Do you lift with your knees straight? You should bend from the knees and hips and hold the load close in to the body and equally in both hands.

● Are you pregnant? You should wear flat shoes, avoid standing for long periods and keep within normal weight limits (see pp. 194-5).

Correct posture: to balance your spine correctly, stand with your feet slightly apart and your weight evenly spread between toes and heels. Pull in your buttocks and push up the crown of your head as far as you can. Keep your shoulders relaxed and your abdominal muscles taut. The aim is to maintain, but not exaggerate, the natural forward curves at the neck and the base of the spine, to avoid aching muscles and nerve damage.

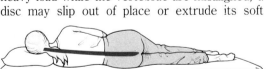

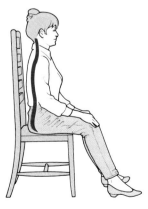

When lying down, *your back should remain as straight as possible. If you lie on your side, do not bend your knees or your arms more than 90°. When lying on your back relax your arms by your sides. Support your pelvis with a cushion when lying on your stomach.*

Sit well back *in a chair so that it bears your weight. Avoid bad habits such as twisting your arms and legs or leaning forward with your chin jutting out. Keep your knees slightly bent and your feet flat on the floor.*

centre. A slipped disc is a condition that needs medical treatment. More important is its prevention by proper care and use of your back and regular exercises to keep the necessary muscles toned up (see pp. 104-5).

Furniture for healthy backs

Over one-third of your life is spent in bed, so ensure that your mattress is comfortable but firm enough to support the weight of your body without distorting its natural curves. A mattress should be replaced every 10 years, or when it starts to sag or get lumpy. To test a new bed, lie on it in several positions, and if you and your partner's weight and choice conflict, consider buying individual mattresses which can be zipped together. If you wake up aching and stiff, try an 'orthopaedic' bed. These give excellent support, although a board placed between the mattress and the base of a bed may produce the same benefit. Always give your neck sufficient support to keep it in line with the rest of your spine.

The fashion for low, soft seating has done much to increase the misery of back sufferers. When buying a chair, look for firmness and support for your back; if you have to struggle getting in and out, it is probably too low.

When working at a table, try to have the surface at elbow-height to allow your back to remain straight and unhunched. When typing, sit up straight. Some excellently designed posture chairs, which automatically put the top half of your body in the correct, upright position, have recently come on the market. With your thighs at an angle of 45°, your lower legs bend back virtually into a kneeling position, so your spine cannot easily slump.

Always flex your knees when bending, and keep your back straight. When stooping to lift, distribute your weight evenly between both hands and hold the object close to your body.

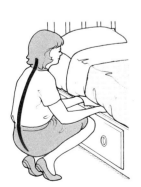

What to do about back pain

If acute backache suddenly strikes:
● Lie flat on your back on the floor.

● Try to retain the forward curve of your lower spine.

● Crawl or roll yourself to the telephone to call for help from a partner or neighbour.

● Ask someone to bring you a painkiller such as soluble aspirin or paracetamol.

● As the pain eases, move slowly, but keep the spine correctly curved. You may need to go to bed for a few days' rest. Torn muscles will heal in time, but they benefit from gentle movement. Hot baths, hot water bottles and infra-red lamps give some relief.

● If the pain persists or radiates away from the back, see your doctor, in case it is more than a simple strain.

● If you experience numbness or difficulty in urinating, seek medical help *immediately*.

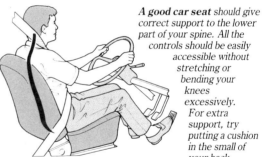

A good car seat should give correct support to the lower part of your spine. All the controls should be easily accessible without stretching or bending your knees excessively. For extra support, try putting a cushion in the small of your back.

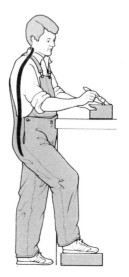

Working surfaces: try to ensure that the working surfaces in your home are at a comfortable height and do not force you to stoop. For ironing and other activities demanding the application of pressure, the height should be a little lower than normal.

Most people are born with perfect feet, but four out of five develop some foot trouble later in life. Since the average pair of feet walks around 1,900 km (1,200 miles) a year, often in badly-fitting shoes, socks or tights, few manage to escape discomfort.

When you are standing on two feet, each bears half your weight, but when you are walking or running, your whole weight is transferred alternately to each foot. The longitudinal arch, which transfers this weight from heel to toe, provides most of the upholding strength; while muscles, ligaments and joints give the foot spring and elasticity. The big-toe joint is particularly vulnerable to stress, especially when the heel is raised by high-heeled shoes and when the sole of the shoe is rigid.

Shoes for children

Children's bones are soft, and if young feet are squeezed in to ill-fitting shoes, they may become mis-shapen for life, so toddlers should not be put into shoes until they are walking well. When a baby first starts to walk, bare feet give the best grip on the floor.

Pram shoes may weaken the muscles of the foot and reduce flexibility. Socks or all-in-one stretch suits must be large enough to accommodate the foot comfortably and should be checked regularly for size. If necessary, the foot part of the suit can be cut out and socks worn instead. Children should have the width and length of their feet measured approximately every 3 months; it is recommended by specialists in foot care that shoes should be selected with a growing space of 18mm ($\frac{3}{4}$ in).

Adult footwear

Shoes need to be flexible to promote a springing step; they must be supple, especially where the toe joints bend, but they should be firm in the arch. Shoes with laces or an adjustable strap are best because they hold the foot firmly to the back of the shoe, so preventing the foot sliding forward and cramping the toes.

Adults should look for shoes that *fit*. They should be at least 1 cm ($\frac{1}{2}$ in) longer than the feet, to allow the toes to move freely, and must be wide enough to allow toes to lie square, without forcing them to the side. When buying shoes, always walk around in them in the shop and try

standing on tip-toe — if the heel slides off easily, the shoes are unsuitable. Shoes with low heels impose less strain than those with high heels because they distribute weight more evenly over the foot; varying the height of heels from day to day helps prevent aching feet. Heels over 6.25 cm ($2\frac{1}{2}$ in) high impose a great strain, so they should be worn for only a short time to avoid damaging the feet.

Nylon socks, tights or stockings may prove harmfully constricting, since nylon does not stretch to adjust to foot movements. For this reason, choose them with care. Always wear the correct shoes for sport. They must be roomy enough to allow the foot to expand when hot, and firm enough to prevent any injury through slipping.

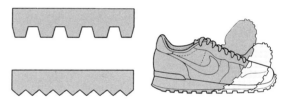

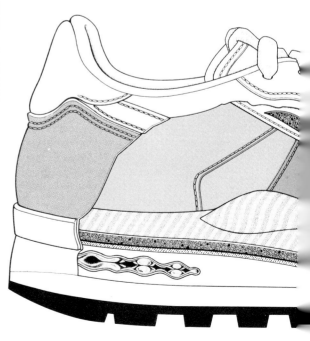

Chiropody, pedicure and foot exercises

Chiropodists are trained to identify and treat common foot ailments and provide a useful service, particularly for the elderly or infirm, who may be unable to look after their feet themselves.

A professional pedicure is a real treat and can prevent the build-up of hard skin on the soles of the feet. Correct care of the toe nails is equally important; always keep the nails short and cut them straight across to avoid ingrowing nails. Regular exercises are also beneficial; try spreading and curling the toes alternately, then flexing and pointing the whole foot. To improve the circulation and strengthen the small muscles of the feet, try rotating the whole foot, then turn the soles inward and outward. Remember to walk barefoot as often as possible without risking any kind of injury.

A pair of running shoes should endure about 1,600 km (1,000 mls) of running. Before you buy, test shoes with the socks you will wear. Choose shoes with tops made of natural materials such as leather or canvas, and layered cushioned soles, as shown. If you usually run on a road or pavement, a waffle-patterned tread (far left, top) *helps to cushion the impact that travels up the legs to the spine. A shallow zigzag (far left, below)* is better for running on softer surfaces. To ensure sufficient support, the sole must be flexible at the ball of the foot, not the arch (near left). The heel back needs a firm collar to prevent sideways slip, while being flexible enough to avoid chafing.

Common foot problems and what to do about them		
The Problem	**The Cause**	**What to do**
Athlete's foot:	A fungal infection between the toes, causing itching, soreness and peeling. May also affect nails.	Wash the feet with soap and water once or twice a day. Dry carefully between the toes and use anti-fungal powder or cream. Change socks and stockings every day and wear cotton, not nylon. Wear open sandals when possible.
Bunions:	The fluid cushion around the big-toe joint, becomes inflamed and thickened through wearing ill-fitting shoes. A tendency to bunions may run in families.	Wear shoes that do not crowd the toes. An operation will relieve the pressure.
Corns:	Painful pads of thick, hard skin on the soles of the feet and toes especially the little one. Caused by tight shoes.	Avoid tight shoes and change footwear often. Corns on children's feet are alarming signs of damage caused by shoes. Corn pads and plasters relieve pressure, but if a corn persists, see a chiropodist.
Ingrowing toe-nails:	Pain, discomfort and sometimes infection caused by a nail growing into the flesh at the sides of the toe.	Avoid tight shoes and socks. Never cut the nails away at the sides. Can be removed by a simple operation.
Verruca (wart):	An infectious wart on the foot. Common in children. Wear special covering 'verruca socks' at a public swimming pool.	Try using special wart-removing preparations. If it persists, see your doctor or chiropodist.
Sweaty feet:	Overproduction of sweat by sweat glands. A common problem.	Keep the feet clean and dry. Change socks or stockings daily. Avoid nylon socks and tights, and buy all-leather shoes. Choose sandals or open shoes if possible. Apply foot powder.

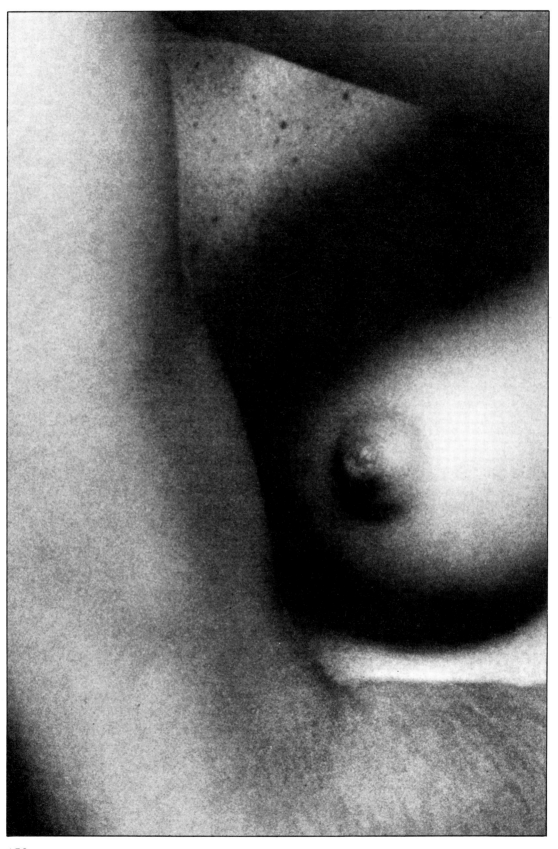

YOUR SEXUALITY

We all have the potential for a healthy and fulfilling sex life. Yet developing and maintaining it is not always a simple matter. When things go wrong — as, inevitably, they sometimes do — many of us are at a loss about what the next step should be.

Problems arise for a variety of reasons, including lack of understanding about sexuality and the sexual response, feelings of guilt when desire outstrips 'propriety', insecurity about technique, ignorance about contraception, stresses that spill over into relationships, general ill health and much more.

An ailing sex life can be revived and, with a little care and effort, improved both physically and emotionally. This chapter explains how. It examines the development of sexuality during childhood and adolescence, when attitudes are formed, and follows the years through to the menopause. Sexual activity, appetite and experience evolve with the years, in tandem with changing emotional attitudes. With knowledge and understanding, these changes can be welcomed not dreaded. Essential information on sexual functions, contraception, health screening and problems that may impair sexual satisfaction are also included.

A rewarding sex life is one of the ingredients of a continuing sense of well-being. Through happier, more fulfilling sexual relationships, the quality of our lives can be improved.

The teenage years are a time of great change and upheaval. The self-consciousness and self-centredness characteristic of adolescence are exacerbated by the inner conflict created by a child struggling to assert independence while he is still acutely aware of the need for emotional and financial support from parents. Attitudes formed toward sex and relationships at this time, however tentative, have profound repercussions later, so tolerant parents can be a great help.

The physical changes

Male puberty usually begins internally at around the age of 9, at least three years before any bodily changes are visible. The pituitary gland at the base of the brain begins to secrete gonado-trophins, which stimulate the testes to produce androgens and, later, sperm. After about a year, the adrenal glands release the male hormone, testosterone, which triggers the growth of secondary sexual characteristics.

The rate of sexual development in boys is highly variable. The growth spurt may begin at 13, but is more usually delayed until 16, and full height is reached by 18. Once the legs have grown to full length, followed by the torso, the muscles begin to strengthen and the figure broadens. Meanwhile, the facial features become more pronounced and the voice 'breaks', in response to a thickening of the vocal cords and enlarging of the voice box cartilage.

Another aspect of puberty is hair growth. Coarse hair begins to appear around the base of the penis and in the armpits, while a fine down sprouts on the upper lip and chin, becoming a coarse moustache and beard when shaving is necessary. Chest and sometimes back hair grows, the extent depending on heredity. The skin and hair become more oily and body odour develops.

The greatest source of concern for boys, however, is the maturing of the genitals, while the testes enlarge and begin to produce sperm. The penis gradually grows toward its full size and becomes more erectile. At this stage, boys may experience nocturnal discharge of semen, and they are capable of fathering a child as soon as the sperm are fully formed. The onset of sexual maturity can be worrying, particularly for 'late developers', and parents should be both sympathetic and informative.

Mental and emotional changes

Becoming a man is not easy. While coping with the havoc the hormones create and with physical metamorphosis, the teenage boy has to grapple with social pressures and search for an adult identity. Some boys have to undergo a public confirmation of their manhood, when they are emotionally far from being men. Jewish boys, for example, celebrate their Bar Mitzvah at 13, regardless of their sexual, mental or emotional maturity.

Inevitably, conflicts arise between parents anxious to retain control and adolescents striving for independence. The revolt against authority manifests itself in many ways. Experimenting with smoking, drugs, extreme politics, wild music and clothes, and petty crime and other anti-social behaviour, are common means of conforming to peer-group pressure.

Crushes on older boys may develop, and

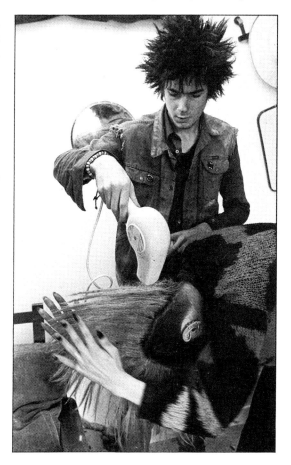

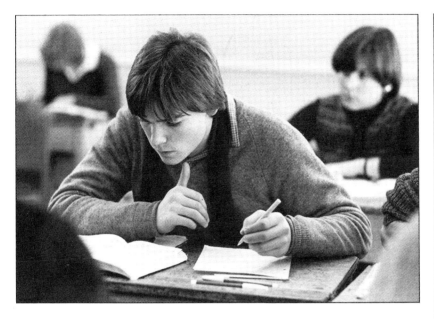

The teenage years are often dogged by examination pressure (above). For some boys, study is an excuse not to socialize and can lead to unease with girls in later life. Others are hopelessly distracted from work by sexual thoughts and may jeopardize their career prospects. A reasonable balance between study and a social life is, thus, important.

Adolescent rebellion against authority often finds expression in extreme fashion, such as punk (left). Frustration, confusion and peer-group pressure drive many teenagers into aggressive non-conformism. Compulsion to attract the opposite sex also leads to obsessive concern with appearance. This experimental phase, however, is generally short-lived and most young people soon find less extreme hallmarks of identity.

strong sexual feelings for girls are often hidden behind an affectation of disinterest. Not surprisingly, the psychological stresses imposed by so many changes often lead to violent mood swings and emotional insecurity before a mature male identity can be found.

Discovering sexuality

Sexuality is neither inherited nor instinctive, it has to be learned. From the age of 3 or 4, boys and girls are aware of the differences between the sexes and enjoy touching their bodies. Since the male organ is more accessible than the female one, males are more familiar with sexual feelings, however confused they may be.

In adolescence, as the sex drive increases, sexuality becomes an anxious preoccupation, and masturbation the rule not the exception. Sexual thoughts and masturbation may result in guilt feelings, unless it is explained that they are normal and *not* a sin nor a perversion, nor a threat to health, eyesight or mental stability. Curiosity and awakening sexual instincts will fire an increasing interest in the opposite sex. Experimentation invites the risk of rejection, confusion and ridicule, so it is most important for parents to show understanding and to create a liberal, though defined, moral climate. If parental signals are negative, the adolescent may associate sex with guilt, which may cause problems in adult life.

What you should tell your teenage son

Sex education is now taught in most schools, but many questions remain unanswered because of the sheer embarassment of asking them.

If at all possible, ensure that your son is familiar with the basics of male and female sexual anatomy, sex, reproduction and contraception *before* the confused knowledge of friends muddies the waters.

Remind him gently of the implications of getting a girl pregnant, contracting a sexually transmitted disease and the effect of alcohol on both male and female sexual behaviour.

Do not scorn or ignore the subject of masturbation, but place it in the context of normal sexual drives.

The onset of puberty and adolescence is as testing for girls as it is for boys. Although it is often hard for parents to be sympathetic, teenagers must be treated with understanding, both to ensure that healthy sexuality is achieved and to ease the painful transition to adulthood.

Physical and mental changes

Sexual development spans almost a decade — from the age of 10 to 18 — for both sexes, but tends to begin and end earlier in girls than in boys. Female puberty begins about two years before the onset of menstruation, when the pituitary gland begins to secrete sex hormones. These stimulate the ovaries to release oestrogen, the female hormone that triggers the growth of secondary sexual characteristics.

The rate of development for girls is enormously variable. Throughout childhood, girls are, on average, 1.25 cm ($\frac{1}{2}$ in) shorter than boys, but their growth spurt takes off sooner, at around the age of 11, so that by the age of 13 girls are usually 2.5 cm (1 in) taller than boys. A year later, most girls have finished growing, when boys are just beginning their growth spurt.

The most significant landmark in a girl's sexual development is menarche, the first menstrual period. Promoted by the gonadotrophic hormones, the ovaries release the two hormones oestrogen and progesterone, which control the menstrual cycle. Menstruation usually starts at 13, but can often begin at 11 or may be delayed until the age of 17 or 18.

A girl is not fully mature, however, and able to conceive until a few months after menarche, when ripe eggs are released and the ovaries have enlarged to sustain the monthly emission of eggs. At this stage, the uterus has enlarged sufficiently to house a future foetus, and vaginal fluid can be secreted to facilitate sexual intercourse.

Some girls welcome the menarche as the arrival of womanhood, others seek to withdraw into childhood, hence the prevalence of anorexia nervosa — slimming to extremes — among teenagers, with its attendant flat chest and absence of menstrual periods.

Most parents and teachers would deny that they sex-type children, yet adolescent girls are still subtly programmed into traditional female outlooks. This idea of 'becoming a woman' conflicts with an evolving social climate and creates

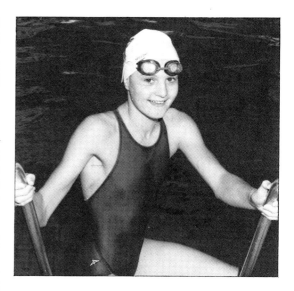

extra difficulties for an adolescent girl who is seeking an identity in an inconsistent world. A few cultures, however, acknowledge the modern view, which is reflected in the liberal Jewish Bat Mitzvah ceremony for girls.

Like boys, adolescent girls are plagued by uncertainties, conflicts and guilt but, unlike boys, they thrive in a climate of approval. Thus when they do rebel it is usually within 'approvable' limits. The most popular way of dealing with accumulating insecurities is to conform to the peer group. Some also become prey to short-lived crushes on members of their own sex. Many adolescent girls become obsessed with moulding themselves into enticing 'relationship material'. This often causes them to relinquish their academic lead over boys at this point, and may be a significant reason why many girls tend to be under-achievers and never manage to develop their full intellectual potential.

Discovering sexuality

As children, girls are less curious than boys about their bodies. Studies have shown, for example, that while 56 per cent of boys under 14 have masturbated, for girls the figure is only 30 per cent. After puberty, however, girls soon become aware of their sexuality and mature rapidly. As with boys, they need to work out a sexual identity that conforms to their wishes and the prevailing moral climate, and to learn how much to succumb to peer-group pressures. In so doing they can

Many girl swimmers (left) *reach their peak of performance during adolescence. This maximum seems to coincide with, or follow soon after, the last growth spurt, which brings them to their adult height. For all girls, sport should be encouraged and not regarded as in any way unfeminine.*

Idolizing the stars at a pop concert (right) *can provide teenage girls with the chance to relieve their sexual frustrations. Such occasions are also an opportunity to 'escape' from the parental lifestyle and to dress in the style currently favoured by a girl's peer group.*

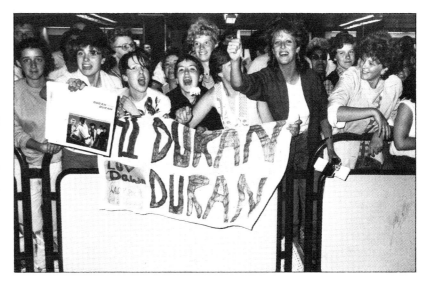

suffer great anguish, which then colours ensuing experimental sexual encounters.

Devising a personal sexual code demands more maturity than most young girls can muster. Some will deny their sexuality and become obsessed with 'neutral' interests, such as horses; others express their frustration by mooning after pop stars or become sexually promiscuous at a young age, often through anxiety and confusion about sex, and the pressure of peer groups. The way in which a girl responds to her sexual awareness also depends on the sexual and moral attitudes expressed at home.

What to tell a teenage daughter

Do tell your daughter about menstruation well before she begins sex education lessons at school so that periods will not come as a shock to her if she is an early developer.

Explain also the male pubertal changes, the basics of sex and reproduction and the various methods of contraception so that she is properly informed and able to make sensible choices for herself when the time arrives.

Remind her gently of the implications of getting pregnant, contracting a sexually transmitted disease and the inhibition-releasing effect of alcohol on both male and female sexual behaviour.

Try to encourage her to feel responsible for her own body and to discuss sex openly with her parents; it may help her to sort out her own sexual code and standards.

Sex and the formation of relationships are essential to well-being in both men and women. The differences in attitudes and approach depend on the nature of sexuality in the mature male and the mature female.

The sex organs

The penis, the most obvious of the male sexual organs, consists of a shaft of spongy, erectile tissue. Its sensitive tip, or glans, is covered by a fold of skin, the foreskin, but in circumcised males this is surgically removed. The testes, contained in the scrotum outside the body, produce the male sex hormone testosterone and sperm cells. In the mature male, sperm production is a continuous process. The sperm is either ejaculated or, when no ejaculation takes place, reabsorbed into the system.

During intercourse, masturbation or other sexual stimulation the sex organs change in a series of phases. In the arousal phase, there is a reflex rush of blood to the penis, making it firm and erect. The skin becomes more sensitive and breathing deepens and quickens.

In the plateau phase, the penis reaches its maximum size and the testes enlarge. Drops of seminal fluid (which can contain sperm and could lead to pregnancy) may appear on the head of the penis. During orgasm the sperm are mixed with fluids secreted by the seminal vesicles and prostate gland to form semen, which is forced out of the penis in a series of rhythmical contractions. In the resolution phase, the system returns to its non-aroused state.

Sexual display and arousal

All human relationships are motivated, to some extent, by the libido or sex drive. But how men go about attracting women, and what makes a man sexually aroused, are largely the result of cultural influences, learned associations and individual preferences and needs.

Sexually, males are much more easily aroused than females. They are extremely sensitive to sexual cues and stimuli — mental, visual and tactile. This is partly a result of their high arousal state from the male sexual hormone, partly from the immediate sensitivity of the penis and partly from the learned pleasurable association most have from masturbation.

In most societies, men are conditioned to be independent, assertive, competitive and sexual. Thus their means of attracting women is by presenting themselves and by highlighting their positive attributes. Women look upon this self-advertisement as attractive; what many do not realize is that the male advance is, whether consciously or not, primarily sexually motivated. It is only secondarily that the woman herself is singled out as 'special'.

Finding a partner

Although most people meet and become couples through friends' introductions, there are many other avenues of approach. These include computer dating, small advertisements, bars, social clubs, evening classes and all kinds of sport and cultural activities.

It seems that men prefer short-term relationships when young — the liberal sowing of wild oats is still a part of the male image — but once that phase has passed, most wish to make long-term commitments, to satisfy the urge for regular sexual activity and to provide a sense of security. Even in today's climate of 'shared homemaking', many also wish to have their needs catered for by a woman.

Stabilization of relationships

The type of relationship a man may seek depends greatly on his attitudes, his age, his career, his financial commitments, his needs and the availability of women. Most men are polygamous: they like many partners (in fact or fantasy), regardless of whether they are single, have a live-in lover or are married. This is not to say that men do not desire serious, stable relationships. Rather, being more outwardly directed than women, and more interested in sex for its own sake, they are apt to take care of the business of life before they become emotionally entangled or, if they do become emotionally involved, to allow the business side of life to take precedence.

Nevertheless, the possibility of forming a relationship with a woman can prove elusive. Men whose adolescent experiences were painful or inconclusive may be socially immature and unable to give the commitment a relationship demands. Others may use work as an excuse for not having the time to spare for a relationship. The truth is that relationships take constant care and nurturing — they do not just 'happen'.

Myths and truths of male sexuality

Myth: masturbation is harmful.
Truth: it has no negative effect and can be an excellent outlet for sexual frustration.

Myth: penis size is in direct proportion to female satisfaction.
Truth: penis size is not relevant; the vagina can accommodate any size and gain satisfaction.

Myth: once impotent, always impotent.
Truth: impotence is mainly a psychological phenomenon caused by external stresses. Once these have been removed, potency usually returns.

Myth: men know intuitively how to satisfy women.
Truth: few men do. It would be more satisfying to their partner if they asked what she enjoys.

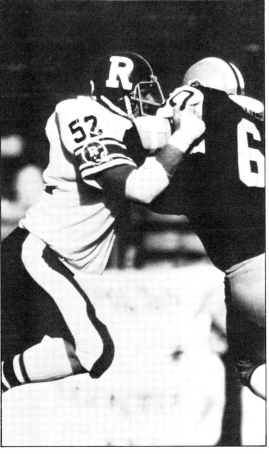

The continual demands of a sport or hobby may prevent men from becoming social beings, and prevent them from forming mature, lasting relationships with women. It is thus important for both men and women to balance all aspects of life with the goal of long-term emotional security in mind.

Safety rules for healthy sex

● If you do not want your partner to get pregnant, use or make sure she is using a contraceptive.

● Guard against sexual disease, if you sleep with many (casual) partners, by wearing a sheath.

● Sufferers from any sexual disease must inform their partners and not have sex until they are cured.

● Remember that violent sex can hurt women.

Self help for the sex organs

● For comfort and protection, shield the testes with a jock strap when playing sports.

● The tip of the penis and foreskin make a lubricant, smegma. This tends to accumulate, so should be washed away regularly.

In their sexual relationships, many men are troubled by the thought that their behaviour may not be normal. Such worries are a result of guilt, poor sex education, lack of experience and lack of communication with a partner. In fact 'normal' sexual behaviour varies widely. The decision as to whether an activity is right or wrong should rest with each couple. Simply tell your partner what you like, ask what she would like and try to come to some compromise.

For homosexual men, however, women hold limited sexual attractions. Although many men experiment with homosexual relationships in puberty, for some this is the preferred style for mature relationships. This should not be a matter of shame, nor regarded as something for which there is a 'cure'. A homosexual struggling to come to terms with his sexuality should be given the support and help of family and friends.

THE MATURE FEMALE

The mature woman's approach to sex and to relationships is determined both by cultural influences and her own sexuality.

The sex organs

The visible part of the female sexual system consists of the highly sensitive clitoris, which is covered by a small flap of skin, and the vulva, which consists of inner and outer lips. Within the body lie the vagina, the cervix (the neck of the womb) and the womb or uterus itself.

As with males, there are four phases in the female orgasmic cycle. In the arousal phase, a reflex action causes the sex organs to fill with blood, both externally and internally. The vagina expands both in length and width, and the vaginal walls produce a lubricant which facilitates intercourse. Breasts may enlarge and nipples become erect. The skin, particularly that around the erogenous zones, becomes more sensitive. Breathing deepens and quickens, and a pink flush may appear on the chest and neck.

In the plateau phase, the vagina entrance narrows to grip the penis. The clitoris becomes fully erect and draws back into its hood. If a woman is sufficiently aroused and is receiving clitoral stimulation, orgasm may occur. An orgasm begins in the clitoris and radiates outward, while the muscles surrounding the vulva, vagina and anus go into a series of contractions. In the resolution phase, the sexual organs return to their normal state, as the blood that swelled them drains away. Breathing slows, and the flush disappears.

Sexual display and arousal

In spite of the slow shift toward self-assertion, most women are still passive, dependent, receptive and far less sexually direct than men. In general they prefer to be approached rather than to make the first move — a reflection of cultural influences and conditioning. The way in which they go about attracting men is an extension of their adolescent interest in external feminine appearance. Women like to think of themselves as attractive to the opposite sex and send out body signals, often through sexy or provocative dress, which are designed to elicit some response in men. Many women send out these signals and are then shocked by unwanted approaches, which points to a dilemma between the desire to be appreciated and the desire to reveal the 'real

woman' only to those members of the male sex whom they choose and trust.

At the same time, women are aroused more slowly than men. In theory, women have the same capacity for a sex drive as men, but convention has instilled in them a more inhibiting pattern of response. Moreover, a woman's relationship with her body is much more tenuous sexually, since her body's purpose is bound up both with reproduction and with the need to feel loved and reassured in an intimate situation. Levels of arousal are partly influenced by pheromones, (odours that evoke a powerful sexual response), but more so by the point in a woman's menstrual cycle; each woman has her own 'high point' at which she is most easily aroused. Studies also show that worrying about sex inhibits arousal; as one psychologist noted, 'a woman is sexiest when she thinks least and feels most.'

Like men, women have very real worries about the parameters of their sex lives, and these are compounded by a wide range of socially conditioned inhibiting factors. Furthermore, women tend to place a higher value on their partner's sexual enjoyment than on their own. The change in sexual climate has helped to increase recognition that women can enjoy a satisfying sex life, yet a more relaxed attitude is still needed to free women from feelings of guilt, fear and abuse.

Finding a partner

The pressure on women to marry young has eased, but the imperative to form relationships remains. The avenues that are open to women are the same as for men, but since they feel more strongly about having a man in their life, they are quicker to seize opportunities. Although women see long-term relationships, particularly marriage, as desirable, they are becoming more flexible about short-term flings. The 'one-night stand', once viewed as certain ruination for a young woman's reputation, is seen as a means of relieving sexual frustration, with a veneer of intimacy but no commitment. The sixties' permissiveness, allowed by the contraceptive pill, is now on the decline. The fear of pregnancy has, however, been replaced by the fear of herpes; and most women still seek motherhood within a legally sanctified relationship.

For women, as for men, there are some individuals who prefer homosexual rather than

Myths of female sexuality

● Women are insatiable.

● It is allowable for men to masturbate but not for women. In fact, both sexes can release tension and frustration and derive sexual satisfaction from it.

● Women who have children are no longer sexual beings.

● Simultaneous orgasm should be the goal for couples. In fact, despite their efforts, it is rare for a couple to get the timing just right.

● Women always have orgasms. This is also untrue: many women are, sadly, not sufficiently aroused during foreplay to experience orgasm and often fake it for the sake of the male ego.

Truths of female sexuality

● To achieve an orgasm, a woman needs clitoral stimulation, by herself or her partner, in addition to intercourse.

● The late 30s and early 40s can be the times of greatest potential and satisfaction.

● Women do enjoy sex, especially if it is bound up with love, but most would feel more satisfied if more time were spent on foreplay.

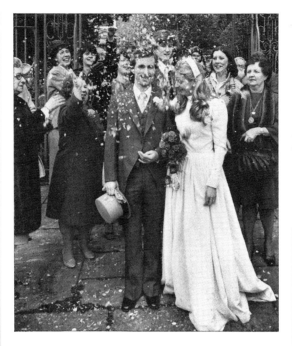

The romantic ideal of marriage remains firmly fixed in the female mind and, however mistakenly, many women still consider themselves 'failures' if they remain single. This is despite the fact that women are becoming more career orientated and are increasingly opting for trial marriages before committing themselves finally.

Self-help

● Wash the vaginal area every day, especially if you have an active sex life.

● Choose underpants with a cotton gusset.

● Remember, any unexplained pain, bleeding or discharge needs *immediate* attention or treatment.

● Vigorous exercise can affect breast tissues, so wear a good supporting bra.

● Beware of exercising to extremes, it can cause amenorrhoea — delayed or absent periods.

heterosexual relationships. In some such partnerships, children are even conceived, with one member of the pair having intercourse with a man simply with this aim in mind. As with male homosexuality, understanding rather than alienation should be the attitude of outsiders.

Stabilization of relationships

From a young age, women are relationship orientated and many place far greater social value on establishing bonds with men than on furthering their education or starting a career. While men may think of establishing a stable relationship at some unspecified point in the future, many women are more concerned with love and bonding in the here and now and with the possible future of any relationship. Many women, regard the 'business' of life as merely marking time. Such a woman waits for 'real life' to begin when a man asks her to marry him.

Evidence suggests that most women are now trying to establish their own identity to avoid becoming simply extensions of their partners. The marrying age has risen, giving women time to study and begin a career. More women, too, are becoming sceptical about enduring marriages and are opting for trial marriages before making a serious commitment.

IMPROVING YOUR SEX LIFE

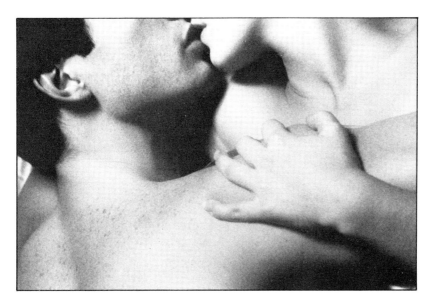

If making love becomes sporadic or boring, then it is time for a change of attitude. *Use your imagination to discover more about your partner and to devise new ways of making love, and discuss any problems or grievances openly and honestly.*

When sex is no longer a pleasure for one or both partners, it can become a source of tension that spills over into other areas of life. Today there is no need for couples to 'just live with it'. An ailing sex life can be revived and difficulties overcome.

Self-help

An ailing sex life is one that has either lapsed into a stale routine or is so limited that it leaves one or both partners dissatisfied. This does not simply happen overnight; it is a result of two people getting so used to each other that they fail to appreciate the subtleties of their needs and desires and the fact that these can change over time. Sex then ceases to be a 'special' experience, and instead becomes relegated to merely one of those necessary rituals in life—such as brushing your teeth.

Putting life back into sex involves a shake-up of attitude, both toward sex with its ever-changing horizons, and toward the partner. Each member of the partnership must again see the other as an individual, whose personal qualities were once a source of attraction. Neither the partner nor the sex act should be taken for granted. This means starting afresh and reopening lines of communication that have been broken.

When sex becomes a problem, it is important for partners to be frank and honest with each other, to express dissatisfaction in a non-hurtful way and to consider ways of remaking a sexually

successful partnership. A simple airing of frustrations, stresses and discontents can do much to bring a couple closer and to emphasize that only joint effort will bring sexual happiness. In this more relaxed atmosphere, both partners will be ready too enjoy what they have and to add variety and depth to their sexual relations.

When imagination fails, this should not be regarded as a personal failure, rather as a spur to resolve a situation that has developed into a problem. Books may help with specific difficulties and give hints for positive improvement. A general practitioner may be willing to answer questions and provide counselling, or may recommend marriage guidance or sex therapy, for advice, support and reassurance.

Although most of the sex aids on the market have little practical value and are often highly priced, some can loosen inhibitions or add a charge, or some humour, to love-making. Vibrators, for example, can help a woman achieve orgasm, either alone or as an extra stimulation during sexual intercourse.

Sexual problems

Nearly half of all married couples experience some sexual difficulties at some time. Many of these problems are occasional, for instance when a man has had too much alcohol and cannot achieve an erection, or a woman has had a tense day and cannot become aroused. More enduring

168

How good is your sex life?
Do any of the following apply to you?

● I cannot tell my partner what I want him/her to do in love-making.

● Our sex life is so predictable, I always know what is coming next.

● Our sex life lacks passion or tenderness.

● Other people enjoy sex, why don't we?

● I wish my partner would try something new.

● There must be more to making love than this.

If two or more of the above are true for you, it is time to inject new life into sex.

sexual problems can be a serious source of guilt, worry and self-analysis if nothing is done about resolving them.

Most sexual problems arise from a subtle and complex mixture of psychological causes, attitudes, upbringing and tension in daily life or in relationships. The most common problems in men are impotence: the inability to obtain or sustain an erection; premature ejaculation; and ejaculatory incompetence, that is, the inability to release semen into the vagina.

In women, the most common problems are painful intercourse; the clamping of the vaginal muscles, or vaginismus; and orgasm difficulties. Other problems include lack of interest in sex and the inability to become aroused.

Finally, there exists the problem of non-consummation, when a man cannot sustain an erection for full penetration to take place, or when a woman is so tense that her vaginal muscles go into spasm and prevent penetration. This often occurs as a result of intense fear on the part of either or both partners. In rare cases, non-consummation may result simply from lack of knowledge. A few sexual problems have medical causes. An overtight foreskin, for example, can make intercourse painful, while an undescended testicle may cause embarrassment; both can be treated surgically. Some illnesses and drugs, particularly those prescribed for depression or high blood pressure, can affect sexual response, particularly in men.

During the midlife transition, men often experience a drop in sexual appetite and performance. In women, painful intercourse may accompany gynaecological problems such as ovarian cysts or vaginal infections. The menopause may reduce the lubrication in the vagina; the contraceptive pill may affect some women's sex drive, and vaginal soreness after childbirth can make intercourse uncomfortable.

Obtaining help
If self-help remedies, doctors, marital counsellors or sex therapists cannot help, they may be able to refer you to a variety of other therapies available, from the highly effective behavioural techniques pioneered in the USA by Masters and Johnson, to more unconventional methods. With perseverance, there is no reason why any couple should not enjoy a happy sex life.

Getting the most out of your sex life
● If your love-making follows a routine pattern, vary the order of events and time spent on each.

● Put romance back into your life with flowers, soft music and a candle-lit dinner. Seduce each other.

● Vary the amount of sex you usually have; if it's twice a week, try it twice in one day.

● Treat sex as fun and add a touch of unpredictability.

● Try making love in different surroundings.

● Speak to your lover during sex and express your desires or simply say you like what they are doing.

● Say 'yes' to sex even if you do not feel like it, then make the effort to enjoy yourself.

● Treat each sexual encounter as if it were your first and seek to discover something new about your lover's sexuality every time.

● Tell each other why you like/love each other.

● Set aside a whole evening just to touch, stroke, caress and massage each other.

● Say 'thank you' once in a while.

No contraceptive has yet been found to be 100 per cent reliable, suitable, practical and without side effects or possible health risks. However, controlling reproduction is any sexually active, fertile adult's responsibility, and it is impossible not to be able to find at least one appropriate method. Single people should accept the responsibility as their own, but with couples, married or unmarried, the responsibility needs to be shared. Contraception and its implications are subjects that parents should discuss fully and openly with their teenage children.

A tremendous breakthrough was made with the oral contraceptive pill, but since the mid-1960s the question of its safety has given rise to much controversy. Since other birth control methods are not ideal, extreme remedies, such as male and female sterilization have recently gained popularity to relieve the burden of birth control, particularly for couples over the age of about 35 who are satisfied that their families have reached completion.

The contraceptive pill
The pill is one of the most reliable and reversible methods of birth control, and its release on to the market in 1960 transformed the sex-life of millions of women. There are two main types: the combined pill, which uses two synthetic hormones, progestogen and oestrogen, to stop ovulation; and the mini-pill, a progestogen-only pill, which alters cervical secretions to impede the sperm's journey to the womb. Although the pill is still the first choice as a contraceptive for the majority of women, a succession of 'pill scares' has led to some caution.

Just how safe is the pill? Early on, the high oestrogen levels in the combined pill were found to encourage blood clotting, which in turn may cause thrombosis (blood clots) and circulatory problems. Since this made women more vulnerable to heart disease and strokes (although they are still five times less vulnerable than men of the same age), the oestrogen levels were lowered. If they are too low, however, breakthrough bleeding (bleeding between menstrual periods) occurs and the pill may be ineffective in preventing pregnancy.

Opinion is now divided about the safest strategy to use. Some doctors say that with the new low-oestrogen formulations, women run only a small risk of thrombosis. Others recommend that all women over 35, and those over 30 who smoke, should either stop using the combined pill or switch to a progestogen-only pill. In view of such disagreement, it would appear that for ultimate safety, a woman in her twenties should have her blood pressure and blood cholesterol monitored frequently, stop smoking, and plan to discontinue the combined pill and use an alternative method of birth control or consider sterilization at around the age of 30 or 35.

Areas of research
The 'scares' of the early 1980s centred on two separate pieces of research that tried to establish a causal relationship between the pill and breast and cervical cancer. The first study, published in Britain in the *Lancet* in 1983, was directed by Dr Malcolm Pike. With his co-workers, Pike proposed that long-term use (5 or more years) by women before the age of 25, of the combined pill with a progestogen potency of 5mg and above, led to four times the risk of breast cancer. This risk did not appear among women who had started the pill after the age of 25 or had taken low-progestogen pills. The research was strongly criticized, largely because Pike used a progestogen potency table that was 20 years out of date, and in that time the progestogen levels had been markedly lowered.

American studies have both proved and disproved the link between breast cancer and the pill. The safest strategy, therefore, is for women under 25 to use a low-progestogen combined pill, to give themselves a breast examination every month, and to have a specialist medical examination every three years which may include a mammography (see pp. 180–1).

The second piece of research, also published in the *Lancet*, was conducted at the Radcliffe Infirmary in Oxford, England by professor Martin Vessey. The theory put forward was that long-term use of the pill increases the risk of breast cancer and carcinoma of the cervix (although other studies have shown that the pill may even protect against cancer of the ovaries and womb).

All types of pill were implicated, and the risk was increased with time. Vessey's research was also criticized, mainly because it did not take into account other factors associated with cervical cancer, such as multiple sexual partners and

Male sterilization

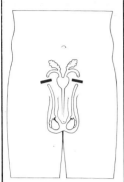

Male sterilization involves cutting each vas deferens to block the sperms' path from the testes. The operation, under local anaesthetic, usually takes about 10 minutes, but contraceptive precautions are needed for the next 3 months, until all stored sperm is ejaculated

Female sterilization

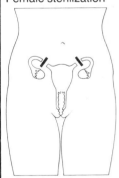

In women, sterilization is performed by cutting or clamping the Fallopian tubes. Operations to remove the ovaries or womb also result in sterilization. These operations are usually conducted under general anaesthetic and take effect immediately.

sexually transmitted diseases. Thus the safest recommended strategy is that women on the pill should have regular cervical smears taken every 3 to 5 years.

Both reports remain unconfirmed and more research is needed before the pill can definitely be linked to breast or cervical cancer. Meanwhile, women who take the pill must take into account that there may be health risks.

Permanent solutions: sterilization

For those who do not wish to have any more children, sterilization provides a permanent solution to the problem of contraception. The decision to have a sterilization operation should not be taken lightly, since there is little chance of reversing the procedure. In men, each tube (the vas deferens) that carries sperm from the testes to the penis, is cut in the scrotum and then closed off at the ends. A vasectomy will not inhibit sex drive, nor the secretion of male hormones, but contraceptives must be used for about 12 weeks, until laboratory tests show that the seminal fluid is sperm-free.

The most common operation for women is carried out on the Fallopian tubes, which carry eggs from the ovaries to the womb. The tubes are either cut, clamped or pulled through a tight plastic ring. In rare cases the tubes may rejoin, sperm may 'swim' through a clamp, or an ectopic pregnancy, in which a fertilized egg is trapped in a Fallopian tube, may occur. Periods will continue as normal or may be slightly heavier than usual after the operation, and menopause occurs at the natural time.

If the ovaries are damaged or diseased, the operation to remove them also means sterilization and may precipitate the menopause. The third method is a hysterectomy, or removal of the uterus, which is usually considered only if a woman has other gynaecological problems demanding hysterectomy.

Sterilization, which takes effect immediately in women, should not affect a woman's weight or sex drive and may even improve sex, once the fear of pregnancy is removed. Nevertheless, counselling is advisable before any decision is made, and sterilization should never be performed at the same time as an abortion because the emotional turmoil of a pregnancy termination may force an over-hasty decision.

Contraceptives of the future

Contraceptive developments in the future remain uncertain, since current research into birth control is confined to refinements of old methods. The most revolutionary foreseeable change is a vaccine that would make the female body reject sperm, but this is unlikely to be perfected until the 21st century. The male pill needs to contend with the problem of halting the ever-moving production line of sperm, and of male resistance to the idea.

Today, a contraceptive sponge for women, at present only 85 per cent efficient, is being developed in the USA and the UK. Available soon may be oestrogen rods injected under the skin, which would be effective for 2 years.

Other modern methods yet to be evaluated include Contracap, a cap made to fit the cervix exactly; hormonally impregnated intra-uterine devices; a nasal contraceptive spray that suppresses ovulation; spermicide-releasing vaginal rings, and a valved diaphragm that needs no spermicide.

'Assuming you don't want to give up sex altogether, you've no alternative but to find an alternative,' so one contraceptive advertisement warned. With so many birth-control methods available, most people can find at least one type of contraceptive appropriate to their age and family circumstances, and to their liking.

The chart lists the main contraceptives (apart from male and female sterilization, which are discussed on pp. 170-1), with an analysis of their effectiveness, safety and convenience. Additional information can be obtained from family planning

Method:	The combined pill
Reliability:	Almost 100 per cent
How it works:	Synthetic progestogen and oestrogen hormones mimic those of pregnancy. Since no message is sent out for an egg to be released, no ovulation takes place. Combination and triphasic pills are taken for 21 days, followed by 7 days of dummy pills or 7 pill-free days.
Advantages:	Easy and convenient to use. Regularizes periods. May reduce menstrual bleeding, period pain and premenstrual tension. Does not inhibit love-making. Protects against cancer of the ovaries and body of the womb.
Disadvantages:	Possible initial side-effects of nausea, headache, sore breasts, water retention, breakthrough bleeding, depression and loss of libido. Possible risk of thrombosis, and possible link with breast and cervical cancer.
Comments:	Not recommended for smokers over 30, those with a family history of heart disease or strokes and some diabetics. Safest have low progestogen/oestrogen formulation. Additonal precautions are needed to counteract vomiting or diarrhoea, with some drugs and if a pill is taken more than 12 hours late. Regular blood pressure checks, cervical smears, and monthly breast examinations advised, as for any other woman.
Method:	Mini-pill
Reliability:	98 per cent
How it works:	A progestogen-only pill, taken every day. It thickens mucus in the cervical canal, inhibiting sperm entrance and implantation of the egg in the womb.
Advantages:	Easy and convenient. Safe for older women. Less risk of heart problems. Suitable while breast-feeding.
Disadvantages:	Same initial problems as combined pill. Higher risk of ectopic pregnancy. Most effective 4 hours after taking. May cause breakthrough bleeding and irregular periods. Possible link with cervical cancer.
Comments:	More suitable for women over 35 who wish to stay on the pill. *Must be taken at the same time every day; if more than 3 hours late, extra precautions and checks needed, as for combined pill.*
Method:	Condom (sheath) lubricated with spermicide
Reliability:	97 per cent, *with careful use*
How it works:	Worn over the penis during intercourse to block the sperm.
Advantages:	Easy to use. Allows the man to take responsibility for birth control. May prevent passing of sexual disease. Lots of fun colours.
Disadvantages:	Interrupts love-making. May slip off or tear. May impair sensitivity.
Comments:	Must be held in place until withdrawal is complete. Never re-use. Lubricate with a specially formulated jelly.
Method:	Intrauterine device (IUD/ Coil/Loop/Copper 7/ Copper T/Multi-loaded Copper 250/Novagard/Nova T)
Reliability:	96 to 98 per cent
How it works:	Made of plastic or copper on plastic. How it prevents a fertilized egg from implanting or developing in the womb remains unknown.
Advantages:	Effective immediately (unless you are already pregnant). Especially suitable for those over 35 and those who have completed their families. Does not interfere with love-making.

clinics or from your doctor. Remember that, without contraceptives, pregnancy can occur while breast-feeding, without a female orgasm, sometimes without full penetration and despite douching. It is always better to be safe than to risk an unplanned conception.

Although there are risks and failures attached to the use of contraceptives, it should be emphasized that most of them work safely for most of the time. And even if a woman takes the pill, the risk of heart disease, for example, is five times less than merely being a man of the same age.

Disadvantages:	Initial pain, heavier periods, spotting, backache possible. Coil may be expelled within the first 3 months. Some men complain they can feel the string. Possibility of pelvic infection, which may cause infertility. Slight chance of ectopic pregnancy.
Comments:	Unsuitable for women with heavy periods. Effective for 2 to 3 years or more. Must be removed before starting a family. A morning-after IUD is also available. This is an emergency measure, fitted within 72 hours of intercourse, if unprotected during love-making.
Method:	The Diaphragm (Cap) with spermicide
Reliability:	97 per cent *with careful use*
How it works:	Three types: Dutch cap (rubber); smaller cervical cap (rubber); vault cap (plastic or rubber). Inserted into vagina so that it covers the cervix, up to 3 hours before intercourse. Cap and spermicide together prevent the sperm meeting an egg.
Advantages:	No side-effects, no health risks. May even protect against cervical cancer. Can be used at any age.
Disadvantages:	May inhibit love-making. Creams and jellies can be messy, and more must be added if intercourse occurs more than 3 hours after insertion or on a second occasion. In rare cases causes vaginal irritation or cystitis.
Comments:	Must be inserted correctly so that the cervix is covered. Must be left for at least 6 hours after last intercourse, then washed, dried, powdered and stored in a cool place. Check for small holes and renew every year, after a birth, miscarriage or termination, or a loss or gain of 6·5 kg (14 lb) in weight.

Method:	Safe period (rhythm method)
Reliability:	Calendar method – 53 per cent; Billings method — 85 per cent; Combination method — 85 to 93 per cent, *with careful use.*
How it works:	The calendar method entails working out the pattern of menstrual cycles to predict safe days. The temperature method indicates a slight drop in temperature just before ovulation. The Billings, or mucus, method relies on detecting changes in cervical mucus near ovulation. The combination methods include muco-thermal (temperature and mucus recording) and sympto-thermal (temperature recording plus symptoms of ovulation, such as backache and depression).
Advantages:	No side-effects except sexual frustration. Partners share the responsibility.
Disadvantages:	Demands great restraint. Calendar method is unsuitable if the cycle is irregular. Unsuitable during times of change. Temperature method may be unreliable. Billings method is difficult to learn.
Comments:	The only methods approved by the Roman Catholic Church. Can be unreliable.
Method:	Coitus interruptus (withdrawal)
Reliability:	Unconfirmed
Comments:	Inefficient and unsatisfactory for many. Used successfully in some cases, but requires a cooperative man.
NB	**Abortion should not be used as a primary method of birth control.**

RELATIONSHIPS UNDER PRESSURE

No marriage or long-standing relationship can ever hope to be perfect all the time; nor can a couple's sex life. Certainly, we all start out with great expectations and a grand passion — but the pressures of life inevitably intrude. It is possible, however, to identify problem areas and in doing so to look at ways in which relationships can be effectively revitalized.

All in the family — children

The family is a demanding, delightful and dedicated unit; at best it can enliven life, at worst it can enslave its members. From the moment the first child is born, to the day the last child leaves home, a parent's life is limited by the demands of seemingly more needy people.

The arrival of children precipitates a dramatic shift in roles and relationships. Despite the current vogue for shared parenthood, most mothers are still the caretakers of their children. The sexual split between partners begins with the exhaustion of childbirth, the demand of the new bond and, for many women, the belief that they are no longer sexual beings.

However, as time goes on, the demands on both parents, but particularly on the mother, begin to grow, and a parent may be pulled in conflicting directions. Common sense dictates that allegiances lie with the most vulnerable party, but a man or woman may not be any less in need of attention than a child. Many children learn to play off one parent against the other, reinforcing the emotional split between them, and a parent may use a child as a weapon or a hostage in a troubled relationship.

The presence of children also militates against privacy. Love-making becomes constrained by late nights, locked doors and whispers of pleasure, particularly when the family is living at close quarters. Indeed, many adults hide their sexuality and displays of affection from their children, so that once they grow older and start to be sexually aware, many young people view their parents' love-making with scepticism or disgust, or even doubt that it exists.

To alleviate some of the pressures inherent in their relationship, parents need to share the load honestly, so allowing enough time and energy for a fulfilling emotional and sexual life. Parents have to learn to be selfish enough to insist on being partners too. This may mean making a concerted

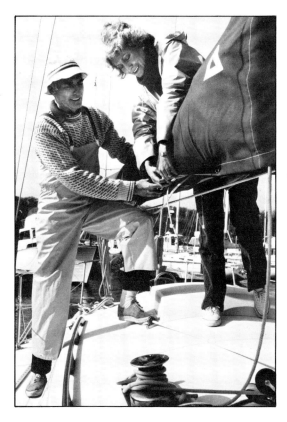

An activity holiday, away from all the aggravations of everyday life may be just the tonic your relationship needs, since stress and tiredness are the twin enemies of libido. Choose, by mutual agreement, the type of holiday that you will both fully enjoy.

and deliberate effort to set aside the demands of parenthood from time to time. Couples may find it helpful to allocate a particular evening each week on which to go out together, or to take occasional breaks away from home without the children.

All in the family — parents

The addition of an ageing, single parent imposes unexpected strains on any family. Even the most thoughtful and sensitive couple cannot foresee how roles and relationships will be revised. Settling-in problems may arise, especially if the parent comes from a different city or town and is used to an independent life, routine and long-standing friends.

Conflicts and guilt inevitably result when one partner slips back into a childhood role, allowing the parent to drive a wedge between man and woman, or stands back while the grandparent takes over the role of bringing up the children or gives advice from the sidelines. In such a tense situation, particularly if physical space is also limited, relaxed love-making will cease.

Adaptation calls for great patience, strenuous efforts and a smoothing over of divided loyalties, if the couples' loving and sexual relationship is to survive despite the problems.

The world of work
Work puts enormous pressure on a couple's relationship because of its inherently stressful nature, its energy-sapping qualities and the amount of time it claims. Too tense, too tired and too busy for sex, was once the cry of male partners, but it is now echoed by many working women. Furthermore, with breadwinning increasingly shared, conflicts arise about the division of family responsibilities. There may also be jealousy about financial contributions, success, independence and absence from home. It is all too easy for a couple pursuing their personal ambitions to become two separate, exhausted adults who happen to live under the same roof and share the same bed.

The only way to revive a 'work-sick' sex life is to revise priorities and to compromise; to care about work without allowing it to supercede the needs of the relationship. Work is best left and done, outside the bedroom door.

The lure of sex
The choice of casual sex outside marriage or a more serious affair, is up to the individual partners. Some people feel the need for sexual variety, the thrill of secrecy and extra emotional support, and a few relationships thrive on such sexual uncertainty.

Many relationships, however, simply cannot survive the strain of extra-marital affairs. It may go against the partner's moral upbringing, dispel their trust, shatter their security and repel them. Infidelity rarely rests quietly without causing heartache. Even if the marriage persists, there will always be residual distrust and fear that infidelity could happen again. The outcome depends on the strength of a couple's commitment to one another, the limits of tolerance and love, and the belief each has in the value and the lasting worth of the bond.

THE PREMENSTRUAL SYNDROME

Five out of every ten women may suffer some physical and emotional distress during the two-week interval between ovulation and menstruation. Dubbed the premenstrual syndrome (PMS), or premenstrual tension (PMT), the condition is now recognized and treated medically.

PMS is most prevalent in women over 30, after the birth of the first child, and it is most severe in highly-strung, highly-stressed women.

Physical symptoms of PMS include:
● Bloated abdomen and fingers.
● Swollen, tender breasts.
● Weight gain: sometimes up to 3kg ($6\frac{1}{4}$ lb).
● Headaches, often on one side.
● Aching back, legs, shoulders, knees and ankles.
● Craving for sweet, high carbohydrate foods.
● Spots, boils, spontaneous bruised, clumsiness, dizziness or faintness.
● Exacerbation of asthma, epilepsy, migraine, conjunctivitis and contact lens irritation.

Among the emotional symptoms of PMS are:
● Tension anxiety, depression, tearfulness, forgetfulness, lack of concentration, irritability and inability to make decisions.
● Violent mood swings.
● Lethargy.
● Some loss of confidence and disinterest in sex, work and social life.

Causes and treatments

No single cause for PMS has yet been identified. A number of theories, however, have been proposed, and have led to successful treatments.

One theory is that PMS is caused by an imbalance of the hormones oestrogen and progesterone. Oestrogen levels normally rise until ovulation occurs, then fall, but research at St Thomas's Hospital, London has shown that in 40 per cent of PMS sufferers, oestrogen levels remain high in the second half of the cycle, while progesterone levels are abnormally low. The treatment consists of doses of progesterone, which reduce fluid retention, breast tenderness, headaches, spontaneous bruising and nausea and also relieve many of the emotional symptoms.

Another theory is that women with PMS suffer from low levels of pyridoxine (vitamin B_6), which works on many parts of the body, including the brain and the pituitary gland — the menstrual trigger — and on the body's response to stress. The effect of this deficiency is to lower the output of progesterone and oestrogen. Advocates of this theory treat PMS with vitamin B_6 tablets from three days before the symptoms start, up to menstruation. In some women, it has been effective in relieving depression and headaches. An alternative theory, however, is that stress and anxiety are, in fact, the cause not the effect of hormonal imbalance.

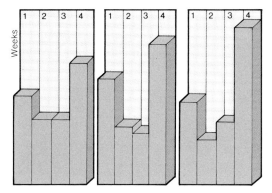

Women with PMS have a higher proportion of car and factory accidents and visit their doctors more often during the week before and after the onset of menstruation. Suicides also peak at this time, when emotional control is at its lowest ebb. Loss of efficiency during PMS can upset a promising career.

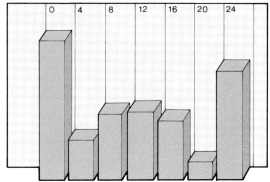

Almost half the crimes committed by women occur during the 4 days before and after the onset of menstruation. Child and husband battering are more common during PMS and it has become the centre of controversial legal debate in the courts in the USA and in Britain.

Other theories and treatments

In the USA, there is strong support for the theory that an excess of prostaglandin hormones cause nausea, moodiness and water-retention. Anti-prostaglandin drugs, such as mefenamic acid or indomethacin, have achieved good results.

A recent theory is that PMS is caused by a deficiency of essential fatty acids, particularly gammalinolenic acid. The seed oil of the evening primrose, *Oenothera biennis*, a natural remedy used by the American Indians, has been given to PMS sufferers where other treatments have failed, and research at St Thomas's Hospital in London has demonstrated a good success rate.

Other treatments include synthetic diuretics, which help to relieve water retention, tranquillizers, anti-depressants and treatment with the pill. These last three, however have made symptoms worse in some cases.

Sometimes more than one treatment must be tried; but with trial and error, a great measure of relief can usually be found.

A plan of action

Self-help is also possible and has brought relief to many women. Use a chart such as the one below to establish your personal pattern of symptoms then treat them as follows:

● Plan your life so that you do not put yourself under unnecessary strain premenstrually.

● Reduce water retention by eating less salt and drinking less.

● Don't worry about the temporary weight gain, you will lose retained water naturally during the menstrual period.

● Keep food cravings in check; weight gained by eating large quantities of chocolate or other sweet foods will not be so temporary.

● Take vitamin B_6 supplements.

● Lift your mood by planning a visit to the hairdresser or beautician.

● To relieve tension, take up yoga, relaxation or meditation.

● Take extra care if you are prone to accidents, dizziness or fainting.

● Take some vigorous aerobic exercise such as running or swimming.

● Alert your family, friends and perhaps workmates, so that they are likely to deal with you more tolerantly.

● Wear a more supportive bra to protect sensitive breasts.

● Try a herbal remedy.

● Make a real effort not to behave irrationally; exert more self-control.

If you believe you are suffering from PMS and have been unable to find relief with self-help measures, consult a doctor, who may refer you to a specialist or PMS clinic.

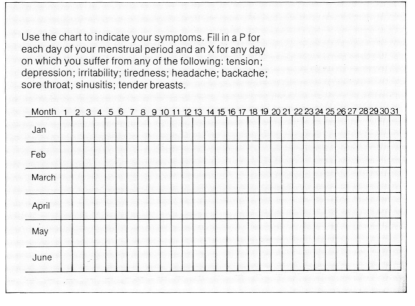

The way to find out if you are truly suffering from PMS is to keep a record of your symptoms. Use a chart, diary or calendar, such as this one, to note when, and how badly, you suffer specific effects. If after 3 months you see a regular pattern emerging, try the self-help measures suggested. If these are not effective, consult your doctor.

Use the chart to indicate your symptoms. Fill in a P for each day of your menstrual period and an X for any day on which you suffer from any of the following: tension; depression; irritability; tiredness; headache; backache; sore throat; sinusitis; tender breasts.

Month	1	2	3	4	5	6	7	8	9	10	11	12	13	14	15	16	17	18	19	20	21	22	23	24	25	26	27	28	29	30	31
Jan																															
Feb																															
March																															
April																															
May																															
June																															

Despite the current trend toward fitness and well-being, many women still do not take enough care of their bodies. Far too often they assume that good health means an absence of disease, or that female complaints are the necessary evils of their sex. These assumptions are incorrect, often dangerously so. Cervical cancer, which may be symptom-free in its early stages, has a death toll in Western countries of about one in 5,000 women. Pelvic infections, if left untreated, may cause sterility.

The range of tests

Most women shy away from gynaecological examination. But no matter how unpleasant it may be, every woman should make regular screening part of her health programme, since cervical smears and breast examinations are crucial to early detection of disease.

All sexually active women should have a full gynaecological examination once a year. Women should have their breasts examined by a doctor or specially trained nurse every year, especially if they are taking the pill or over 35. In the USA, cervical smears are advised once every six months to one year. In the UK the recommended interval between tests is 3 to 5 years. Women on the pill should have their blood pressure monitored regularly. These tests take only a few minutes and they may make the difference between life and death.

A full gynaecological examination begins with the taking of your medical, personal and gynaecological history. It is helpful if you have to hand details of previous tests and problems, dates of your last few periods, any premenstrual symptoms that you may experience and any other facts you may think relevant, including your method of contraception.

The gynaecologist examines your breasts and, if necessary, takes a mammograph (X-ray) and gives instruction in breast examination (see pp.180-1) — all with the purpose of detecting abnormalities that may give early indication of breast cancer.

A pelvic examination will then be carried out to reveal any signs of disease, abnormal growths, damage or infection in the womb, or in the cervix or vagina.

A cervical smear (also called a Pap or cytotest) — a routine of all gynaecological examinations and

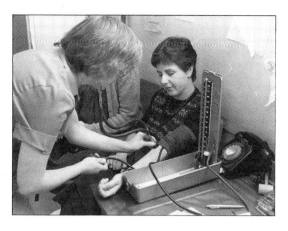

undertaken separately by general practitioners, family planning, antenatal and well woman clinics — is then taken. The procedure is painless and entails lightly scraping off some of the cells of the lining of the cervix (neck of the womb) with a wooden or plastic spatula. The sample is then sent to the laboratory to be examined for possible malignancy. Cervical pre-cancer, if detected in its earliest stages before it becomes invasive (it can take up to 10 years to develop) can be treated simply and with complete success. If it is left untreated cervical cancer can be fatal.

Women who have abnormal discharges are tested for vaginal and cervical infections by taking a sample for laboratory culture. In this way, thrush and venereal diseases can be diagnosed and treated.

Additional tests for blood pressure, anaemia, urinary infections, diabetes and rubella may also be taken where appropriate. After the examination, when the doctor discusses his findings, do not forget to ask any questions you may have.

Menstrual problems

Women's menstrual periods vary enormously, but the average monthly loss of blood is only 80 ml (2 fl oz). Irregular, painful or heavy periods are not unusual, but should not be tolerated unquestioningly. A proper diagnosis should always be made by your doctor or gynaecologist.

The worst symptoms of menstrual problems can be alleviated through self-help or medical treatment. Irregular periods (metrorrhagia) may be caused by emotional upsets as well as physical disease or the onset of menopause, and may be light or heavy. If treatment of the cause is not

Blood pressure measurements, (left), are an integral part of well woman screening. They are particularly important for women who are on the pill, since the hormones this contraceptive contains may lead to high blood pressure.

A cervical smear or Pap test consists of a scrape of tissue taken from the cervix (neck of the womb).

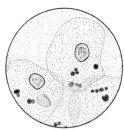

Healthy cells, stained and seen under the microscope are large with small, dark nuclei (above).

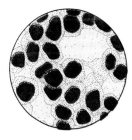

Cancer cells from the cervix are small with large, dark nuclei almost filling them.

The regularity of cervical smear tests is essential, since cervical cancer can be prevented if pre-invasive changes are detected early.

successful, hormones may be given until the cycle is regular again.

Absent periods (amenorrhoea) not caused by pregnancy require specialist investigation. This may be due to emotional upsets, anorexia nervosa, stopping the contraceptive pill or even too much exercise. Painful periods (dysmenorrhoea) may be primary (spasmodic acute cramps, common in women before their first pregnancy) or secondary (congestive, dull aching and heaviness, usually coupled with the premenstrual syndrome and spanning the later years up to menopause). Severely painful periods arising from medical causes are treated with drugs and sometimes with surgery.

Any type of period pain may be relieved by self-help treatments including painkillers, curling up with knees on the chest or with a hot water bottle. Exercise such as swimming, dancing or jogging, both before and during a period, is also effective. Medical treatment is available if self-help measures are unsuccessful.

Extremely heavy periods (menorrhagia) are common in the early menstrual years, but are not acceptable. Any sudden change to heavier periods is a cause for concern, since it may be symptomatic of a serious complaint, and should be reported to your doctor. However, women with IUDs (see pp. 172–3) often have heavier periods in the first few months.

Investigations of menstrual problems

Menstrual problems that do not respond to self-help treatments often demand more thorough medical investigation. One of the commonest of these is the D and C which stands for dilatation (of the cervix) and curettage (of the womb). In a D and C the womb lining is cleared under general anaesthetic and a sample of tissue taken for examination. Often the clearing alone is sufficient to solve the problem; if not, drug treatments may be required.

Sexually transmitted diseases

Venereal diseases such as syphilis, gonorrhoea, herpes and urethritis are not uncommon. If you think there is a chance you may have such an infection, go at once to a special VD clinic attached to a hospital and tell your partner or partners immediately. Except for herpes, treatment is usually quick, simple and successful.

Check list
● Have you had a full gynaecological examination in the last year?

● Have you had a professional breast examination in the last year?

● Have you had a cervical smear in the last 2-3 years?

If you answer 'no' to any of the above, make an appointment *now*.

● Have you recently suffered a sudden change in your periods?

● Have you noticed a recent change in your breasts?

● Do you think you may have a disease or disorder?

If you answer 'yes' to any of the above, see your doctor as soon as possible.

Breasts are a symbol of femininity. Yet it is a cruel fact that breast cancer affects one in every 15 women, and that this is the single commonest cause of death in women between 35 and 54.

Although it cannot actually be prevented, breast cancer stands a good chance of being cured if detected in its earliest stages. This is why it is *essential* for women make a habit of examining their breasts every month and of having regular clinical screenings. Remember: one fifth of all cancer deaths is due to breast cancer.

Breasts undergo subtle and normal changes throughout a woman's life. The rise and fall in the levels of the female hormones, oestrogen, progesterone and prolactin, contribute to breast changes during the menstrual cycle, during pregnancy, when breast-feeding a baby and at the time of the menopause. The contraceptive pill may also cause changes. Every woman needs to distinguish these normal changes from new lumps. **Most are benign; only one in ten will be cancerous**.

Who is at risk?
The cause of breast cancer is not yet known, although according to some researchers the contraceptive pill may be a contributing factor, possibly by delaying the first pregnancy. The Western way of life is another contributory factor. Those most at risk are women over 35 years old; childless women; those who had their first child after the age of 30; those with previous benign breast problems and those closely related to someone with breast cancer.

Self-examination
All women, from puberty onward, should examine their breasts every month. This should preferably be done immediately after each period (because the breasts may feel tender and lumpy in the week before menstruation) or, after the menopause, on the first day of the month.

The crucial signs to watch out for when you examine your breasts are: a lump in the breast or local lumpy areas; unusual increase in the size of one breast; one breast unusually lower than the other; puckering or dimpling of the breast skin; turning in of the nipple; fluid emerging from one nipple only, especially if it is bloodstained; a rash on the nipple; swelling of the upper arm; enlargement of the lymph glands in the armpit.

If you notice any abnormality, **see your doctor immediately**. Breast disorders, such as chronic mastitis, cysts and benign tumours are fairly common, but their symptoms may mimic cancer.

In chronic mastitis, the breast feels swollen, lumpy and painful, particularly before and during menstruation. This condition is most common in women between 30 and 50 but can occur at any age. Cysts, small sacs in the breast tissue which become filled with liquid, are most common in women in their mid-thirties and forties. Cysts may cause pain, discomfort and a discharge from the nipple and may need to be removed surgically or aspirated. Often innocent lumps in the breast are clumps of fibrous tissue which may swell and cause pain. They are usually permanent and may require surgical removal.

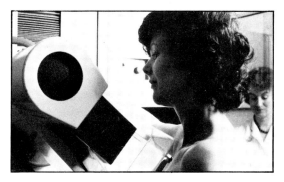

Mammography can detect signs of breast cancers before they become noticeable through physical examination.

Breast screening
Regular screening entails examination of the breasts by a doctor, together with a breast X-ray, known as a mammography, which reveals any malignancy as an irregular opaque patch on the resulting image. The procedure can detect about 92 per cent of cancers. Although not always comfortable, mammography is not painful. It should however, be avoided if you are pregnant or suspect you may be so.

An additional diagnostic test is a needle biopsy which involves inserting a needle into the lump. If liquid is aspirated and the lump disappears, the problem is due to a cyst. If the lump is solid, a few cells can be drawn into the needle. Laboratory tests will subsequently distinguish between malignant and benign disease.

How to examine your breasts

The aim of self-examination is to get to know your breasts and to be able to detect any abnormal changes in them that warrant further clinical examination. Most growths are benign, but all changes in the breast tissue should be investigated at once. Only by detecting abnormalities early can cancer be fully cured.

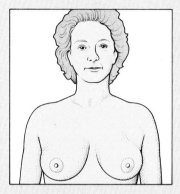

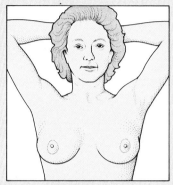

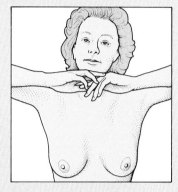

Sit in front of the mirror stripped to the waist. Sit completely straight, then carefully study your breasts. Look for any marked change in size and see if one breast has recently become lower than the other.

Examine the nipple. Has it drawn back or turned in since your last examination? Inspect the inside of your bra for any signs of discharge. Look at the skin of the breast for any puckering, dimpling, rashes or changes in texture. Lift the breasts to examine them underneath. Raise your hands above your head and see if there is any swelling or skin puckering on the upper breast or around the armpit.

Lower your arms and raise them to chin level. Have both nipples moved upward to the same extent? Lean forward and examine each breast for unusual changes in outline, dimpling or retraction of the nipple.

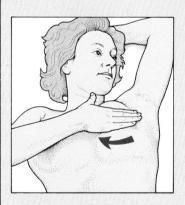

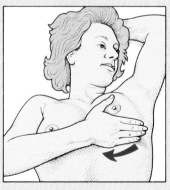

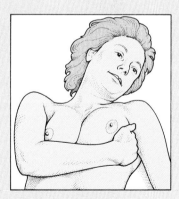

Lie down in a relaxed, comfortable position, either on a bed, with your head on a pillow and a folded towel under your left shoulder blade, or in the bath. Put your left hand under your head. Examine your left breast with your right hand. Use the front part of the flat of your hand and keep your fingers straight and close together.

Slide your hand above and below the nipple, from the armpit to the center of the body. Press gently to feel for lumps.

Pass your hand from the bottom of the breast, across the nipple and upward to the armpit. Slide your hand sideways and diagonally across the breast and over the nipple, making sure you have felt all parts of the breast. Feel for any lumps in the armpit or the top of the collarbone. Now examine the right breast with your left hand.

The midlife transition strikes many men hard. Although there are no sudden hormonal changes as in women, men may feel abnormally stressed —a feeling that often results in some dramatic alteration of behaviour.

Awareness of the implications of the midlife transition makes it easier to cope and to develop a more positive attitude. For midlife is *not* the end of life, and it certainly does not signal the end to a man's sex life, particularly if he pays careful attention to his health.

Health screening for men

Sexual health is part and parcel of whole body health. If a man does not feel well in himself, is constantly overtired or under pressure, is suffering the effects of drink excesses or drugs or is prey to a debilitating illness, his sexual appetite and performance will decline. Although routine health screening should have become part of every man's health programme before he reaches middle age, during middle age it is more imperative, since there is an increased risk of cancer, strokes, and heart, lung and liver disease.

A comprehensive screening, which tests blood pressure, heart and lung function and analyses the blood for fat content and liver, kidney and metabolic disease and tests the urine for diabetes, should be able to detect diseases and disorders. Further, since such tests build up a comprehensive picture of a man's health, suggestions may be made for alterations in lifestyle and habits. Cutting out smoking, reducing drinking, a healthier diet, more exercise and adequate holidays and outside interests will all contribute to improved fitness, which in turn are reflected in a more vital sex life.

Within this context, there are only a few conditions that actually inhibit a man's sexual performance and comfort. Aside from physical defects, which require surgical treatment, the main problems include urinary infections, enlargement of the prostate gland, sexually transmitted diseases, drugs and alcohol. Any infections demand immediate treatment and abstinence from sex until they have cleared up. With anti-depressant drugs, often prescribed to combat the emotional problems, there is often a loss of sexual appetite, which may deepen a man's distress and make him feel guilty.

A partner must be reassuring to avoid a complete breakdown in sexual relations, and men may gain closeness and pleasure from sexual contacts other than intercourse. Alcohol, with its depressant qualities, is often the reason for incapacity. After a number of failures, a man may become psychologically impotent, thus exacerbating his physical failure. Less alcohol and a realization of its effect will do much to restore a man's potency.

The midlife transition

Middle age has a curious way of stealing up and catching you unaware. For a man suddenly confronted with this *fait accompli*, the physical facts of ageing can be traumatic. As a result, many men develop uncharacteristic vanities and attempt to recapture their youthful appearance to little effect.

Many men feel pressurized into a reappraisal of their lives, and those who are already insecure, anxious and defensive may become distressed about the future, their financial status, the looming end of their career advancement, domestic pressures, health and much more. All this self-obsession leads to the typical midlife symptoms: tension, depression, irritability, resentment and a concern for their male image. Such turmoil may create problems for a man's partner, who may herself be undergoing a similar rethink of her life, as well as coping with the physical symptoms of the menopause.

Strangely, some men may experience physical symptoms such as hot flushes, insomnia, palpitations, loss of memory and so on, similar to those experienced by women during the menopause, although there is no evidence of a diminished hormone output in men of this age group.

Many men regard the dwindling sexual powers of the middle years as an affront and as a threat to their masculinity. The solution for some is to seek out younger women, who they hope will restore their virility and self-image; some achieve satisfaction in this way, others do not.

Improving relationships

Reduced sexual interest within a marriage can be upsetting for both partners, and the woman may feel she no longer inspires affection or desire. She then suppresses her own desires until the man also feels rejected, and the resulting tension spills over into other areas of the relationship.

It is important for a man to realize that his

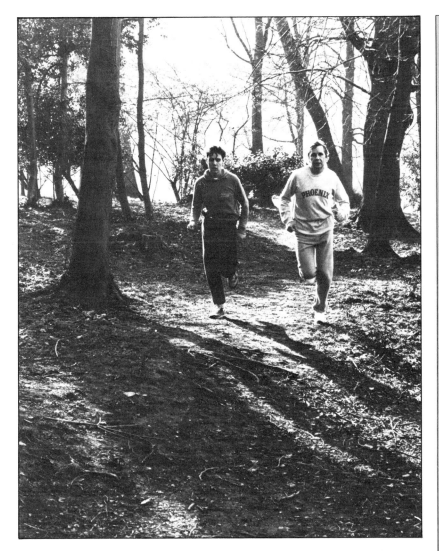

Regular exercise can do much to revitalize a man's middle years. It will not only give him more physical and mental energy, but will help to counteract the effects of stress. At a time when teenage children are beginning to grow away from their parents, a shared activity such as running can help promote the development of a caring, adult relationship between a father and his sons or daughters.

sexual prowess and appetite will decline as he ages. This is a fact of mature sexual life. There will be a gradual curtailment of libido, a lengthening of the time taken to achieve an erection and a decline in orgasmic potential. If the physical quality of sex wanes with ageing, the emotional pleasure and intimacy may still remain. It is, therefore, essential that couples take time to reopen lines of communication and reassure each other about their continuing affection, attraction and sexual abilities.

Middle age should not be an end. There are many years ahead, and there is no reason why sex should not be an integral part of them.

When your sex life suffers:

● Try reducing your alcohol intake to improve potency.

● Have a urinary test if you suspect an infection.

● Lose some weight to improve general fitness and vitality.

● Take more exercise to increase energy.

● Consult your doctor for a change of drugs or other advice.

● Have a complete health screen.

● Take a holiday with the woman you love.

● Try having sex in the mornings and at week-ends, not on nights during weekdays when you are tired after the working day.

THE MIDLIFE TRANSITION

The menopause marks the end of a woman's reproductive life. It can be a difficult time for many women, since it involves not only adjusting to the psychological fact of lost fertility but coping with physical symptoms caused by hormonal changes, which may be unpleasant. In the past, the 'change of life' was dreaded as the beginning of a steady decline. Now, however, women view the menopause more postively, and with self-help and medical care, they can expect an easier passage to a new and fulfilling life.

What is the menopause?

The menopause is a stage in life that lasts a year or two. It is not an illness. The cessation of regular menstrual periods marks the menopause. The ovaries become resistant to instructions from the pituitary and stop maturing the eggs that have been present in them since birth. Since the stock of eggs has been depleted over 30 to 40 years, progressively fewer eggs are released. This interrupts the cyclic production of the hormone progesterone, which in turn prevents the release of sufficient oestrogen from the pituitary to trigger the growth and shedding of the womb's lining (menstruation).

The end of menstruation can occur at any time between the ages of 36 and 56, though the median age seems to be 48. There is some truth in the old wives' tale of early puberty/late menopause and late puberty/early menopause, but it is difficult to predict. Sometimes menstruation stops abruptly. More commonly, however, a few months of irregular bleeding are followed by normal losses, then there a few more months of irregular bleeding until it ceases altogether. A year without bleeding in a woman under 50, or 6 months in a woman over 50 can usually be taken as the end of menstruation. Contraceptive precautions must be used during the entire menopause since there is still a slight chance of pregnancy occurring.

Surgical menopause

A surgical menopause consists of the removal of the ovaries and Fallopian tubes of a premenopausal woman. This kind of surgery may be necessary for many reasons, including: cancer of the tubes or ovaries; damage due to pelvic inflammatory disease; or large fibroid tumours. With the removal of the ovaries, menstrual periods and

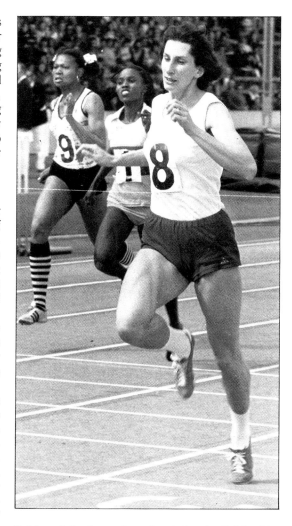

Gold medal winner Irena Szewinska, *the Polish 400m runner, now approaching midlife, continues to compete successfully against girls 20 years her junior.*

ovarian hormone production cease at once and for this reason oestrogen replacement therapy is usually prescribed.

Problems of the menopause

Women suffer menopausal problems to different degrees. The three major physical symptoms are hot flushes, night sweats and loss of lubrication in the vagina. All are believed to be caused by low oestrogen levels.

Hot flushes can occur frequentlyor infrequently either during the day or night, and leave a woman feeling chilled. Some women never have them, others endure them for years, but most experience them spasmodically for a few months. Night sweats often cause insomnia, a reason in itself for exhaustion, irritability and depression during waking hours.

One of the most troublesome symptoms for sexually active women is loss of lubrication of the vagina, caused by reduced oestrogen levels. The lining of the vagina also becomes thinner, which may make intercourse uncomfortable. It may also make a woman vulnerable to vaginal and urethral infections, which can cause bleeding and ulceration of the vaginal walls. The resulting disinclination for sex may fit in well with the ageing male partner's loss of sexual interest or capacity, or may become a source of friction between two people whose sexual desires no longer coincide.

During the menopause, women's bones may become more brittle, through loss of calcium, so exercise is important to prevent fractures. Women also complain of other symptoms, including irritating dryness of the nasal mucous membrane, headache, palpitations, dizziness, weight gain, abdominal pains, nausea, vomiting, swollen ankles and loss of memory and concentration. As yet there is no established link between the menopause and these symptoms, and according to one study only 20 per cent of women suffer them severely enough to cause any disruption of life. Symptoms should not be endured — they can be treated, so seek expert advice.

Emotionally, the menopause is a highly charged time and, for some women, it is difficult to separate physical from emotional symptoms. The end of childbearing can be traumatic for those who equate worth with motherhood, particularly if the menopause coincides with the time when children start to leave home. Many women believe that the menopause signals the end of their sex lives; most feel they must take stock and find this reassessment painful and disquieting. The stress of so many midlife problems can lead to depression as a woman struggles to achieve a new role and meaning in life.

Yet the 'change' can be a change for the good. Positive rethinking is crucial to 'life after youth'. With the burdens of menstruation and fear of an unwanted pregnancy lifted, women should search for new interests and work and continue to enjoy a full sex life.

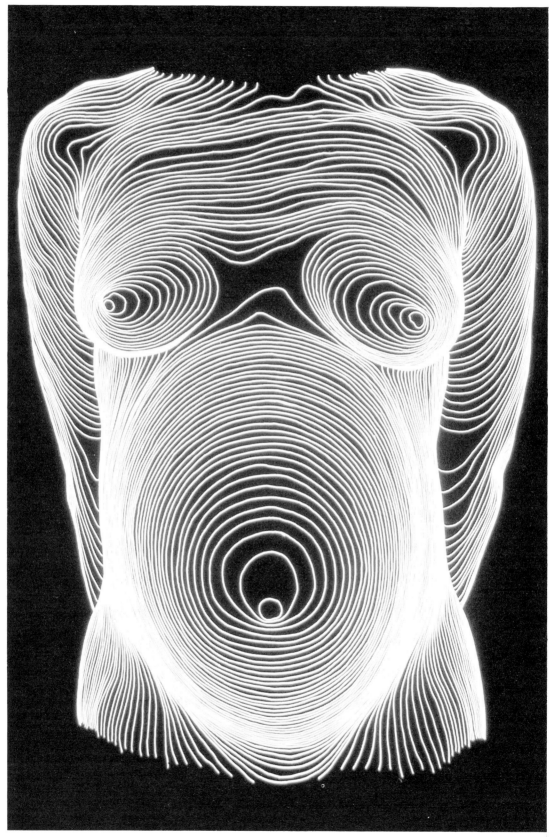

PREGNANCY AND BIRTH

The discovery that a baby is expected is one of life's most exciting moments. During the next few months, especially if it is a first baby, both parents-to-be will experience a wealth of new feelings, from exhilaration to fright, and all of them ultimately rewarding.

Increasing self-awareness and concern for healthy living has produced an enormous change in attitudes over the last half century. No longer are women confined, quite literally, during their pregnancy; some 75 per cent work outside the home until ten weeks before the birth. Diet and exercise, and giving up cigarettes and alcohol, are now considered as important a part of antenatal care as medical checks. A corollary of this is the growing movement toward encouraging prospective parents to look at, and if necessary reform, their lifestyles even before a baby is conceived.

Technology, working toward safer births and improved health of mothers and babies, has made enormous strides. But it has also presented the expectant mother with many more choices. At the least, she may be able to decide on the position she prefers for labour. At most, she may have to decide between the life and death of her unborn child.

From the mine of information and advice that exists on pregnancy, the chapter that follows distills the essentials, to provide parents with the basic information they need about fitness and well-being during pregnancy, labour and birth. This is done in the knowledge that, in most cases, a healthy mother means a healthy baby and a healthier start to life.

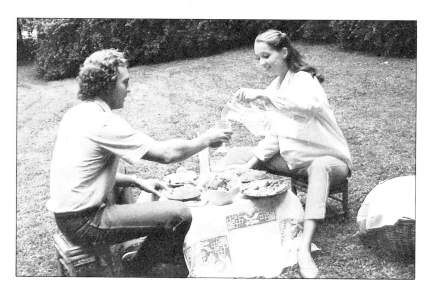

Both partners should start to eat well before conception is considered. Do not eat high-protein foods to the exclusion of fats and carbohydrates. Choose fresh foods for preference and avoid foods preserved in sugar. Unrefined foods contain more desirable ingredients. Proteins, vitamins and minerals such as calcium and iron are needed for body building and prevention of illness or complications during pregnancy.

Pregnancy is a time in a woman's life when it is important for her to be as fit as possible. Increasingly, doctors are also stressing the significance of health care and fitness during the months prior to conception for both the potential parents. If you are already pregnant, then do not worry about what you should or should not have been doing until now. Whatever stage you are at, it is not too late to begin working toward a healthier lifestyle for the rest of your pregnancy, and it is important that you do not feel guilty about what is already past.

A healthy way of life adopted before conception may lessen the risks to the growing baby during the crucial early weeks of development, when a woman may be unaware that she is pregnant. The baby's spinal cord develops between $4\frac{1}{2}$ and $6\frac{1}{2}$ weeks, the arms during the same period, the legs between $5\frac{1}{2}$ and $7\frac{1}{2}$ weeks, and by the eighth week of pregnancy, the foetal heart is beating.

Preconceptual care

If you are planning a baby, then first you must stop contraception. If you are taking the pill, you should switch to a barrier method for at least three months to allow time for the natural pattern of hormone production and egg release to be re-established. And remember that it takes one in eight couples longer than a year to conceive successfully.

If you and/or your partner smoke, then you should try to stop, or at least cut down. Reduce your alcohol consumption as well — even an occasional binge is not a good idea. Diet is also important. Your doctor may prescribe iron and folic acid supplements. It is wise to pay attention to your weight before conception. While overweight is not ideal, excessive slimming can reduce fertility. You should not attempt to go on a reducing diet once you are pregnant, but you can make sure that you are at an ideal weight before you conceive (see pp. 76–7).

There are several other matters that call for medical guidance. Ask your doctor to check that you are immune from German measles (rubella). If you need immunization, continue to practise birth control for at least two months afterward, for while the vaccine is taking effect it may damage a growing baby.

Discuss with your doctor noxious chemicals you or your partner may have contact with at work, and any potentially harmful drugs you may be taking. Some antibiotics, steroids and anti-cancer drugs can harm a foetus. For safety, it is advisable to do without any drugs, even aspirins, if you can. Any drugs of addiction or habituation are definitely harmful to the baby.

If you are concerned about handicaps and diseases passed on in the family of either potential parent, ask your doctor if he knows of a genetic advisory centre. Alternatively, refer to any large hospital in your area. A genetic counsellor will be able to advise you and your partner of the risk of your baby being affected.

The menstrual cycle is governed by hormones and operates so that an ovum or egg is released from the ovary approximately once every 28 days, a process known as ovulation. The cycle also ensures that the uterus is prepared to receive and nurture the egg if it is fertilized by a sperm. If fertilization does not occur, then the uterine lining is shed as the menstrual period. If the ovum is fertilized, continued hormone production ensures that menstruation does not take place.

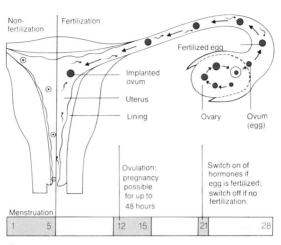

Days

Smoking and alcohol

Nicotine, carbon monoxide and alcohol are poisonous substances that damage the placenta, thus reducing the amount of oxygen and food reaching the baby. This raises the foetal heart rate, leading to foetal distress. Congenital problems also result from nutritional deficiencies at an early stage of foetal development.

A woman who continues to smoke during pregnancy has a 30 per cent greater chance of miscarrying or losing the baby through complications at birth. The baby is more likely to be premature, have a low birth weight and run a greater risk of infection. Even moderate drinking may affect the foetus, particularly its heart, limbs and face.

It is as well to be aware, however, that many genetic abnormalities cannot be detected by screening before conception. Down's syndrome, for example, which produces 'mongol' babies, can occur because of defective chromosomes in either parent, but more often in the woman. It can also happen randomly at the time of conception. The chances of giving birth to a Down's syndrome baby increase with the mother's age: by 46 she has a 1 in 40 chance. Spina bifida, in which the spinal cord develops abnormally, is also more likely in older mothers. Both can be detected during pregnancy (see p. 192).

Problems of infertility

Despite preconceptual care, many couples experience problems of infertility. One in 10 couples is thought to suffer some degree of infertility, with the causes split roughly equally between the partners. The causes are many and varied, and some are easily treated although others demand complex treatments. Artificial insemination, *in vitro* fertilization and adoption are the last resorts of the infertility counselling clinics.

With little effort, it is possible to increase your chances of a healthy pregnancy and a healthy baby. Organized preconceptual care is rapidly becoming widely available in the USA, but Britain and Europe lag behind although the situation is improving. On both sides of the Atlantic research is also being carried on into why pregnancies fail or go wrong.

Preconceptual checklist

Before you try to get pregnant:
● Stop contraception: if on the pill, switch to barrier method for 3 months first.

● Stop smoking: 5 cigarettes a day is a reasonable target if you cannot.

● Reduce consumption of alcohol: 2 glasses of white wine a week is a good target.

● Eat a healthful diet.

● Start an exercise programme or take up a sport.

● Check with your doctor about rubella and other infections.

Sport

If you have never exercised or played a sport, then pregnancy is not the time to take up vigorous activity. A brisk walk every day is excellent exercise, and swimming is one of the best forms of all-round exercise you can get. Some women, however, if they are already fit, successfully continue playing tennis or other sports until well into their pregnancies.

Inherited diseases

Many inherited abnormalities are 'recessive', that is, they do not appear in the baby unless the defective genes are carried by both of the parents. An example of this is cystic fibrosis. Other conditions appear if there is only one dominant gene, for example, Huntingdon's chorea.

Once you suspect you are pregnant, you will want confirmation as soon as possible. A missed period may well be the first indication, but there are other 'symptoms' that could give you a clue. Your breasts may feel tender and swollen; you may urinate more frequently; you may feel tired and listless for no apparent reason; you may experience nausea, find certain foods and drinks distasteful or lose your desire for alcohol and cigarettes. The feeling of being pregnant is so distinctive that many women in their second and subsequent pregnancies realize that they have conceived within a matter of days.

Pregnancy testing

You can do your own pregnancy test or use the services of a pharmacist; both of these methods are reasonably reliable. Most testing requires a urine sample. If you are pregnant, it will contain the tell-tale hormone, human chorionic gonadotrophin (HCG). A urine test is reliable 6 weeks after the start of your last period. A blood test will confirm pregnancy earlier, but the service is not always available. Alternative means of obtaining a pregnancy test include family planning clinics, health centres and pregnancy advisory services.

These may often be able to provide you with a result more quickly than a busy hospital or general practice.

Once your pregnancy is confirmed, your doctor will calculate when the baby is due. Pregnancy lasts, on average, 266 days from conception, but since few women know exactly when they conceive, 280 days are added to the date of the first day of the last menstrual period, to give an estimated delivery date. This, in fact, adds up to 9 months and 7 days, but a full-term baby could arrive 2 weeks before or 2 weeks after the estimated delivery date.

Your doctor will make arrangements for your antenatal care once your pregnancy is confirmed. He may refer you to the hospital where your baby will be born for all your antenatal check ups, or he may see you during most of the pregnancy, and you will visit the hospital for special tests and to have the baby. Alternatively, you may have home care from your doctor and a midwife, with a home delivery. However, few first babies are born at home in Britain. In some countries, such as the Netherlands, home births are more common; in others, including Canada and the USA, they are almost unknown.

Antenatal checks

Some time before the end of the third month of pregnancy, your doctor will arrange for you to attend the hospital antenatal clinic to be booked in. Routine antenatal checks will be initiated, and you will be asked many details of your personal medical history and that of your partner. He will also enquire about your work and lifestyle, and that of your partner, to pinpoint any danger areas. Do not forget, however, that this is *your* opportunity to ask questions, too.

From then on, you will attend a clinic every month until the 28th week of pregnancy, after which visits will be every 2 weeks until the final month, during which you should attend every week. Regular attendance at these clinics is essential. The results from tests carried out at your first visit are the yardstick against which all subsequent findings are compared. Any fluctuations in readings that might be significant to the health of either the mother or the baby should be carefully monitored at all stages of pregnancy to reduce the risks as much as possible.

Routine tests on urine and blood enable checks

Home testing

To avoid ambiguous results, follow the instructions in a home pregnancy testing kit carefully. Always use the first urine of the day, since it will have the highest hormone concentration. If you are pregnant, the chemicals in the test-tube will react with the hormones in the urine. The result will vary with the kit, but in many, a positive result is indicated by a dark ring. Remember that the approach of the menopause can give false positive results.

Positive   Negative

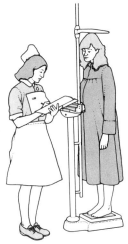

Measuring height and weight. On your first antenatal visit your height will be noted. This gives a clue as to the size of your pelvis. Your weight will also be checked at this and subsequent visits.

By feeling, or palpating, the abdomen, a doctor can detect the position of the baby.

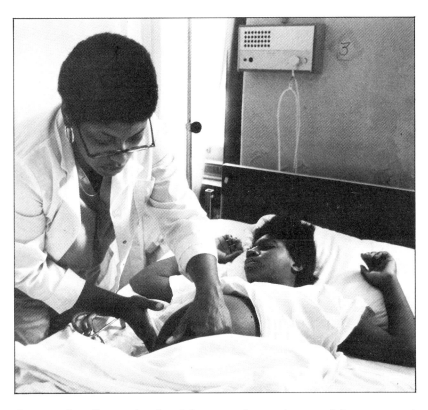

on several counts. The urine sample will reveal any kidney infections (many of which normally go unnoticed but cause complications during pregnancy) and diabetes. The urine protein level is also tested, since later on in pregnancy its rise can indicate pre-eclampsia, a serious condition which puts the baby at risk.

A blood test will reveal your blood group. If you are Rhesus negative and your baby inherits a different blood group from his father, you can build up antibodies which may harm subsequent babies. Tests on the blood will also measure the level of iron (and hence whether you are anaemic). They will also show whether you are immune to rubella and will reveal the presence of infections harmful to you and the baby, such as hepatitis B and syphilis.

Blood pressure measurement is part of the antenatal routine. Blood pressure tends to increase in 20 to 25 per cent of pregnancies and can indicate serious conditions such as pre-eclampsia, which need careful medical management if they are not to harm the baby.

At each antenatal visit, the doctor will palpate the abdomen to locate the top of the uterus and the position of the baby. This gives a clue to the stage of your pregnancy although only an ultrasound examination (see p. 192) will give an accurate estimate of this. Initially you will have a vaginal examination to enable the doctor to feel the uterus and check for pelvic abnormalities, but further internal examinations will not come until later on in your pregnancy.

Self-help routines
The establishment of a routine of antenatal care goes hand in hand with your own self-care, now you know that you are pregnant. The common-sense practices recommended in preconceptual care, such as giving up smoking and drinking (see pp. 188-9), are now essential to maintain maximum fitness and health during pregnancy. The correct diet and exercise, as well as regular check-ups, will give your baby the best chance of a healthy start to life. They will also prepare you in the best possible way for the impact — both physical and psychological — of the months before and immediately after the birth.

TESTS AND THEIR TIMING

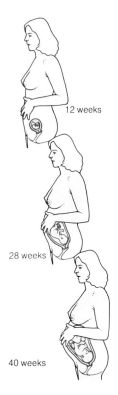

12 weeks

28 weeks

40 weeks

As well as routine antenatal checks, your doctor may advise certain special tasks. If deformity is found in tests such as these, parents may take the decision to terminate the pregnancy. Tests for alpha feto protein (AFP) are routine in many hospitals. If the baby is suffering from an abnormality such as spina bifida, AFP enters the mother's bloodstream. It can also indicate multiple pregnancy. AFP tests are usually carried out at about the 16th or 17th week of pregnancy and are routine if the mother has already given birth to a spina bifida child or if she has a family history of the abnormality.

Amniocentesis to detect Down's syndrome involves the insertion of a needle (under local anaesthetic) into the womb. Some of the amniotic fluid surrounding the growing baby is extracted, and its cells studied for chromosomal and other defects. At the moment, this test cannot be carried out until the 16th week, although it may soon be possible much earlier. It carries with it the risk of spontaneous abortion of approximately 1 in 50. It is usually recommended only for women over 37 — at 35 there is only a one in 300 chance of having a Down's syndrome baby.

Ultrasound safety
Ultrasound gives instant results with no risk of miscarriage.
Between the 12th and 16th weeks of pregnancy, a scan can estimate the age of the growing baby by measuring it. At this stage, a scan will reveal twins or other prospective multiple births and some abnormalities.
Between 30 and 36 weeks, a scan can assess foetal maturity and thus confirm the delivery date. At this stage a scan will also reveal the position in which the baby is lying, which may have implications for the delivery. The position and condition of the placenta can also affect the passage of the baby down the birth canal.

At 12 weeks, the baby is about 5 cm (2 in) long and all major organs have formed. By 28 weeks the baby is often head-down, ready for delivery. It would have a slim chance of survival if born now. At full term (40 weeks), the abdomen may appear to get smaller as the baby's head enters the pelvis.

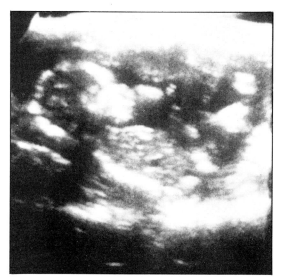

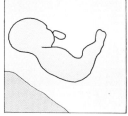

An interpretation (above) of an ultrasound scan taken at 18 weeks (left) shows the development of the unborn baby to be remarkably advanced. The head and body are clearly visible and one leg, with a well-formed foot attached, can also be distinguished.

An ultrasound scan involves bouncing ultrasonic sound waves off certain body tissues to reveal an image of the baby on a screen (above). The image is often fuzzy and unclear and can be interpreted only by someone with a trained eye. But the operator will point out the baby's limbs, its head, the placenta, and certain organs such as the heart or stomach. Most prospective parents find the experience both exciting and reassuring.

STAYING FIT IN PREGNANCY/1

Staying both fit and healthy during your pregnancy may seem an unrealistic goal if, like 70 per cent of women, you feel tired, nauseous and emotionally at sea during the first 2 or 3 months. Hormonal changes are responsible for this miserable state of affairs, and also for a host of other possible discomforts.

To combat sickness, eat little and often and stick to bland food. Have a plain biscuit and a cup of tea before you get out of bed in the morning, and keep a stock of easily digestible, nutritious 'nibbles' by you during the day. Avoid greasy foods, but do eat potatoes, pasta and bread. You will probably feel worse if you become overtired. It is best, however, to take anti-sickness pills only as a last resort.

Another unpleasant side effect of early pregnancy is constipation, since hormonal changes slow bowel movements. Drink plenty of water and eat generous amounts of high fibre food — including fruit and vegetables, wholemeal bread and cereals. A constant need to pass water may prove an embarrassment and inconvenience, while vaginal discharge may lead to irritation and an increased susceptibility to thrush. You may also experience vaginal bleeding. Always treat this as serious and consult your doctor.

You are most unlikely to be subjected to all the possible discomforts of early pregnancy, and you may not be affected by any of them for long or at all. After the 12th or 14th week you may develop the 'bloom' of pregnancy, with shining hair, a clear skin and a general glow of well-being. In any event, you will probably feel at your best during the middle 3 months but you are likely to feel fitter if you are maintaining a healthy diet, if you are cutting out alcohol and cigarettes and taking some exercise every day.

On the debit side, the middle months are the time when you are likely to experience trouble with your teeth and gums. When you brush your teeth, the gums may bleed easily and be subject to ulcers and the infection, gingivitis. Your teeth may also suffer from calcium depletion as the baby's bones are built. It is advisable to have your teeth checked at least once during pregnancy. Ask the dentist to scale your teeth to remove plaque and keep up the good work with a meticulous hygiene routine (see pp.150-1) and by eating plenty of crisp, raw vegetables.

Twins

Your chances of giving birth to twins vary considerably according to the part of the world in which you live. In some regions of Africa, 1 birth in every 30 results in twins; in the Western world it is about 1 in 70; in the Far East it is about 1 in 140. You are more likely to have twins if you are aged between 35 and 40 and if you already have children (especially twins).

Identical twins are formed when one egg splits into two. Non-identical, or fraternal, twins occur when two eggs are fertilized at the same time. The identical twinning rate is constant between races and unaffected by inheritance, but a woman who is the daughter of the mother of fraternal twins is almost twice as likely to have twins as a woman with no twins in her family.

The position of the womb can be the earliest clue to twins. With a singleton, the doctor can feel a firm lump behind the pubic bone by the 12th week of pregnancy — with twins this may be evident as early as the 8th week. If the doctor thinks you may be carrying twins, an ultrasound scan will confirm or deny his suspicions any time after the 12th week.

You are more likely to become anaemic if you are carrying twins and your doctor may prescribe more than usual quantities of iron and folic acid tablets to counteract this. The 'burden' of a multiple pregnancy increases more quickly, but twins rarely go to full term (40 weeks). Studies vary, but generally show that between 23 and 44 per cent of twins are born within 37 weeks, compared with 4 per cent of normal pregnancies. Hospitalization for rest is often recommended, since mothers are more at risk from high blood pressure.

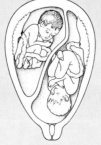

Fraternal twins   Identical twins

STAYING FIT IN PREGNANCY/2

More and more women continue to work outside the home during pregnancy, and they also work until nearer the birth than their mothers did. However, it is wise to know and respect your limitations at this time. If you feel tired and nauseous during the first three months, access to a rest-room will be an advantage.

Try to rearrange your hours of work so that you do not travel at the height of the rush hour, and avoid excessive strain and tiredness. If you are working, rest for an hour with your feet up when you get home. If you are not going out to work, make relaxation part of your daily routine. Rest in a way that is likely to be most beneficial to your body (see below).

If you work with children or in a hospital, beware of infections, especially any virus infections to which you are not immune. This includes rubella (see p.188). The possible effects on the

unborn child of many industrial chemicals is unknown, but if you work with such substances, you should explore the possibility of transferring to another department for the duration of your pregnancy. Avoid, especially, any unnecessary X-ray examinations during pregnancy.

Exercises

Pelvic exercises are important during pregnancy. You should be particularly aware of the muscles of the pelvic floor that control the vaginal and anal openings. Practise tightening and releasing these muscles (see opposite), then learn to do this exercise while sitting, walking and standing. Also learn to tilt your pelvis by tightening your abdominal and buttock muscles to support your trunk. You can also rock and circle your pelvis – dancing is a good way of putting such exercise into practice, but should not be too vigorous.

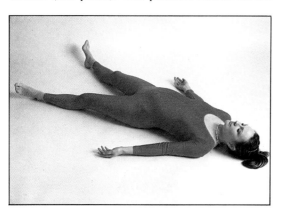

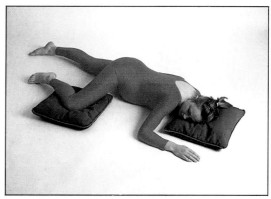

Relaxation techniques learned during pregnancy will improve your well-being and help ease the pain of labour. Practise daily, so that eventually you can relax at times of stress. Lie flat on your back on the floor (above), then order each part of the body to tense or stretch, then to relax, concentrating hard on the changes that are taking place. Learn to relax parts of the body that are particularly prone to tenseness, such as the neck and shoulders. This may also be a good position for sleep.

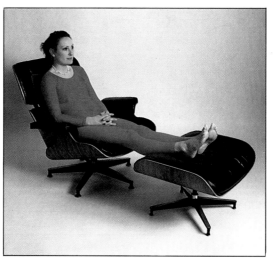

Lying on your side, with all parts of your body supported (above), is another good position to relax in. You may find this a comfortable position to adopt during the early part of labour.

When you sit down (left) make sure your back is well supported (use cushions if necessary) and put your legs up, especially if you have varicose veins. Never sit with your legs crossed.

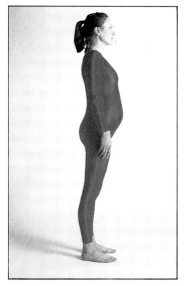

Tailor-sitting (below) *helps strengthen the back, loosen the groin and hips and improve circulation in the lower half of the body. Sit like this while watching television.*

Squatting (below) *is a position which is helpful for labour and which you might choose for giving birth. Strengthen the leg muscles by squatting when you do anything at floor level.*

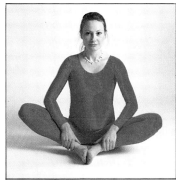

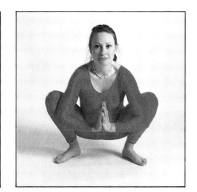

Good posture is important (above). *Use your tummy muscles to straighten your spine. Tuck your bottom in and keep your shoulders down.*

Test your abdominal muscles (right): *Place your fingers just below your navel. Breathe in. As you breathe out, raise your head and shoulders. If you can feel a bulge of flesh between taut muscles, your abdominal muscles need toning up. Do this by repeatedly raising head and shoulders. Exercise your pelvic floor muscles in this position, with your head supported.*

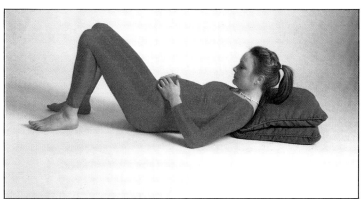

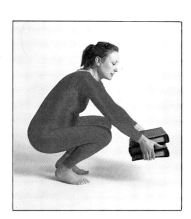

When you are lifting, always *bend your knees* to avoid back strain. *This is especially important if you already have small children.*

Diet
In no circumstances should you 'eat for two' during pregnancy. Follow the guidelines of the healthful diet (see pp.52-85) but remember the following points:

● Dairy products are nutritionally valuable, but ideally choose low-fat varieties.

● Meat, fish and poultry are all good sources of protein, but trim off any fat. Liver is a particularly good source of iron and vitamins.

● Green vegetables and fruit provide vitamins, iron, folic acid and fibre and can be eaten in large quantities.

● Avoid salty, sugary and fried foods.

Check your weight gain
There is no hard and fast rule about weight gain during pregnancy. Some doctors maintain that you should put on no weight at all, but most consider a gain of 9-13 kg (20-30 lb) acceptable if not ideal.

As a rough guide, you will put on about a quarter of your total weight gain between about 12 and 20 weeks, half between 20 and 30 weeks, the remaining quarter after that. Many women stop gaining weight after about the 36th week, and some start to lose weight in the days before birth.

Remember that it is notoriously hard to lose excess weight after the birth, so try to keep your weight in check without slimming.

There is no hard and fast evidence that exercising during pregnancy reduces the pain or length of labour; but there is no doubt that it can reduce fatigue, stress and insomnia, improve your circulation, relieve physical discomforts, strengthen your muscles and train you for the hard physical exertion of labour.

A question related to exercise is whether it is safe to have sexual intercourse during pregnancy. Except in special circumstances, for example if there is a risk of miscarriage, there is no reason why intercourse should not be safe. However, you may feel uneasy about it during the first three months or during the last two or three weeks. Do not attempt to have sexual intercourse once you have had a 'show' (see p.198).

You will probably have to adopt a slightly different position for love-making as the 'bump' grows. Do not be alarmed to feel uterine contractions after intercourse — this is a natural part of female orgasm.

During the second half of pregnancy, you may wish to start massaging your breasts and nipples ready for feeding. This may be especially necessary if you have flat or inverted nipples. Draw them out with your fingers or wear a plastic nipple shell inside your bra. Your breasts will be heavier throughout pregnancy, so a well-fitting bra is essential for comfort and support.

If you wish to use the exercises shown on these pages, consult your doctor to make sure it is safe to do so.

Use the exercise routine shown on these pages to help you keep fit in pregnancy.

Sit cross-legged on the floor (right). Stretch your right arm toward the ceiling and bend your elbow so that your hand reaches down your back. Bend your left arm behind you and grasp your left hand. Hold for 20 seconds, breathing normally. Repeat, reversing your arms.

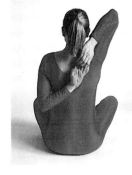

Sit with knees bent and with the soles of your feet touching. Bring your feet as near to your body as you can, holding on to your ankles (below). Lean forward, keeping your back straight, and hold for 20 seconds. Breathe normally throughout. Repeat 5 times.

Return to the cross-legged position, take hold of one leg at the knee and pull it in toward your body. Rotate the foot to the left and then to the right, breathing normally (above). Repeat with the other leg.

Stretch your legs out straight in front of you (below). Pull your toes toward you, exercising right and left feet alternately, and breathing in as you push each foot away.

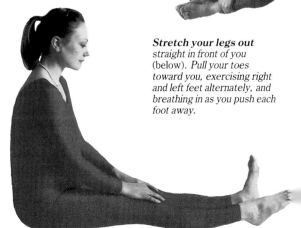

Breathing

While exercising and relaxing, and during labour, it is important to breathe properly. If you hold your breath or breathe irregularly, you will tire faster. Practise breathing like this: breathe deeply; expand the chest and abdomen as you inhale, and aim to breathe 4-6 times a minute. Next breathe just from the chest. Then practise shallow panting, which is used for strenuous exercise and at the peak of contractions. Keep your mouth slightly open and rest your tongue on the floor of your mouth. During labour, exhale while muscles are contracting and inhale when muscles are relaxed.

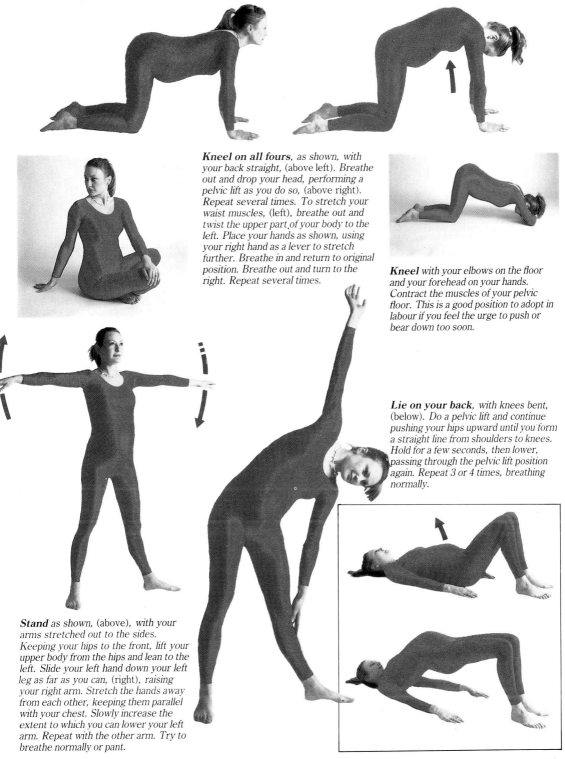

Kneel on all fours, as shown, with your back straight, (above left). Breathe out and drop your head, performing a pelvic lift as you do so, (above right). Repeat several times. To stretch your waist muscles, (left), breathe out and twist the upper part of your body to the left. Place your hands as shown, using your right hand as a lever to stretch further. Breathe in and return to original position. Breathe out and turn to the right. Repeat several times.

Kneel with your elbows on the floor and your forehead on your hands. Contract the muscles of your pelvic floor. This is a good position to adopt in labour if you feel the urge to push or bear down too soon.

Lie on your back, with knees bent, (below). Do a pelvic lift and continue pushing your hips upward until you form a straight line from shoulders to knees. Hold for a few seconds, then lower, passing through the pelvic lift position again. Repeat 3 or 4 times, breathing normally.

Stand as shown, (above), with your arms stretched out to the sides. Keeping your hips to the front, lift your upper body from the hips and lean to the left. Slide your left hand down your left leg as far as you can, (right), raising your right arm. Stretch the hands away from each other, keeping them parallel with your chest. Slowly increase the extent to which you can lower your left arm. Repeat with the other arm. Try to breathe normally or pant.

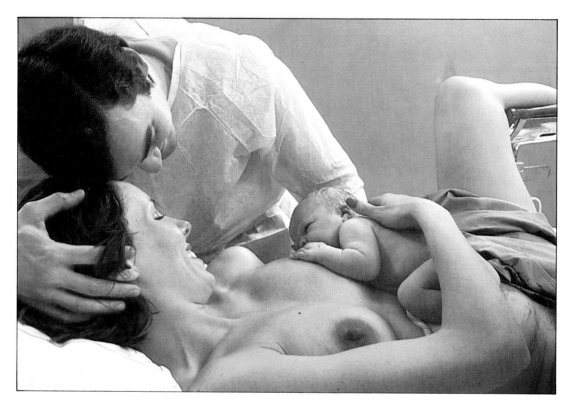

Adopting routines of relaxation and breathing will help you during labour and birth. Many women worry that in labour they will forget all they have learned beforehand, but this is where your partner comes into his own. Fathers are now widely accepted as an invaluable source of support during labour, but a close relative or friend may accompany you if you wish. If your partner is unable to attend antenatal classes, repeat any instructions to him when you get home, and practise together.

Signs of labour

Strong, regular contractions may herald the first stage of labour, which is to dilate the cervix, but their intensity and frequency may vary. They usually start at the rate of 6 to 7 per hour. When the cervix (the neck of the womb) is fully dilated, then the second stage of labour begins, and it ends in the birth. The third stage is the delivery of the placenta.

It is best to move around at home during the first stage of labour for as long as you can, but remember that second and subsequent labours are often shorter than the first. You should think about going to hospital when the contractions are coming at about 5-minute intervals and lasting for 40 to 60 seconds. You should go to hospital in any case if the fluid-retaining membranes around the baby break, which may be before you get contractions. Alternatively, labour may be preceded by a show, as the mucous plug from the neck of the womb is passed out. This alone is not sufficient reason to go to hospital.

Relax during the build-up of a contraction and breathe as regularly as you can. Try to conserve energy by remaining calm, and try to stay upright. Positions you may find comfortable are squatting, supporting yourself in front with your arms, or sitting the wrong way round on a chair, leaning forward on a pillow. Alternatively, sit the right way round and lean on your partner. In either position he can massage your back to assist relaxation and pain relief. In hospital, keep mobile if you wish.

The method of childbirth you choose will depend on your preference and your medical history, and will be modified by hospital facilities and

The presenting of the baby straight to the mother's breast before the cord is cut (left) is part of the philosophy of 'birth without violence', advocated by Fréderick Leboyer. Calm and quiet are also essential, he maintains. A similar stance is adopted by the French doctor Michel Odent. His patients have the option of a birthing pool in which they can relax and into which the baby may be born.

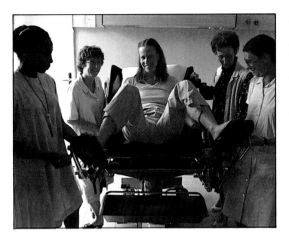

A modern version of the old-fashioned birthing chair is now used with great success in many hospitals. Giving birth in an upright position means that labour is assisted, rather than hindered, by the force of gravity. To encourage an atmosphere of calm, hospitals are also installing birthing rooms, in which a couple can make themselves reasonably comfortable during labour.

attitudes. Supporters of 'active' birth believe that a woman should be free to determine the conduct of her own labour and should not automatically be confined to bed, to give birth in a recumbent position. They reject the increasing use of drugs and foetal monitoring in favour of more natural methods, although these are not necessarily safer for the mother or the baby.

Whatever your preferred method of childbirth, you may find that your medical history or the progress of the labour demand medical intervention. The baby's heartbeat may be monitored to detect any signs of distress, for example, if you have suffered from high blood pressure. If the doctor suspects a risk to the baby he may advise you to have the birth induced through the administration of hormones or by rupturing of the fluid sac around the baby.

Induction of your labour will probably be recommended if you have experienced weight loss recently, if the doctor suspects that the baby may be at risk from the inadequate functioning of the placenta; if there is a marked reduction in the baby's movements, or if you are late for your dates. A Caesarian section (cutting through the abdominal wall) will be necessary if the placenta is blocking the neck of the womb (placenta praevia); if the baby is in an awkward position, bottom down (breech) for example; if your baby is too large for your pelvis or if you are suffering from the venereal disease herpes.

Pain killers
During labour and birth, you may feel the need for pain killers and should not feel guilty about this. A

mixture of gas and air can be breathed in through a face mask. This has the instant effect of making you feel light-headed and can be used to help you over the worst of each contraction. It has no side effects. Pethidine, administered in the form of an injection, takes about 20 minutes to work and lasts about 2 hours. This drug is normally safe, but may make you feel sick and may possibly hamper the baby's breathing if it is administered too late in labour.

You may also be offered an epidural, that is, an anaesthetic injection into the spinal cord that numbs all sensation in your lower abdomen and birth canal. An epidural depends upon the availability of a trained anaesthetist and it necessitates a medically controlled labour and birth. If you have an epidural, you will have to lie on your side throughout; you will need a drip and a catheter, and the baby's progress will be monitored throughout your labour.

A few women suffer a blinding headache after an epidural, and the baby's ability to suck may be temporarily affected. However, an epidural can be a boon in a long labour and may also be used for a Caesarian so that you can see the baby being born. If you do not like the idea of drugs you may prefer hypnosis or acupuncture as means of pain relief (see pp. 278-9, 290-1).

Whatever happens, do not attempt to stick to your original preferences come what may, and remember that the hospital staff are there to help you. At all times during labour and birth, feel free to ask what options are open to you and to discuss the reasons for the recommendations that are made by the doctor or midwife.

For about 10 days after the birth of your baby you will need special care and attention. Whether the birth was at home or in hospital, a midwife or doctor will attend you daily for this period, doing routine checks on blood pressure and temperature and examining your womb and any stitches.

Vaginal bleeding continues for up to 2 weeks. This may turn into a white discharge which can last for 6 weeks. If the blood remains bright red and the flow is heavy, if there are clots in it or you are aware of an offensive smell, report it to your doctor or midwife.

If you have been stitched for a cut or tear, a salt bath is immensely soothing. Constipation is a common complaint after the birth. Do not expect a bowel movement for a few days and try to overcome your natural reluctance. A high-fibre diet and plenty of liquids should help. If you experience painful contractions from your uterus breathe through them as you did in labour.

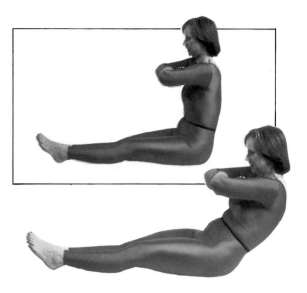

Feeding your baby

Most women are able to breast-feed their babies if they so desire. You should not feel guilty if this is not your choice or if your milk supply is inadequate. What is more important is the closeness between parent and baby at feeding time, and the bond that this establishes.

Sometimes large amounts of milk are produced from the time the milk comes into the breasts 2 or 3 days after the birth, but breast-feeding often takes a week or two to become established. And it may also take the baby a while to get used to sucking. If your nipples are sore, let the air get to them or apply a proprietary cream or spray.

Once you start to supplement breast feeds with a bottle or cup, your milk supply will probably start to dry up. It is important to pay meticulous attention to hygiene when bottle feeding and to follow the manufacturer's instructions exactly.

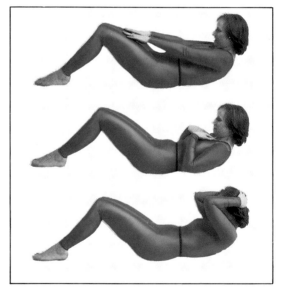

Pelvis and abdomen
You can start your pelvic floor exercises as soon as you feel like it. These will help healing and start toning your muscles. The abdomen also needs attention during the first few days: begin with the first exercises you did to strengthen the abdominal muscles (see p. 195). In no circumstances start to do sit-ups in your eagerness to tone up your sagging stomach. Little and often is the key and gently does it. Stop if you begin to tire or feel sore. Start also with abdominal breathing (see pp. 196-7) and, after a few days, pelvic lifts (p. 194).

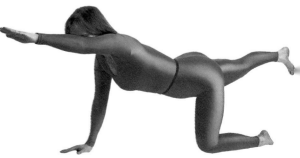

Curl downs: *after about 2 weeks, sit on the floor in the position shown* (left) *and breathe in. As you breathe out, do a pelvic lift: pulling in your abdomen, lower your chin and lean back until you feel your abdominal muscles tighten. Hold for a few seconds, breathing normally, then sit upright. Repeat about 6 times at first. Gradually build up the number of repeats to 20 and increase the holding time.*

Feeding your baby

The advantages of breast-feeding are:
● Colostrum, produced in the first few days, and breast milk contain antibodies that protect the baby against gastrointestinal and respiratory infections and allergies.
● The baby is less likely to get fat or develop nappy rash.
● Breast milk is always available, suitable for the baby, sterile and at the right temperature.
● Supply meets demand, and flow varies according to the baby's degree of hunger.
● Physical contact encourages bonding.

The advantages of bottle-feeding are:
● People other than the mother can feed the baby.
● It is easier to keep track of exactly how much the baby is eating.
● No embarrassment of feeding in public.
● The baby is not affected by drugs the mother is taking or her diet.

● The baby is not so affected by the mother's state of mind.
● Bottle feeding is less tiring to the mother.

Check your progress
Weight: unless you were overweight before the birth, you should not have difficulty losing weight afterward if you eat a healthful diet (see p. 54 ff). Breast-feeding aids weight loss.

Diet: do not go on a reducing diet if you are breast-feeding. Your food requirements will not differ from those during pregnancy, but you may supplement your milk and whole grain intake. You will need 500 calories (2,100 kJ) a day more than a non-pregnant woman to produce enough milk. Drink plenty of liquids (other than milk) Note: cigarette smoking suppresses milk production; oral contraceptives may be passed on in breast milk.

Exercise: start gentle exercises as soon as you wish but do not begin the exercise programme given here until 2 weeks after the birth.

Curl ups: *once you can do curl downs easily, lie on the floor as shown* (left) *and breathe in. Breathe out, raise your head and shoulders and reach for your knees. Progress by doing this with your hands on your chest and then behind your head. Again, build up the number of repeats from 6 to 20 and increase the holding time.*

Trunk stretches: *lie on the floor with legs straight and arms outstretched* (left). *Raise your right knee toward your chest and then take it over to your left side to touch the floor* (below). *Keep your right shoulder on the floor and hold for 20 seconds. Return to the original position. Repeat with the left leg.*

Cat stretches *(for the pelvis): kneel on all fours and breathe in. Breathe out and stretch your left arm and your right leg* (left). *Breathe in and let them down. Repeat with the right arm and left leg. Stretch the fingers and heel each time. Gradually increase the number of repetitions.*

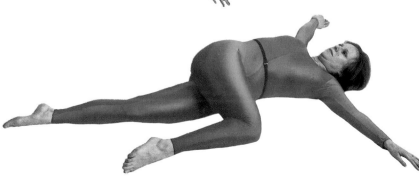

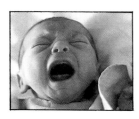

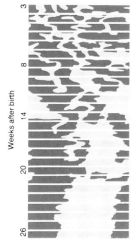

Weeks after birth

A baby is not instinctively aware of the pattern of night and day. Experiments show that in the first few weeks after birth, there is a shifting pattern of sleep (blue) and waking (pink). First to emerge is a 25-hour rhythm between 5 and 25 weeks. Shortly afterward, this reduces to a 24-hour rhythm, with most hours of sleep during the night.

With the birth of a baby, especially if it is your first, you embark upon a new phase of your life — one that will be both challenging, and rewarding. However, the days and even weeks, after birth can be time of conflicting emotions for a mother and may prove confusing or distressing for a new father, who may himself be experiencing a wealth of hitherto unknown and disturbing feelings.

After the initial joy of the birth, you may come down to earth with a bump: many women experience the 'baby blues' on about the fourth day after the birth. This mood will not usually persist but you may feel in low spirits for a while and cry a lot for no reason.

Postnatal depression that lasts after the first week or so, affects some 40 per cent of women to some degree, although relatively few seek help. Symptoms can include chronic lethargy, backache, headache, poor appetite, loss of interest in sex, sleeplessness, tearfulness and irrational fears about the baby's health. Do not be afraid to consult your doctor about the problem if necessary, but also help yourself by making sure you get some rest for each part of the day, by not neglecting your diet and by taking regular aerobic exercise of some kind.

Getting into routine

Your daily routine will be dictated by your baby's needs. Any sleeping and feeding patterns established in the early days may change suddenly and inexplicably. Alternatively a baby who was initially contented may suddenly cry a lot and be difficult to placate. The problems become easier to solve as the baby gradually settles down to a more regular pattern of eating and sleeping, as you are able to sleep more and as you begin to be able to distinguish between the cries that mean hunger, pain, frustration and so on.

Sex may well be the last thing on a woman's mind at this time. Her stitches may only just have healed, and sleepness nights may mean she has barely enough strength to cope with her baby's needs, let alone her own or those of her partner. There is, however, no time limit upon the resumption of love-making, but pentration is not advisable until you are sure that any stitches have healed and until all vaginal discharge has ceased (see p.200).

At about 6 weeks after the birth, you should return to the hospital or visit your doctor for a

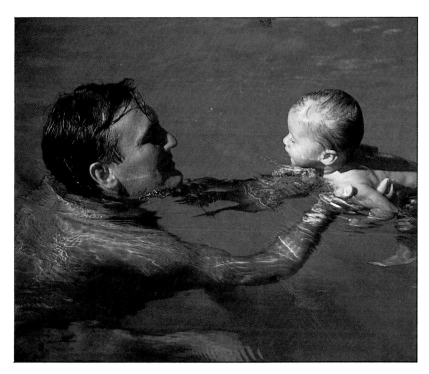

Resuming leisure and *sporting activities as a family is important to postnatal health and well-being. Swimming is not only good exercise for both parents but is an activity that a baby can enjoy. Doing things together is even more important once one or both parents have returned to work.*

postnatal check up. This will involve an internal examination of the condition of your uterus, a cervical smear test (see pp. 180-1) if it was not done at the antenatal clinic and a check that all has healed well. Your breasts and abdomen will also be checked to make sure that everything is normal.

If you are returning to work, it is probably best from the baby's point of view if you do so at between 3 and 6 months, and in any case not before you are well healed and rested. It is also essential, of course, that you make arrangements for the baby to be looked after. Do not feel guilty about either returning to work or not working. Your decision is bound to be a complex one based on your financial and your emotional and intellectual needs. Only you can decide what is the right balance for you.

Contraception after birth

If you are bottle-feeding, your periods (and hence fertility) will return 5 to 8 weeks after the birth. With breast-feeding, periods may not return until after the baby is weaned, but breast-feeding is *not* a reliable contraceptive. You may need to revise your contraceptive method: use the following for guidance.

The pill: may be unsuitable, especially if you are breast-feeding, had high blood pressure or varicose veins in pregnancy or suffered postnatal depression. Discuss with your doctor.

Condom: your vagina may be poorly lubricated after birth. Use a proprietary lubricant, such as KY jelly, as necessary.

Diaphragm: you will probably need a larger size, but fitting cannot be done until 6 weeks after the birth of your baby.

IUD (coil): can often be fitted and retained less painfully after childbirth. Fitting time is as for the diaphragm.

Rhythm method: not effective until your menstrual cycle is regular once more.

Coitus interruptus: unsatisfactory and unreliable in most circumstances and not conducive to the re-establishment of love-making.

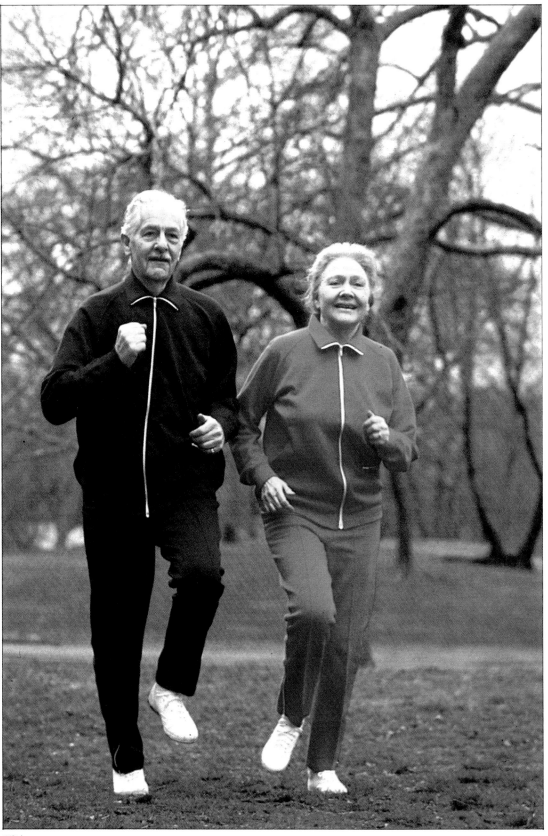

GROWING OLD GRACEFULLY

Old age still receives a bad press in Western industrialized societies. The reason why is not entirely clear, since there is ample evidence that old people today are more numerous, fitter and have more to offer than at any time in the past. All the official statistics are negative, unadorned chronicles of bad news. We hear how many people become ill or are bundled into homes to die, but rarely how millions of people enjoy a happy and healthy old age.

How refreshing it is, therefore, when we read of the long-lived peoples of the Caucasus — fit and active centenarians some of them — who have not even begun to feel old. Or that, on the eve of his seventieth birthday, the French cellist Paul Tortellier attributed his manifest youthfulness and vigour to the belief that we should aim to die young but to delay doing so for as long as possible.

Many creative people, and musicians in particular, seem to outlive the rest of us, surviving to a fruitful old age. There are plenty of precedents: Verdi sat down to write *Falstaff* when he was approaching 80; Casals, Stokowski and Picasso were all still engaged with their art at 90; Goethe finished *Faust* when he was 81 . . .

The longevity of some creative artists may be due to the fact that they never retire. But the rest of us would do well to regard retirement as a bonus, not a burden. In fact, with perhaps a quarter of our lives still to live, we should think more in terms of a renaissance than a general running-down. We should be embarking on a well-planned transition to a less pressured existence, when, free at last from the constraints of earning a living, we can do exactly as we please.

Looking forward with enthusiasm, the potential to grow, keeps the vital spark ignited. The challenge is to keep mentally and physically stimulated like the artists. Perhaps the signal of success in retirement is the wonder that there was ever time to go to work.

AGEING AND ATTITUDE

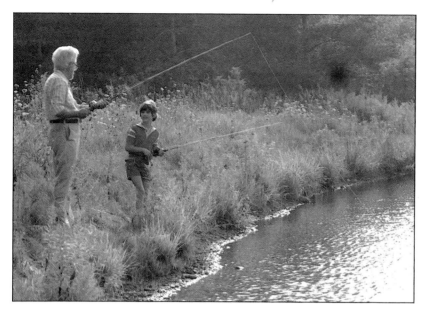

Young and old *can often bridge the generation gap with consummate ease. Grandfather and grandson find no difficulty in communicating or in sharing pursuits and pastimes such as fishing. It should be our aim to extend this sort of attitude to the elderly across all sectors of society, and both inside and outside the family, so that the aged are not vunerable to physical and mental attack and are not written off as a useless burden to society.*

The fate of old people today and in the future may be determined by society's attitudes toward them, and it is these attitudes — often harshly negative — which urgently need revision. In an age neurotically obsessed with youth, old is unfashionable, unattractive, sometimes even frightening, despite the fact that as many as a quarter of the people in some Western countries are over retirement age. Old age itself is mutely approximated to some chronic disease. However, old people themselves, however unknowingly, frequently invite disinterest by refusing to make an effort with younger generations. In countries with a long history of state benefits, they may also expect to be looked after and so make little effort to fend for themselves.

A place in society

The media does not help, with its double standards on advancing age. At one extreme, the 'now' generation is exalted for its strength, beauty, success, sexual prowess and all the associations of youth. At the other end of the scale, we are served up depressing and sometimes mawkish items on society's neglect of the old. Nobody documents the progress of the mass of elderly folk, who, far from drawing pathetic figures, enjoy constructive and rewarding later years. The fund of knowledge and wisdom accumulated with age is largely ignored.

This is particularly true of industrialized nations, in which the position enjoyed by the old in traditional societies has been undermined. The socially divisive practice of compulsory retirement probably lies at the heart of this problem. For while statesmen, clergymen and the like can remain at the helm indefinitely, enjoying continued self-respect, the mass of the working population must step down at 60 or 65. Sadly, for many working people, the biggest challenge of retirement is to avoid becoming a non-person.

Primitive societies do not put their elderly people out to grass, and so benefit from their abilities to the end. Yet in the West, we are rendered obsolete on the night of our retirement. As Dr Alex Comfort has pointed out: 'We may even, by the same token, make the elderly physically old, for mind, body and society interact in a degree that can still amaze us.'

So we become officially unproductive — a burden — something most old folk are at pains not to be. Far from being venerated, the village elders become the urban community's cast-offs, euphemistically dismissed as 'senior citizens'.

Responses to the elderly

This negative stereotype of old age as a rehearsal for death permeates all levels of society. At the point of daily contact, people's responses to the elderly are shaped by the firm belief that old is

How do you treat the elderly?

Take an honest look at the way you approach older people. If the answers reveal a negative attitude, stop and think. The old are human beings just like the rest of us, with the basic human needs for warmth, understanding, support, dignity and company.

Do you?
● Avoid them.

● Look through them or talk over their heads.

● Address them as 'dear' or 'grandad', even if you are not related to them.

● Fuss over them unnecessarily.

● Try to run their lives for them.

● Get impatient with them.

● Make allowances for their age and mobility.

● Go to them for advice.

● React enthusiastically to their plans.

● Keep a discreet eye on them.

● Involve them in your activities.

The ageing process

The physiological changes brought about by age are inevitable. The rate and extent of change, however, follow no set timetable and vary from person to person. The effects include the following:

Skin and hair
A gradual loss of elastic tissue (and of fat beneath the skin) causes the skin to sag and wrinkle. Changes occur in pigmentation and the hair loses colour. Weakened blood capillaries often cause the skin to bruise more easily, and harmless burst blood vessels may produce red patches on the hands.

Skeleton and muscles
Old people lose height because of the 'shrinking' of the discs between the vertebrae. Loss of elasticity in the connective tissue causes the joints to stiffen and enlarge. The bones become more brittle, and muscles lose some of their bulk and tone.

Heart and circulation
Arteries harden and thicken inside. This means the blood circulates less freely. There is some reduction in the supply of oxygen to the tissues, and a poor response to any sudden demand for an increased burst of energy.

The heart, which becomes less efficient with age, has to work even harder to pump blood through the narrowed arterial pathways, and this may cause the blood pressure to rise. These circulatory changes, combined with the changes in the skin, mean that old people feel the cold more.

Lungs
The tissues of the lungs lose elasticity with age so that breathing is less efficient. This, too, is a factor in reducing the supply of oxygen throughout the body.

Abdominal organs
The capacity of the abdominal organs is less, and they are less ready to process vast quantities of food. The kidneys, too, are slower to filter impurities from the blood.

Brain and nervous system
The brain shrinks with age: the significance of this is unknown, since intellectual powers are usually not affected, but short-term memory fails. The main threat to the brain is shortage of oxygen, due to the impaired blood supply. The reaction time of the nerves increases, making responses slower.

Senses
Some sensory loss is to be expected, but not a total shut-down. The two most common effects are a reduced ability to focus on nearby objects and a degree of hearing loss (particularly for the higher tones). Taste, smell and touch are diminished to some degree, and the mechanisms of balance become less accurate.

inevitably decrepid. Consequently, instead of being treated as people, old folk may find that they are stage-managed, bullied, treated like retarded youngsters or cosseted to an extent that severely cramps their style.

Such awkward approaches often conceal unresolved fears of growing old, particularly among those who, due to the break-up of the extended family, rarely come into contact with old people. Although you can expect about 20 years of life after retirement, it is important as you grow older to recognize and come to terms with the unavoidable physical effects of ageing. By keeping active, interested in life and philosophical about what is to come, it is possible to enjoy the later years and to inspire a more friendly attitude in younger people. Many youngsters relate well to the elderly, but some are openly antagonistic. It could be that it is not their years that make old people vulnerable, but the frailty of their status in society.

Many of us add to the sense of isolation experienced by the elderly by thoughtlessly failing to acknowledge them, by excluding them from conversation or patronizing them.

Resilient as well as wise, many elderly people can endure such insults. Yet we should remember that we devalue them at our own cost; for we too could face some of these same indignities in years to come, if society's attitudes to the elderly do not change for the better.

The elderly population of the developed world is at an all-time high, and the indications are that more people alive today will survive to a ripe old age than ever before. Since the elderly now represent an increasingly influential and vocal section of the community, governments are finally being forced to revise their ideas of old age.

The 'greying' of nations

Three major factors have brought about this progressive 'greying' of industralized nations: a falling birth-rate; a drop in the infant mortality rate; and increased life expectancy.

One of the most dramatic examples of this ageing trend is Japan, where, following the post-war baby boom, the fertility rate went into steep decline. When a head count was taken on Japan's Respect for the Aged Day, in September 1982, the over 65s (11,320,000 people) were found to account for 9.5 per cent of the population. This is a relatively low proportion alongside, Britain's 14 per cent or the 11 per cent of the USA.

Yet, by the year 2025, an estimated 21.3 per cent of the Japanese population will be over 65 — the highest proportion in any advanced nation. By this same year, West Germany will be populated by 20 per cent of old people, Britain and France by 18.6 per cent and the United States by 15.8 per cent. Moreover, this increase will be most marked among the over sixties, as the comparative chart (right) shows.

The French are so concerned at the social, economic and political implications that, in 1981, they nominated a Secretary of State for the Ageing — the first such cabinet appointment in history. His objective, he declared, was 'to allow the ageing the freedom to choose as long as possible, their way of life and fulfil their existence with dignity.' A similar spirit emerged from the 1982 World Assembly on Ageing. Here it was agreed that steps should be taken to help the elderly remain fit and well-integrated in the community, for as many as possible of their remaining years of life.

A more sophisticated approach to the needs of the elderly was suggested by Professor Bernard Isaacs, a leading British geriatrician, who pointed out that: 'the numbers of old people who are not incontinent, who have never had a stroke, a fall or a pressure sore, who are not housebound, chairbound or bedbound run into millions.'

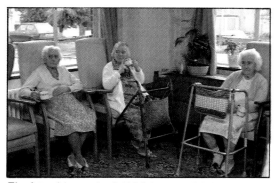

The fate of thousands of old folk is to spend their days in sedentary occupations. Enlightened approaches to the care and needs of the elderly recognize that such a restricted way of life is unfulfilling and often unnecessary. The elderly have much to offer, and should be motivated and encouraged to use their time and energy to the full.

Although the World Assembly generated a number of pious hopes about mobilizing the fit elderly as a productive resource, no government has yet devised a flexible set of proposals. This is not surprising, perhaps, in a situation of high unemployment for populations as a whole.

Significantly, Japan, with its prosperity, low unemployment, and tradition of working into old age, has raised the retirement age from 55 to 60: workers reaching formal retirement are frequently re-employed by the same companies, albeit in a humbler capacity. Similarly the USA has raised retirement age to 70. Some other countries are, however, looking toward voluntary retirement for people in their fifties.

The concept of formal retirement — as a well-earned rest for the workers — arose in the far-off days when average life expectancy was perhaps 20 or 30 years less than it is today. Now that there are moves to pull back retirement age to 60 or lower, most people in the developed world can expect to live well into their 70s. Since the post-retirement phase represents a significant and sizeable chunk of human experience, the Industrial Revolution's notions of retirement have become irrelevant.

The claims of the elderly

In many ways, the elderly have never had it so good. In Britain, the basic retirement pension is available to all retired folk, irrespective of financial status. In addition, those in need may receive help with housing, transport and medical ex-

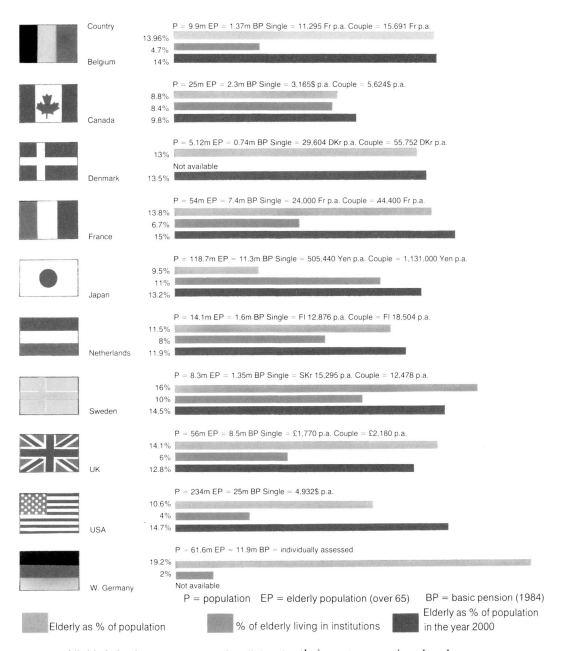

Belgium	Country P = 9.9m EP = 1.37m BP Single = 11,295 Fr p.a. Couple = 15,691 Fr p.a. 13.96% 4.7% 14%
Canada	P = 25m EP = 2.3m BP Single = 3,165$ p.a. Couple = 5,624$ p.a. 8.8% 8.4% 9.8%
Denmark	P = 5.12m EP = 0.74m BP Single = 29,604 DKr p.a. Couple = 55,752 DKr p.a. 13% Not available 13.5%
France	P = 54m EP = 7.4m BP Single = 24,000 Fr p.a. Couple = 44,400 Fr p.a. 13.8% 6.7% 15%
Japan	P = 118.7m EP = 11.3m BP Single = 505,440 Yen p.a. Couple = 1,131,000 Yen p.a. 9.5% 11% 13.2%
Netherlands	P = 14.1m EP = 1.6m BP Single = Fl 12,876 p.a. Couple = Fl 18,504 p.a. 11.5% 8% 11.9%
Sweden	P = 8.3m EP = 1.35m BP Single = SKr 15,295 p.a. Couple = 12,478 p.a. 16% 10% 14.5%
UK	P = 56m EP = 8.5m BP Single = £1,770 p.a. Couple = £2,180 p.a. 14.1% 6% 12.8%
USA	P = 234m EP = 25m BP Single = 4,932$ p.a. 10.6% 4% 14.7%
W. Germany	P = 61.6m EP = 11.9m BP = individually assessed 19.2% 2% Not available

P = population   EP = elderly population (over 65)   BP = basic pension (1984)

Elderly as % of population   % of elderly living in institutions   Elderly as % of population in the year 2000

penses. All this is in sharp contrast to the plight of old people in many of the Third World countries. Yet money does not buy recognition.

Many old people, no longer content to remain a passive lobby, are beginning to press their own claims. In the USA, for instance, today's old people, survivors of the 1930s depression, are much more vocal about political issues than are their contemporaries elsewhere.

At the moment, then, it is sheer pressure of numbers that is forcing governments to start taking notice. But if the American initiative were to be taken up internationally, retired people could be organized into an active political force. Then perhaps they would again be recognized as people in their own right.

FACING UP TO RETIREMENT

For many people, the gold watch traditionally awarded on retirement is a symbolic threat, ticking their lives away. These are people who resist the idea of retirement, seeing it as an end to their purposeful life, and not — as it should be — a rich new beginning.

Leaving aside the minority who never retire — mostly creative people such as musicians, writers and artists — the rest of us would do well to admit that such a negative view of retirement is outdated. For today, as more people are living long enough to spend a quarter of their lifetime in retirement, millions are finding these leisured years as rewarding as their working lives.

The controversial trend toward early retirement has supplied the retired population with a vigorous baseline of active people. Nevertheless, the actual break with working routine is a bereavement which inevitably comes as a shock to the system and requires major adjustment. Most people, as one United Nations report puts it, 'hesitate to prepare for it' and 'become anxious and afraid when it eventually approaches.'

The bonus years

In retirement, the most important problem to be solved is that of developing new interests and activities. These provide purpose and identity that may be lost with retiring from formal work. New interests and activities do not 'just happen'. Experience shows that the key to successful retirement is facing up to it — and well ahead of time. Today, when retirement can extend to two decades or more, we need to review our lives and relationships long before the gold watch is due to make the most of these bonus years.

This is the message of the many organizations set up to help older employees facing retirement. The American Association of Retired Persons (AARP), the largest of its kind, found that, with proper foresight and planning, many problems would never have arisen. So it developed an offshoot called AIM (Action for Independent Maturity) to cater for those people who are coming up to retirement.

In Britain the Workers' Educational Association and the Pre-Retirement Association (PRA) teach people how to retire. The PRA, for example, offers a schedule of public seminars and personal guidance on health, finance, living arrangements, part-time employment, and leisure pursuits.

Both employers and unions are beginning to respond to these programmes and, according to the PRA, an increasing number of employers are accepting retirement planning as one of their obligations to employees. Some large companies have pioneered phased retirement schemes, which involve a progressively shorter working week for the last year or so of working life. But, overall, only a tiny fraction of people reaching retirement has had any kind of preparation for it, and this often only at the last minute.

This leaves the mass of workers to develop some sort of positive philosophy on their own. At 50, says AIM, most people find their family responsibilities easing, and this is when they should start to lay the groundwork for their future comfort, happiness and security.

Money matters

Finance is the first priority, since it can take years to fashion the proverbial nest-egg. Over the 10 years leading up to retirement, you should fulfil the following objectives.

First clear existing debts, overdrafts, bank loans, hire-purchase agreements and, perhaps, pay off the mortgage. Anticipate and realize a major undertaking, such as reroofing the house or financing a move, while you are still on a full salary. If possible, begin to accumulate savings and arrange an investment income to supplement the basic state pension after retirement.

If you are not a financial wizard, seek the help of a bank manager, accountant or investment adviser, who will find the best returns for your cash. Remember, however, that any plan will need to be reviewed at intervals. Budgeting should become progressively easier as retirement day approaches and is a good way of mentally phasing yourself into retirement.

Five years before retirement, you should have formulated some idea of where and how you want to live. One of the most common and miserable pitfalls to be avoided is to move on retirement to completely strange, often isolated, surroundings, remote from family, friends, even public utilities. In this way, you double the bereavement by leaving both work and your familiar surroundings behind.

However, if you do plan to move house, now is the time to decide on your retirement setting. This creates opportunities over the coming years

Don't get carried away by romantic locations when it comes to considering where you will live when you retire. A country cottage with hollyhocks nodding in at the door, will not suit you if you are not really a country lover at heart. A day by the sea on a sunny day may tempt you to move to the coast. But busloads of tourists in summer, and Force 10 gales in winter may be too high a price to pay. Familiar faces and places can be reassuring when your working life changes. A smaller, more convenient house in your present locality may be the best answer.

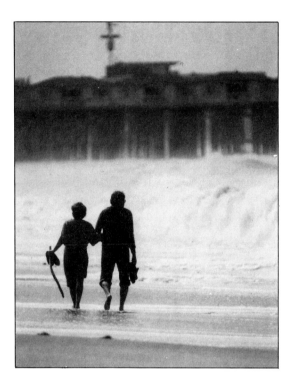

Ten steps to retirement

● Find out about your pension and other entitlements.

● Clear financial debts.

● Reassess your investments.

● Arrange a valuation on your home.

● Check that your insurance policies are adequate.

● Decide where to live.

● Survey public facilities in the area.

● Explore possibilities for part-time work.

● Make a will.

● Develop your leisure interests.

to spend the occasional holiday or spare weekend reconnoitring an area to check out the public transport, hospital and library, which would become increasingly important in later years. These reconnaissance expeditions may also lead to a few new social contacts.

As you get the feel of the locality, you will discover what kind of property comes into your price range. Bungalows are popular with older people, although they tend to be more expensive than houses of comparable capacity. A house with stairs may become difficult to manage in later years while an apartment without a garden may prove too limiting, and so on. Whatever your choice, plan to move well before retirement, so the cost of removal can be borne on a full-time salary. This will also avoid another upheaval later and enable you to strike up new friendships.

For the minority of people who opt for a custom-built home, there are a number of options. These range from residential hotels for the elderly to the no-expense-spared retirement centres, springing up in places such as Florida, California, and Spain. While everything from a laundry service to a golf course is supplied, these centres are unlikely to suit freer spirits.

The blueprint for retirement should begin to take definite shape five years, and certainly no later than two years, before the gold watch is due. This is not a simple question of filling the 2,000 hours a year normally spent at work, but of formulating a comprehensive and practical retirement philosophy, designed to ensure a rounded existence.

In Britain, the Pre-Retirement Association (PRA) bases its courses and seminars on a retirement formula, which includes six crucial elements. An adequate personal philosophy of life, good physical and emotional health, an adequate income beyond subsistence level, suitable accommodation, one or more absorbing interests and congenial associates and neighbours.

At this stage, having already tackled the long-term issues of money and accommodation, you should be resolving practical details of how you want to live. Do you want to embark on a second career, or to look forward to at last having time for leisure interests?

Surprisingly, perhaps, most people want to continue to work. About 30 per cent of retired Americans would like to be working, at least part-time, and no fewer than 75 per cent of those still in employment would like to go to some kind of paid, part-time work. In Japan, the urge to work is even stronger. Although the rate of employment among the elderly has been dropping steadily (in the 1950s it was 42 per cent), in 1980, 26.3 per cent of Japanese were still working beyond the age of 65, compared with 12.3 per cent in the United States; and more would continue if they could. A survey conducted in Japan in the early 1980s revealed that the number of elderly jobless wanting employment had doubled in 10 years, and three-quarters of these hankered after jobs to enrich their lives, not for the cash.

In Britain, the London-based employment agency Success After Sixty (SAS) conducted its own survey of retired job-seekers. This showed that the majority accepted different work from that to which they were accustomed, mostly with less responsibility, and that they sought out re-employment both to cope with the effects of inflation and to keep occupied.

Research has repeatedly shown that work in retirement improves health, morale and life-expectancy; yet it is not always easy to find, particularly in the present climate of widespread

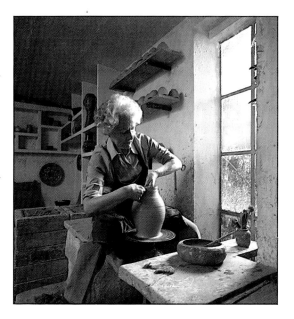

unemployment and strong discrimination against age. It is, therefore, essential to explore new openings in good time if you face compulsory retirement. This is easier said than done, however, in view of the scarcity of employment schemes for the elderly.

Seeking employment

The retirement advisory bureau run by the Institute of Directors may offer a start; meanwhile, SAS not only finds jobs for the elderly but also champions their cause in the labour market, promoting their qualities of punctuality, reliability and conscientiousness. 'Older people have had time to develop those unwritten qualifications of tact, diplomacy and experience. They are rarely concerned with status . . .'

However, the most fruitful approach to job-hunting is probably the personal grapevine. As retirement approaches, it pays to let your contacts know that you will shortly be on the market, if only for a part-time commitment.

Alternatively, older people are often willing, and supremely able, to take on a voluntary commitment. Here, their wisdom and experience is of great value, the work less fraught than it is in paid employment, and there is no age discrimination. Indeed, if it were not for the contribution of the recently retired, the outlook for the underprivileged, 'grand elderly' in hospitals and the

Retirement offers a wonderful opportunity to develop new skills. At last there is time to try your hand at something you have long wished to attempt. Taking a course in pottery, (left) or welding (right) might also allow you to earn some money by selling the objects you produce. Even if this is not the case, there is much to be gained, both socially and intellectually.

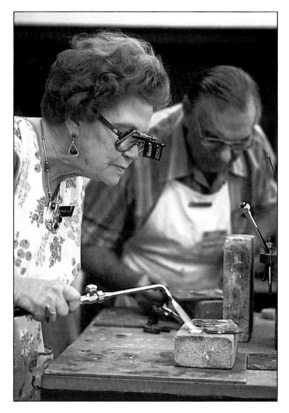

community could be even bleaker.

When making overtures for any kind of work, it helps to have a pattern of service in mind which will leave you time for other things. For now more than ever is the time to balance work with leisure and relaxation.

The answer is to follow your instincts; for, short of winning a gold medal at the Olympics, retired people can enjoy sport as much as the young. Any glimmer of talent at writing or painting, for example, can also be developed with practice and guidance. Academic and technical courses are also available at institutes of further education. The French, for instance, are justifiably proud of their University of the Third Age, a scheme which uses all the facilities of no fewer than 23 universities.

Whatever you choose, the aim is, as a Council of Europe paper puts it, 'to preserve creativity and curiosity, the ability to marvel and the capacity to listen and learn.' Continued mental and physical stimulation are the two essential keys to growing old gracefully.

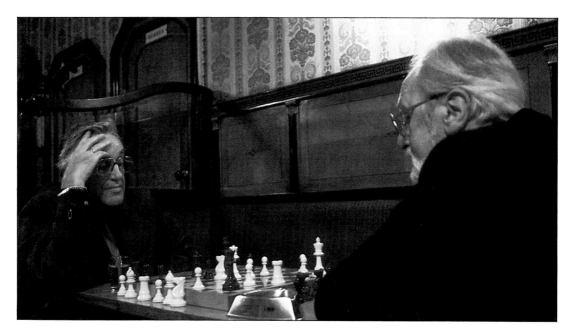

Retirement can provoke an identity crisis every bit as real as the adolescent doldrums or the midlife crisis. Some newly retired people enjoy a feeling of euphoria; others are seized by a compulsion for feverish activity, such as spring-cleaning, DIY or getting the garden straight. Yet many others—men especially—suffer a keen sense of deprivation, even depression. When the farewell speeches are over, a feeling of job bereavement sets in, affecting not only the retiring person but all those concerned with them.

Relationships
All marriages suffer the ripples, if not the full impact, of retirement shock. If both partners are prepared for this and have some positive philosophy for these leisure years, the shock is more readily absorbed. Women are, generally, less ostrich-like than their male partners about the need for reappraisal, and the transition comes more naturally to women who have devoted their lives to the home. However, women must accept that the house will now be used all day.

Partners need to plan their new life together, from readjusting the domestic routine—and hopefully sharing the chores—to agreeing on a list of goals still to be achieved and jointly attending a pre-retirement course. This should be a time of fulfilment, not an embittered siege.

Friendships
Now, more than ever, is the time to cultivate new friendships outside the home. Working life may have obscured a general lack of social contacts, and when business friendships fizzle out on retirement, as most inevitably do, life is at grave risk of becoming dreary. Women are often better at maintaining social momentum, but both partners should concentrate on renewing and cementing old friendships, as well as remaining open to new overtures. New romantic attachments are not out of the question at this stage, as evidenced by the many late marriages, and friendships can be based on long-lived interests, experiences and memories.

Single people living alone are most at risk from estrangement in these later years, although they may have learned the art of self-sufficiency and the value of keeping up with friends. They will know that we all need to work at relationships, so as to fill the vacuum left by retirement, and to continue to look outward.

Younger generations
It helps to gather a good mix of ages around you as many retired Americans do, pursuing their involvements over the years and so making for a more varied and enjoyable retirement—at least in the early stage.

Social contacts in the retirement years are often easily fostered by mutual interest in a game such as chess, (left), or outdoor bowling, (right). The companionship, competition and the stimulation such contacts provide are essential to well-being in the retirement years. Ageing is inevitable, but loneliness is not. It is up to you to seek out others whose company you enjoy.

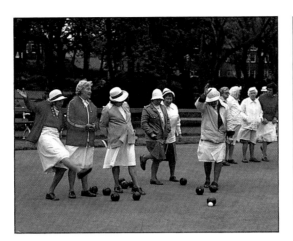

In approaching other generations—children, neighbours or friends—it is as well to realize that younger people are not automatically healthier, wealthier and more carefree than yourself. They, too, have problems; they get lonely, and many like to call on the wisdom of age. In a crisis they will gladly look to your maturity and consoling thoughts learned from past experience.

Sex and the elderly
The main problem with sex in later life is not so much physical as the shadow cast by misinformed beliefs—that sex in the later years is somehow distasteful and not expected, or that older people are 'past it'. True, there is some falling off in libido, although less with those who remain active, but men do not automatically become impotent at 60 nor women lose interest in sex after the menopause.

The important point to remember is that there really is no difference in sex before or after 60 or beyond (see pp.182-5). If you have always had a warm, loving relationship, which finds part of its expression in mutually satisfying sex, it should continue as before. This is particularly true if you make love regularly, with a continued imaginative effort to please, rather than making the occasional perfunctory effort.

Even when older people are no longer able or willing to complete intercourse, they should not draw physically apart. No one is too old for, or immune to, physical warmth and affection. Love-making in these more tranquil years is contact and communication and physical reassurance, in a love that has stood the test of time.

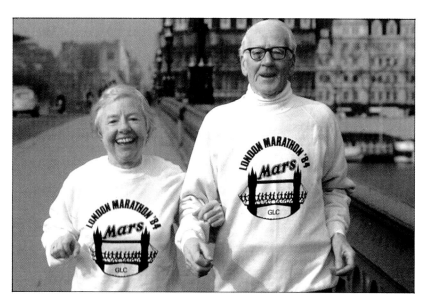

Energy breeds energy and physical activity keeps the body in tune and the mind alert. It preserves your sense of independence and your control over life. A shining example of just what can be achieved by those over retirement age is given by two Britons, Madge Sharples, aged 67, and Robert Wiseman, aged 81, who were among the oldest participants in the 1984 London Marathon.

Medically, old age is an imprecise condition. For practical purposes, however, it can be considered as the time between normal retiring age, that is, 60 to 65, and death. Many people remain fit, alert and vigorous well into their eighties, while others seem to be born middle aged. The boundaries between young and old become increasingly blurred in the later years since there are no clear developmental stages as in childhood, but most people become frail from about 80 onward.

In fact, ageing begins in the womb, for even the most primitive foetal cells divide, multiply serve out their time and are shed. By the time physical growth ceases, ageing is well under way.

Nevertheless, some diseases and disabilities have become symptoms of accelerated ageing. There are, for example, 15 million people in the United States alone suffering from osteoporosis, a progressive thinning of the bones, which is simply a chronic form of a process occurring naturally in everyone, and starting before the age of 50, but particularly in women because of hormonal changes. Likewise, osteoarthritis is a manifestation of the normal wear and tear sustained by major joints.

The cardiovascular system is particularly susceptible to the consequences of age. The arteries slowly harden, and arterial plaque furs up the blood vessels, causing a condition that may lead to strokes and heart disease. The old are more at risk, too, from respiratory infections as the lung tissue loses its elasticity and its resilience.

Older people also contract diseases completely unconnected with the ageing process because their general resistance is low and they have been exposed to harmful factors for a long time. Cancer is a case in point.

Resisting old age

Disease and disability are not, however, inevitably companions of old age, and one of the largest obstacles to health is the widespread tendency to dismiss any symptoms as 'old age'. Often both doctors and patients are hesitant to explore many symptoms that could signify a treatable disease.

The body has a remarkable ability to adapt to the changes that come with age. Illness is no more normal in later years than it is any any other time of life. Old folk should feel as fit and well as the rest of us, even if they are less resilient to sudden stress, and should always seek medical help for health problems.

It can sometimes be difficult for even the most enlightened doctor to know at what point normal ageing shades into a decline caused by self-neglect or depression. Yet the distinction is critical, for most illness or injury can be successfully treated — or at least greatly relieved — at any age. It may take elderly people longer to recover, but they do. Even the extremely old can be treated and comforted and so regain the will to live and pass the time comfortably, to the end.

Common problems

Medicines
The over-prescription of drugs to the elderly is a growing problem. The necessity for drugs should be regularly reviewed, and you should question your doctor to this effect. Almost half of all old folk do not take medicine as prescribed, and many find it difficult to keep track of dosages. To avoid any confusion, a simple schedule needs to be kept for regular medication and occasional remedies marked with the condition they are intended to treat. Do not hoard drugs indefinitely; many have a short shelf-life.

Hypothermia
This condition, in which the body temperature drops dangerously low, is a major cause of hospital admissions and death in old age, particularly in people living alone. The elderly are particularly at risk because of reduced mobility, impaired blood supply and the decreased insulating properties of the skin. Good heating and warm clothing are necessities in the cold months, for if the deep temperature of the body falls below 95°F (35°C) the whole body feels cold — even the abdomen and armpits. Movements and speech slow up. The victim becomes pale, confused and drowsy, eventually losing consciousness. If no help is forthcoming, death intervenes within a few hours.

Memory lapses
Recent memory suffers more than than long-term memory, and lapses from one minute to the next may become distressingly common. It often helps to make lists and to tackle tasks systematically, one at a time, particularly in critical operations such as cooking.

Impaired senses
All five senses are subject to some loss in old age, but it is the cumulative effects that prove most significant to safety, for example, when driving. It is thus important regularly to assess whether you are fit to drive. The two most troublesome effects are difficulty with near focusing and a serious reduction in hearing acuity; both are correctable to some degree. Impaired sense of balance is often ignored and may lead to falls.

Incontinence
This is not an inescapable part of growing old and should not be accepted as such. However, urination and defaecation become more frequent with age, due to the reduced efficiency and tone of the sphincters and ligaments associated with the outlets of the digestive and urinary tracts. Incontinence should always be fully investigated, since it can usually be improved and often cured completely.

The following symptoms are *not* normal consequences of ageing. They need immediate investigation:
- Undue shortness of breath
- Palpitations
- Persistent or recurrent pain
- Constant tiredness
- Double vision
- Ringing in the ears
- Sudden weight loss
- Persistent thirst
- Persistent low back pain
- Loss of power in an arm or leg
- Sudden change in bowel habits
- Bleeding from any source

The desire to extend the human lifespan is almost as old as man himself, but not one that is likely to be fulfilled in the foreseeable future. To a great extent, Western medicine has done all it can in banishing the epidemic diseases that once saw off most people by middle age and, in the last century, has more than doubled life expectancy. But the conquest of further diseases is unlikely to extend the average human lifespan of people in the developed world significantly.

Instead, we are looking to medical science to make old age more tolerable. The main thrust being made by the branch of medicine known as gerontology — the study of ageing — is to establish the factors behind the normal process of ageing, and to distinguish between the effects of age and those caused by misuse or disease. Its aim is to slow the decline in vigour that comes upon the human frame with increasing age.

From research of this kind, it emerges that the foundations of a robust old age are laid in youth; in making a positive investment toward good health through sensible use and care of the body. For there is growing evidence that lifestyle may be a more significant factor in producing degenerative diseases that are among the most common in old age than the ageing process itself.

Many illnesses of old age, then, are attributable to lack of exercise, smoking and heavy drinking in earlier years, to obesity and to unhealthy eating habits. One leading American gerontologist estimates, for example, that almost a third of his countrymen die from chronic overeating. The good news is that, whenever we care to correct any or all these bad habits, there is a bonus to be had in terms of health and well-being. The earlier this is done, the greater the benefits, but experiments have shown that a switch to a more health-conscious regimen can yield positive results, even in people aged 70 and over. On the debit side, there is some evidence that injuries to the skeleton incurred while playing sport during youth can aggravate conditions such as arthritis in later years, but this is a small risk compared with the many benefits of exercise.

It seems that we have seriously underestimated the human potential to lead a full, active life at any age. The cultural expectation that older people should slow down means that many eventually ask too little of themselves, and so give up or grow bored.

The science of gerontology cannot remove the fact of ageing, but it can point the way to replacing dependency with extra years of vigour. It has already given a glimpse of a new era — when it could be thought abnormal for the old to be sick, frail and vulnerable before they become 80. Now it is up to us, in modelling our lifestyles before and during retirement, to recognize that age need not necessarily 'weary, nor the years condemn . . .'

Food and drink

There is a mass of evidence linking unhealthy diet with degenerative disease, including heart-trouble, strokes, hypertension, late-onset diabetes and certain cancers. The two most immediate health problems in the later years are obesity and malnutrition. So check your own diet.

● If your diet is high in fat and low in roughage, change it. To ward off constipation, add wholemeal bread or bran.

● If you are bored, don't resort to food. Take some exercise or seek company.

● If you have lost interest in food, try to tempt yourself with your favourite meals, but keep your menus well-balanced with protein, starch, fat, fruit and vegetables.

● Remember that cooked food is more easily digested than raw food.

● It is a fallacy that elderly people should cut down their fluid intake. The recommended daily intake is 1.8 to 3 litres (3 to 5 pints) and even more in summer or if you are confined to a centrally heated home.

Keeping in motion

Society is at last beginning to recognize that a balance of work, play and exercise is essential at any age.

● A heart attack does not ban you from activity; exercise in moderation is advisable.

● Everyone of retirement age should build some exercise into their daily round. It will pay dividends.

● Make a point of walking or, possibly, cycling to the shops.

● Use the stairs instead of the lift when possible.

● If you have no dog of your own, perhaps offer to take someone else's for a walk.

● Take up something you enjoy, such as golf, dancing, walking, swimming, tennis, gardening, at least 3 times a week and preferably every day. It should be strenuous enough to make you puff with exertion. Use the programmes on pp. 106-15.

● Start an exercise routine to

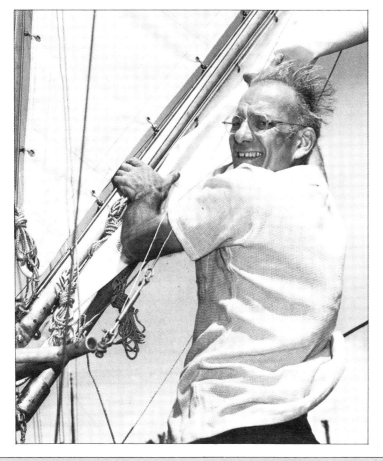

Lone yachtsman Francis Chichester is a perfect example of just what can be achieved in the later years of life. Having made a remarkable recovery from cancer, Chichester set out from Britain on his single-handed round-the-world voyage in August 1966, less than a month before his sixty-fifth birthday. Yachting is one of the many sports and activities open to you when you pass retirement age. With increased leisure hours, you have an ideal opportunity to take up new sports and fitness ventures.

mobilize your joints. Use the warm-up and flexibility exercise on pp. 100-103.

● It is never too late to start.

Routine maintenance

Go for regular health checks, just as you organize maintenance checks for your car; it will either put your mind at rest or uncover any problems at an early stage. Your doctor should be happy to arrange this, or there may be a clinic in your area specializing in preventative surveillance for the elderly. Meanwhile, keep all the ancillary parts in order.

● 'Flu injections may give a degree of protection and at least reduce the severity of an attack.

Vision: the vast majority retain more than adequate vision with a little help all their lives.

● Keep your glasses clean and use adequate lighting for close work.

● Have your eyesight checked every 1 to 2 years: your spectacles may need changing and examination may detect a treatable condition such as cataract.

● Report any pain in the eyes or sudden deterioration in vision to your doctor without delay.

Hearing: deafness is not inevitable in old age; wax accumulates faster, so syringing may help.

● If you cannot hear ordinary conversation, see your doctor.

Teeth: neglected teeth or ill-fitting dentures can make you look older than your years, cause infections and impair digestion.

● Have regular 6-monthly checks if you have your own teeth.

● Dentures should be checked at least every 5 years; they may need adjustment or replacing.

Feet: there is no point in becoming housebound because your feet hurt.

● Treat yourself to some good, supportive shoes — avoid cheap shoes and slippers for daily use.

● See the chiropodist regularly.

Older people have as keen a sense of safety as anyone else. Moreover, they have more experience than the rest of us at anticipating danger and taking precautions to avoid it. However, they are clearly no longer as nimble and alert as they used to be, so situations we all take for granted, such as crossing the road, can become hazardous.

Reduced mobility, and the combined effects of failing senses and reduced nerve reaction times, render the old particularly vulnerable. Most old folk compensate for this by taking life at a more leisurely pace and becoming extra attentive in potentially risky situations. Unable to hear traffic clearly, for example, they are more likely to look to see that the road is clear before crossing.

Accidents and injuries

Falls are the most common calamity for elderly people, with three million a year receiving medical attention for this cause in Britain alone. Women's bones break more easily than men's, and about half the intake to female orthopaedic wards consists of old ladies with fractures caused by falls. Broken hips are especially common and notoriously slow to mend, but many respond well to surgery.

'Drop attacks' also pose a threat to the elderly. These are sudden episodes in which the legs become unaccountably weak, causing the victim to fall to the ground without losing consciousness. Their causes are not fully understood, but they are usually related to a fall in blood pressure or constriction of the brain's blood supply.

Injuries incurred by falls and drop attacks may be compounded by falling against something sharp or hot, such as the corners of cupboards, heating appliances or stoves. There is the additional risk that a person may lie undiscovered for hours or even days. It is essential, therefore, for older people to be alert to these dangers, to guard against falls and to consult a doctor if they should experience a drop attack.

Few people would want to live in an environment so safe and structured that it feels clinical, and the elderly probably manage as well in a place they know as they would in some custom-built home. However, it does pay to invest in safety, as it does for health, by eliminating some of the potential hazards before anyone gets hurt. The illustrations provide examples of some of the helpful gadgets and safety devices available.

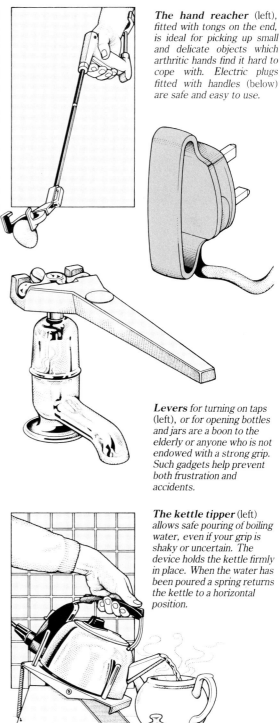

The hand reacher (left), fitted with tongs on the end, is ideal for picking up small and delicate objects which arthritic hands find it hard to cope with. Electric plugs fitted with handles (below) are safe and easy to use.

Levers for turning on taps (left), or for opening bottles and jars are a boon to the elderly or anyone who is not endowed with a strong grip. Such gadgets help prevent both frustration and accidents.

The kettle tipper (left) allows safe pouring of boiling water, even if your grip is shaky or uncertain. The device holds the kettle firmly in place. When the water has been poured a spring returns the kettle to a horizontal position.

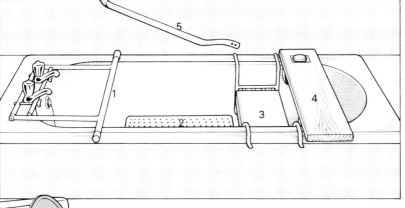

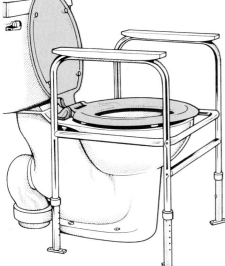

The bathroom, like the kitchen, can be a hazardous place for the elderly. It is wise, as you get older, to fit your bath (above) with hand rails (1, 5) and a non-slip mat (2). A bathboard (4) may be used for support or as a seat. Bath seats (3) allow more of the body to be immersed in the bath water. A toilet fitted with supporting frame (left) is invaluable for many elderly and disabled people. A toilet with a raised seat may also be helpful.

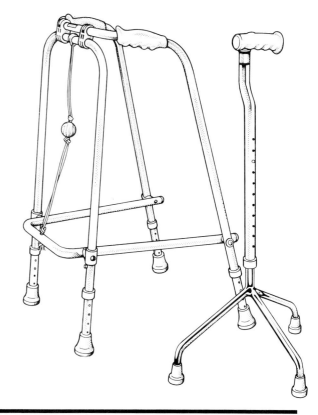

If mobility becomes a problem as you become older it is sensible to use some kind of supportive device to help you get about. It is better to 'give in' to your need for such aids than to be immobile or an accident victim as a result of your own pride. Walking sticks designed to give more support than the conventional staff come in many guises. The tetrapod (far right) gives extra support and stability at the base. Look for a model whose height can be adjusted and whose handle can be altered for use in either right or left hand. A walking frame is cumbersome but a better proposition than being confined to a bed or chair. It should be strong enough to support the entire body weight. Models such as the one illustrated (right) can be folded away for easy storage and transport.

An aim for the elderly

The Nun's Prayer, written in the seventeenth century is now well known across the world. Shot through with humour and compassion, it speaks volumes to us of the patience and restraint for which many people strive with advancing age.

'Lord, thou knowest better than I know myself that I am growing older, and will some day be old.

Keep me from getting talkative and particularly from the fatal habit of thinking I must say something on every subject and on every occasion.

Release me from craving to try to straighten out everybody's affairs.

Keep my mind free from the recital of endless details — give me wings to get to the point. I ask for grace

enough to listen to the tales of others' pains. Help me to endure them with patience.

But seal my lips on my own aches and pains — they are increasing and my love of rehearsing them is becoming sweeter as the years go by.

Teach me the glorious lesson that occasionally it is possible that I may be mistaken.

Keep me reasonably sweet; I do not want to be a saint — some of them are so hard to live with — but a sour old woman is one of the crowning works of the devil.

Make me thoughtful, but not moody; helpful, but not bossy. With my vast store of wisdom, it seems a pity not to use it all, but thou knowest, Lord, that I want a few friends at the end.'

The characteristics and foibles acquired in early life often become exaggerated with the passage of time, so that old age reveals a more fascinating mix of characters than any other age group. Some old folk, however, develop into caricatures of their former selves, becoming mellow and nostalgic or miserably bitter and inward-looking. Yet, mercifully, many remain wonderfully alert, vigorous and unselfish and present a valuable example to younger members of the community.

A positive philosophy

There is no magic formula for achieving a happy and constructive old age, but it is important to seek ways of priming the morale for the coming years. Most important of all is to realize that mental and physical stimulation are both essential and possible. Whatever your age, it is never too late to learn something new.

Another essential of the positive philosophy is to confront your fears about old age and to recognize that, if allowed to get out of proportion, they can prove more diminishing to the personality than the ageing process itself. The four principal fears, common to most people, are loneliness, physical incapacity, senility and death. It may not be possible to banish those fears completely, but you must come to terms with them and not let them overshadow your life. For fear undermines the morale and so saps our vitality and resistance to disease.

Anxiety and depression can occur at any age, but remember, they are reversible. The inci-

dence of total incapacity in the elderly population is surprisingly small and, since most old folk continue to function efficiently to the end — albeit in a lower gear — everyone should look for fresh ways of gaining both experience and achievement in their later years.

Too many people fall into the trap of viewing old age as a waiting room for death and gradually become what society expects them to be — sedentary and submissive. So, instead of falling into unnecessary decline, you must take up the challenge of retirement.

Well-integrated older people capitalize on the advantage of a long life — knowledge, experience, wisdom, memories — and find that these help to compensate for the gradual physiological changes. Such people turn these later years into an Indian summer of joy and achievement. For them, after a full life, death intervenes as Leonardo da Vinci believed it should: as sleep comes after a hard day's work.

An expression of caring

Contrary to popular belief, death is, for most people a calm rather than a painful experience. It is important to allow a dying person to elect their own style of death, and to encourage them to make the most of every living moment that remains to them. Even the dying have much to experience, and much to offer to those destined to outlive them. Thus the proximity of death should add, not subtract from the value of life.

For those with a deep sense of commitment to

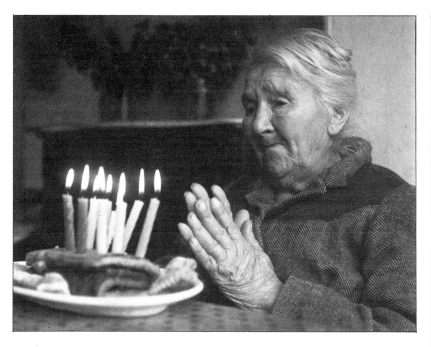

Birthdays are a reason for celebration at any age, but all the more so when, like this lady, you reach the landmark of 90. While the elderly must come to terms with the fact that every birthday may be their last, pride in past achievements and a hope of future fulfilment are the sorts of emotions to cultivate. All joyous occasions are to be cherished, not overshadowed by fears and forebodings.

the people they love, discussion of death and its consequences is an expression of caring and *not* a morbid exercise. Bereavement is hard enough to bear when it comes, and should not be burdened with the problems of trying to resolve practical affairs that could have been anticipated and forestalled well in advance.

Partners should talk together openly about death, so that their wishes and the whereabouts of relevant papers — wills, insurance policies and so on — are known to both parties and to children, other family members or close friends. This helps the surviving partner to cope in the first few disorientating months.

It is hard to be left alone late in life, and feelings of grief may be tinged with resentment, anger and guilt. All these conflicting emotions need to be released, and family and friends must encourage the bereaved partner to talk about the loss, until each successive stage of mourning is adequately worked through (see pp. 260-1).

Grief distorts the human sense of perspective, so it is wise to resist any major changes, such as moving house, for some months after the loss of a partner or a live-in companion, housekeeper or relative. Remember, the bereaved person is at risk, both psychologically and physically for at least a year after the event.

Tips for mental fitness

● Learn to adapt to a lifestyle that is not governed by the need to earn a living.

● Recognize your own strengths and put them to work in new and fulfilling ways.

● Plan for the future and devise plenty to look forward to.

● Set yourself new goals.

● Stay tuned in to the outside world, including current events, the social scene, family life and the arts.

● Hang on to your own identity, no matter what pressures there are to conform to the geriatric mould.

● Maintain standards of dress and behaviour that add to feelings of self-respect.

● Keep self-pity, introspection and any other negative tendencies at bay so that you present a positive and purposeful image to the world.

● Be dignified, not submissive.

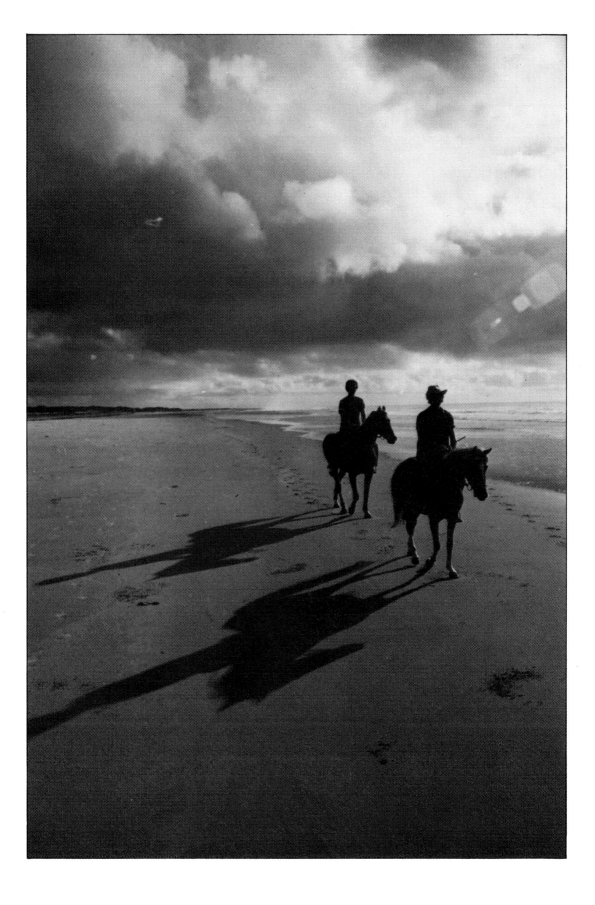

THE
WHOLE PERSON

The human mind and body work together to create the whole person, and, through this complex interaction, we respond to the elements of our environment, including those that are stressful, in both a physical and an emotional way. While we all need a certain amount of stress and challenge to fire us, to keep us alert and well-motivated, too much stress is linked with the development of a variety of illnesses. Thus it is obvious that understanding stress, and learning how to deal with it, need to be an integral part of both preventive health care and of therapeutic medicine.

Sometimes the link between stress and physical symptoms is obvious. We can probably all remember the stomach pains and headaches that once afflicted us before examinations, and the minor ailments we suffered when we had unpleasant lessons to face. These feelings were real enough, but we marvelled — and our parents cynically smiled — when the aches and pains disappeared if the test or the feared lesson was cancelled.

As we get older, the sources of stress in our lives do not decrease. Instead, we get used to expecting some symptoms and living with them. Certainly we begin to master our environment, and some of the events that once engendered panic no longer do so. However, modern life is full of stresses — there is no limit to the circumstances that pressure, frustrate, irritate or anger us. And compared with our forebears, we live life at a faster pace and have much higher expectations of both it and of ourselves.

Life is often problematical, but we too often attempt to escape our problems — or try to resolve them — by using props such as drugs, alcohol or cigarettes. In the short term, these provide some relief, but the costs are high. They may cause more problems than they solve and may also stop us from effective resolution of the original source of stress.

This chapter explains the physical and mental responses to stress and the risks they involve. It will help you to identify the underlying causes, to analyse your reactions and to seek out new, safe and sensible ways of problem-solving and stress relief.

PERSONALITY

Personality is the individual hallmark of every member of the human race. No two people, even identical twins, have the same personality. Your personality gives definition to your life by marking you out as a person in your own right. It also determines many aspects of your life, including the things that please and displease you, the type of employment you choose and the sorts of friendships and relationships you make.

We all vary in the way we tackle the problems that are created by stress. In many ways, our approach is determined by our personality. There are, however, no certain ways of defining personality, and different aspects of personality tend to emerge in different circumstances. Personality is not consistent. It alters with the situation, with your mood and with past experiences. The danger in discussing personality types is to assume that people react in the same way all the time and to all situations.

In labelling personalities, psychologists and psychiatrists attempt to make sense of our experiences, to analyse our behaviour and to work out why we act in the way we do. They gather together behaviours that have something in common and give them a name. If you are, for example, a person who likes to be organized down to the last detail, from the positioning of papers on your work desk to the arrangement of clothes in your cupboard or the positioning of your car in the garage, your personality might be described as obsessive. This does not mean that you are obsessive about everything, nor that you have had any specific experiences in childhood, at school or as an adult. It is merely a convenient type of description.

Personality and fitness
The way in which we *tend* to react to situations has a bearing on the way we cope with stress and, by implication, on our physical and mental fitness. The labels — obsessional, introspective, passive, compliant, aggressive, over-controlled and so on — are a useful shorthand, which helps in the definition and resolution of problems.

Some personalities can, for instance, be described as anxious. Whatever the situation, such people always find themselves with a higher than average level of anxiety. They may feel worried about going to meetings, even if they are on good terms with all the other attenders. They are nervous about going to social events and about asking questions, and often suffer from phobias such as fear of crowded areas, of open spaces or of travelling in lifts.

Anxious personalities are often born with a genetic loading toward anxiety — their parents and close relatives often suffer from similar problems. As children, they are often bed-wetters or nail-biters, are frightened of the dark and are scared of animals and/or people. All children have some of these problems, but anxious children suffer from most of them.

If you are born with a certain level of anxiety, there is little point in trying to overcome it by sheer will power. The harder you try, the greater will be the anxiety about failure. And the greater the anxiety, the worse your performance. It is, thus, important for anxious personalities to be aware of their limitations and to make a careful choice of job, of living environment and the like, so that they do not expose themselves to intolerable levels of stress.

People with other personality types also expose themselves to a potential overload of stress. They include obsessional personalities, who create stress by their meticulous attention to detail and introspective types, who think long and hard about every event and worry about its implications for themselves and others. Thus they tend to find reasons for 'standing still' or for simply doing nothing.

How personality is formed
It is still not clear whether we are born with a certain type of personality or whether our personality is determined by the events we experience throughout our lives. The answer is almost certainly a mixture of the two. You are born with a certain type of personality, and your personality develops as a result of your childhood experiences. Certainly a tendency toward anxiety is inherited. This covers a whole range of personality types, from people who are obsessional to those who are withdrawn because they are unable to cope, for example, with social pressures and decision-taking.

Other types of personality, such as having low self-esteem or being over-controlled, are probably learned. Children who grow up in situations in which they are not allowed to express feelings of anger and frustration find that, as adults, they have an inability for such expression. Children brought up in homes where there is no affection find it difficult as adults to give and take affection; while children from homes in which both parents are achievers find themselves under severe pressure to become achievers themselves — because achievement is the thing that they were rewarded for as youngsters. This aspect of upbringing can have a marked effect on their personalities as adults.

The development of personality can also have something to do with physical factors such as height or weight. A child who is physically small often tries to make up for it by becoming more aggressive and determined to succeed. This may be done in an attempt to acquire some sort of status or authority. An overweight child may act in an extrovert way in an attempt to cope with the jibes of peers and become one of the crowd.

Self-esteem
One of the most important factors underlying stress-prone personalities is self-esteem, that is, the value we place upon ourselves. If you are born with a genetic loading toward high anxiety, this does not do a great deal of damage, provided that you feel worthy and lovable and that you do not need to prove yourself all the time. Problems certainly begin if you have high anxiety and low self-esteem. You may pressurize yourself so much that you become an extreme type A personality (see chart).

As parents, it is important to encourage children to develop a sense of self-esteem. Children should grow up feeling loved and secure. Goals that are set for children should be consistent and attainable. And the goals should not be changed as soon as they have been reached. Children should be told that they are doing well and not made to feel that they are a constant disappointment to their parents.

Children who grow up with self-doubts distrust others, resent injustice and fear betrayal. They continually pressure themselves to achieve, to be more aggressive and competent than others. They find it difficult to form stable relationships, for fear of being betrayed.

Can personality be changed?
Although it is impossible to undergo a complete change of personality, it is possible — within the constraints of the personality that has developed over many years and has been reinforced by people and events — for personality to be modified to some degree.

If you consider that there are aspects of your personality that you would like to change, take a close look at yourself, what you are and the way you think. Notice how you add to your own stresses and difficulties by the way you react. Then use the techniques described throughout this chapter and elsewhere in the book to help you make a change. Things may never be perfect, but by thinking positively and changing some aspects of your life, you can improve the quality and quantity of your life. Never forget that stress, if it is out of control, shortens or depreciates the quality of life, making it generally less pleasant for ourselves and those around us.

In the 1960s, two American scientists, Mayer Friedman and Ray Rosenman, devised a way of classifying personalities that has important implications for the way we deal with stress.

Type A
● Unremitting urge to compete.
● Easily aroused to anger, irritation, aggravation and impatience.
● Aggressive with people who get in their way.
● Cannot bear delays or waiting in queues.
● Speak in a loud, staccato. Tend to interrupt and to finish other people's sentences for them.
● More likely to smoke cigarettes.
● Twice the risk of coronary heart disease and death from heart attacks as type B personalities.

Type B
● Do not feel the constant urge to compete.
● Relaxed, not easily roused to explosive reactions.
● Tolerant toward others.
● Able to wait patiently.
● Speak slowly and calmly, do not interrupt. Good listeners.
● Less likely to smoke cigarettes.
● Half the risk of coronary heart disease and heart attacks as type A personalities.

The implications of these findings is that type A personalities need to learn relaxation to control their behaviour. Physical relaxation and self-talk (pp. 234-5), meditation (pp. 288-9), autogenics (pp. 286-7) and biofeedback (pp. 284-5) are among the many helpful techniques that can be used.

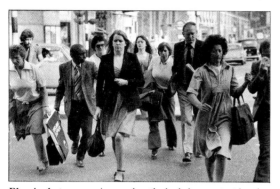

Physical stress, as imposed on the body by constant bustle, poor posture, ill-fitting or inappropriate shoes and by carrying shopping incorrectly, can cause muscle tension. This may provoke stress by activating the nervous system and thus preventing muscle relaxation.

Stress is the response within our bodies that occurs when some kind of external event 'threatens' us. Surprisingly, perhaps, stress is the general response of the human body to any demand made on it, regardless of whether or not that demand is pleasant, and whether it is emotional or physical. The stressful effects of accidents or bereavements, or of simply trying to keep up with the many tasks we have to accomplish during the day, are obvious. But the body's response to happy events, such as getting married, having a baby, receiving an increase in salary or falling in love, are just the same as for unpleasant events.

Is stress necessary?

All living creatures need challenges to keep them stimulated, and man is no exception to the rule. Without challenges he becomes dull and apathetic and loses the will to live life to the full. The 'soft' life is, therefore, not as attractive as it may sound. In fact, it holds as many potential dangers to fitness and well-being as one in which there is a high degree of stress.

For primitive man, the challenges that were posed were largely physical. In modern society, physical challenges are few, and those that do exist tend to be self-created, such as those of sport. Instead, we are regularly faced with challenges that concern our emotions. These emanate from our work and our home life, from the tasks we have to accomplish and from our relationships with other people.

Challenges are not only necessary but are also enjoyable and can raise your performance to unexpected heights. Watching a horror movie, taking part in a high-risk sport or tackling a difficult piece of work successfully, can all provide you with an inner thrill. And anxiety, as long as it is controlled, can help you perform your best in all kinds of tasks, from taking academic examinations to handling business meetings or competing in a club tennis tournament.

Stress thresholds

Overt, damaging stress occurs when the challenges that are imposed on us become, too much to cope with at that time. In this sense, stress is a protective reaction to too much challenge. The effect of too much stress may manifest itself in a variety of ways and cause potentially harmful changes in your behaviour and/or your physical health (see pp. 230-1).

Apart from being deprived of food or sleep, there are no situations or circumstances that are universally stress-inducing. People vary widely in the amount of challenge they can take before adverse effects start to occur. This means that while some people can cope easily with, for example, the demands of a job that involves regular international travel, others find such a challenge intolerable.

Similarly, the threshold at which potentially harmful stress reactions occur in any individual vary with different stresses and in different circumstances. Thus you may find it easy to cope with the stresses of office life but more difficult to cope with the challenges of parenthood, of managing your personal finances or of maintaining a loving relationship with your partner. Or you may find your work easy to cope with when you are alone, but difficult or impossible when tackled in a noisy office.

The factors that determine human stress thresholds are many and varied. They include past experience, personality, self-discipline and the discipline imposed by society and by circumstances. As a rule, however, people whose lives and relationships can be labelled 'successful' are those who have the highest tolerance of all kinds of stress.

The success of such people need by no means be material and may be achieved in any aspect of life, from the family home to the factory floor. These are the people who have learned to cope

The cause of stress
Stress is nothing new, but the 20th century has produced many changes that have increased the amount of stress people experience.

● Any change that upsets our accustomed pattern of life can cause stress.

● Economic changes have increased the pressure on us. In an age of speed and easy, worldwide communication there is much less 'breathing space' than in the past.

● More decisions have to be made nowadays. The average person has a high degree of responsibility and accountability.

● We have a wider range of choices at all levels of our lives, in our work and in our leisure.

● Overcrowding, noise and pollution have resulted from an increase in population.

● We have come to demand higher quality of communication and understanding in all our relationships.

● Technology has affected our work, leisure and relationships. Human contact is decreasing as a result.

● Unemployment, which will be a fact of life in the future, is stressful because we still see work as indicative of success in society.

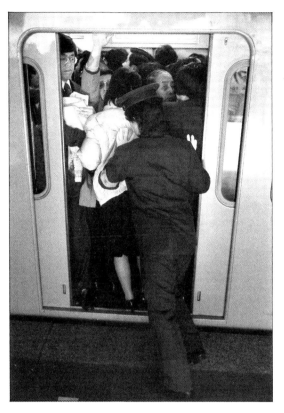

Rush hour travel, with passengers packed like sardines into trains and buses, is just one of the many stressful aspects of modern city life.

with stress and to overcome it, and who have learned how to equate their aspirations and attributes with the reality of life. They may be tired at the end of the day, but their morale is high and their health is not suffering.

Stress and fitness
While the body's general reactions to stress are the same for everyone, the adverse effects do not strike everyone equally. One of the important aspects of dealing with stress is, thus, to know your body and the way it reacts to challenges that are too severe. These adverse effects are automatic and subconscious and may range from being irritable or overeating to coming out in spots, developing migraine or having heartburn. Once you understand the stresses in your life and begin to cope with them, so you will find that it is possible to control your own stress-related symptoms (see pp. 234-7).

Stress and expectation
As long as you feel that there is a good correspondence between the world as it is and the relationships that you have, and the world as you expect it to be, you are unlikely to suffer from stress as a result of the conflict between expectation and reality. But if the reality and fantasy of what life should be are different, stress emerges.

When assessing the role of expectation in your own life, and the amount of stress it provokes, remember:
● Expectations are taught from our earliest childhood. To avoid stress it may be necessary to 'unlearn' some of them.

● The nature of the society in which we live brings with it certain expectations. We are expected to be competent, to achieve, to conform.

● Your expectations are subtly moulded by the media. The expectation of perfection induces stress if you try too hard to live up to it.

● Your feelings of self-worth are likely to depend on whether you live up to your standards or expectations. It is more important to learn to live with yourself (within limits) as you are.

● The beliefs that you accept unquestioningly as truths will lead to increased stress because they blind you to alternative courses of action.

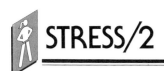
Reactions to stress

Throughout life, all the component parts of the body strive to work together in efficient harmony, reacting constantly to the demands made on them from within and without. Many of these demands pose a threat to the body, which responds to them in a specific way.

This is both universal and primitive. The body's response to threat of any kind is to prepare itself for fight or flight. First, in a reflex action, the muscles become tense. After this, a whole series of reactions comes into operation.

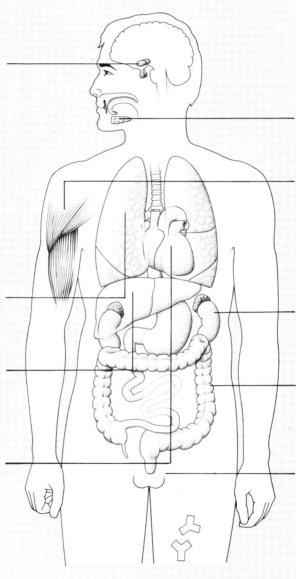

The hypothalamus at the base of the brain becomes activated and stimulates the pituitary gland to release hormones. These then stimulate the adrenal glands above the kidneys to produce further hormones, which have wide-ranging effects on the body. Some body activities are increased, others decreased.

The pupils of the eyes dilate.

Breathing rate speeds up to supply more oxygen to the muscles.

Blood pressure rises.

The liver discharges sugars into the blood to provide muscles with extra energy. It may also produce and release excess amounts of the substance cholesterol.

Heart rate increases to supply more blood to the muscles.

Sweat production from the skin is increased, ready to cool down a body overheated by the exertion of fight or flight.

The skin becomes pale as blood is shunted away from it.

The salivary glands stop secreting saliva, making the mouth feel dry.

Muscles may ache. Pain may also result from the slow mobilization of lactic acid.

Kidneys work less efficiently because their blood supply is reduced.

Digestion ceases or slows down.

Defaecation and urination are prevented by the tightening of muscles. Alternatively, diarrhoea or uncontrolled urination may take place.

The immune system works below its normal level, making a person susceptible to disease or to an allergic reaction.

Physical symptoms of stress
Do you recognize two or more of the following in yourself or someone close to you? If so, the stress problem needs to be tackled immediately (see pp.234-7).

● Have your eating habits changed?

● Has your sleep pattern altered?

● Is your digestive system upset?

● Have you developed any nervous habits such as fidgeting, touching your hair and face repeatedly. (It is changes in behaviour that are significant. If an activity has become ingrained, it is a habit, not a sign of stress.)

● Is your blood pressure raised?

● Do you have frequent headaches, cramps, and muscle spasms?

● Do you feel breathless although you have not been exerting yourself?

● Do you suffer from fainting spells?

● Do you often cry or feel like crying?

● Has your sexual performance, drive and enjoyment deteriorated?

● Are you drinking or smoking more?

● Has a child reverted to an earlier, outgrown habit, such as bed-wetting, temper tantrums or thumb-sucking?

The first reaction of the body to any potentially harmful demands made on it is to prepare itself for action. It gets ready to face danger (fight) or to run away (flight). To understand this process, consider what most usefully happens to a person's body if it is attacked by a wild animal.

Priority areas are the muscles, to make the body ready for physical action, and the heart, so that it can pump more blood to those muscles. The lungs need to provide more oxygen to the muscles for energy and to the brain for alertness. High-energy foods, stored as sugars and fats, are released into the blood, but because of the overriding need of the muscles, the blood flow to organs such as the digestive system is cut off.

When immediate danger passes, this 'gearing up' process is almost exactly reversed. And it seems that the act of fighting or running away actually helps this reversal process. In our everyday lives, however, we encounter many threatening situations in which we cannot fight or flee. Since there is no physical action we can take, the reversal process does not occur, and we stay 'wound up'. This is one good reason why exercise is so effective in stress relief.

Adaptation and exhaustion
When the body is exposed to stress over a long period, the biochemical state of the body—constantly prepared for fight or flight—becomes chronic. Blood pressure is permanently raised and digestive problems arise. Tension in the muscles leads to aches and pains, and disease or allergic responses may occur.

This adaptation stage can last for many years without major mental or physical breakdown. Whether it will do so depends on physical constitution (determined by heredity), on personality and attitudes, on health habits such as diet and exercise, and on social relationships.

Not surprisingly, unless action is taken at the adaptation stage to alter either the stress factors themselves or the body's reaction to them, exhaustion sets in. No longer able to cope, the body collapses into disease or a person becomes helpless in coping with psychological demands.

It is thus essential to be able to recognize the signs of stress. Use the symptoms listed on this page as a guide, but remember that many of them can result from causes other than stress, and that it is *change* that is most relevant.

Mental symptoms of stress
Do you recognize two or more of the following in yourself or in someone close to you? If so, stress is reaching a potentially dangerous level.

● Have you begun to suffer from a phobia or obsession?

● Have you lost self-confidence and self-esteem?

● Have you lost interest in life?

● Do you constantly feel guilty?

● Do you dread the future?

● Have your memory and concentration deteriorated?

● Do you find yourself unable to finish one task properly before having to rush on to the next?

● Do you feel constantly irritable and angry?

● Do you feel isolated?

● Do you fill the day with trivial tasks?

● Do you find it hard to take decisions?

● Does your mind race so that you cannot focus on one task or thought?

● Are you physically hyperactive?

Whether you are a driver or a passenger, travel can be one of the most significant sources of stress in your life. Although many people find that going for a drive can help them unwind when they feel tense or angry, research suggests that driving is, in fact, enormously stressful.

Drivers and passengers

The stress associated with driving is caused by many factors, including noise and vibration, fatigue, the behaviour of the passengers and the traffic. Studies on rush-hour drivers show them to experience marked rises in heart rate, blood pressure and electrical skin resistance — all reliable indicators of inner stress.

The very act of driving also appears to effect a personality change. While aggressive people become even more so when driving, what is more surprising is that people who are normally restrained, calm and unassertive can reveal the same aggression as soon as they are placed behind the wheel of a motor car. It has been suggested that inside the car the driver feels alone and secure and becomes aggressive because he experiences no face-to-face confrontation.

As drivers, our responses to traffic are of mounting irritability and hostility — as if someone has to be 'blamed'. To our own amazement, we feel postively murderous about drivers in front of or behind us and take it as a personal affront if someone overtakes us or prevents us from getting ahead. And these feelings are multiplied if we feel envious or dismissive of either the driver or of the other car. Furthermore, our 'fight or flight' response (see pp. 230-1) will make us try to release our tensions through more aggressiveness and risk-taking. Add to all this the frustrations and exhaustions of a day's work, and your 'stress total' can be excessive.

As passengers in all forms of transport we may fare little better. Frustrations arise as we wait for bus, train or taxi and mount with increased waiting time. The queue is another source of frustration, exaggerated by people who rush ahead of us and will not wait their turn. Anxiety and stress also arise as we worry whether we will arrive at our destination in time for an appointment, and these feelings are made more intense by each delay along the route.

Other passengers are also a source of stress. We may feel resentment — unjustifiable but part of being human — that others have a seat on public transport and we have not. By the end of a journey fraught with difficulties, the behaviour of other passengers, down to everyday actions such as blowing the nose or coughing, can trigger extreme resentment.

Add to such stresses those brought about by bureaucratic procedures, such as checking in at an airport or being woken up in a train for a ticket to be clipped, and it is no wonder that you arrive at your destination harrassed and irritable. And the cup of coffee you are offered on your arrival to calm you down has the effect of exacerbating, rather than reducing, your stress symptoms (see pp. 244-5).

Reducing travel stress

There are many practical ways in which you can reduce the amount of stress to which you subject yourself when travelling, especially when driving.
● Learn to calculate journey times sensibly. Add on extra time for inevitable delays.
● Resign yourself to the fact that there is no way of speeding-up arrival times.
● Sit as comfortable as you possibly can, especially behind the wheel of a car. Check that your shoulders are not hunched, your teeth are not clenched and that your hands are not gripping the wheel too tightly.
● Reduce neck tension with relaxing movements of the head.
● Do not drive for more than 2 or 3 hours without a break. At breaks, take a short walk or a nap and eat a light snack.
● Change your position regularly.
● If children or other passengers create a disturbance, stop the car and explain that it is unsafe to continue.
● Learn to suspend, rather than give in to, frustration. Use your imagination. Try labelling a reckless driver as 'probably someone whose loved one is on the danger list in hospital', the poor driver as 'someone who is on a once-a-year outing'.
● Find a less frustrating means of travel.

Coping with jetlag

Many family holidays and business trips have been marred by jetlag. The reason behind this is that, when local time changes, our body rhythms take several days, or even weeks, to make a

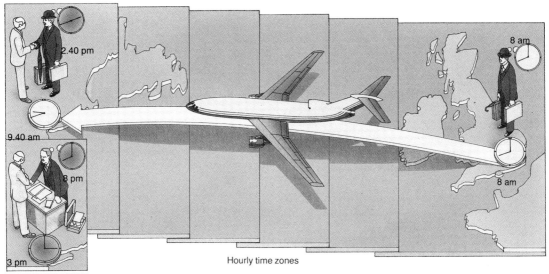

Hourly time zones

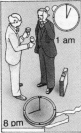

A British businessman leaves London for New York at
8 am. He travels 5,600 km (3,500 mls) across 5 time zones in
6 hr 40 min. He arrives at his destination at 9.40 am, New
York time. His body clock registers 2.40 pm London time.
Arriving at his American office at 1 pm he is in time for a
working lunch, and the serious business is done at 3 pm, when
he is still performing at peak level. At 8 pm New York time,
he goes out to celebrate. By this time he is too tired to enjoy
himself and the drink quickly goes to his head. It would have
been more sensible for him to have eaten a light meal and to
have retired early to bed.

Training for local time

Cope with jetlag by
preparing your body
beforehand.
● Calculate the time
difference between
home and your
destination.

● For a few days before
your journey, start going
to bed an hour earlier or
an hour later each night
(depending on whether
you are travelling east
or west).

● Rise an hour earlier
or an hour later each
morning.

● Adjust your meal
times to the new
schedule.

complete adjustment to the new time zone.

Jetlag should not be ignored in the hope that it
can be surmounted by sheer effort or with sleeping pills. Rather you should adopt the approach
that you will either keep to home time or train
yourself for the new local time before you travel.
If neither of these is possible or practicable, you
should attempt to arrive at the best possible
compromise.

Plan ahead so that events will fit in best with
your own home rhythm, whether these are for
business or pleasure. Plan your flight so that you
make life easy for yourself. A late afternoon or
evening flight from Europe, for example, will
bring you to California in the late evening. If you
have slept on the plane, as your body clock would
tell you to do, you will arrive refreshed and ready
for an evening meal. You should then get some
sleep that night and be reasonably fresh next day.
Sleep will be easier if you take some exercise at
any stops en route and when you arrive at your
destination.

Decision-making

After a long flight:
● Do not make
decisions when your
body clock says you
should be asleep.

● Schedule important
decisions to fit in best
with your body clock.

● Do not make
decisions until you have
had at least one good
night's sleep following
your arrival.

● Do not make
decisions if you have
recently arrived from a
different time zone and
have had a heavy meal.

Two important strategies in discovering how to deal with stress are learning to relax and learning to modify your behaviour so as to alleviate stress or avoid it. Relaxation helps lessen stress by distracting your mind away from stress-provoking thoughts. It may also bring into play those parts of the nervous system that work to counter the effects of the 'fight or flight' reaction (see pp. 230–1). Relaxation is a skill well worth learning, although it takes considerable practice, and mastery comes slowly. To help you, use the hints and tips given in the chart below.

As an alternative to physical relaxation, try the positive use of your imagination. Imagine, for example, a pleasant or peaceful scene; concentrate on all the colours, smells and sounds, and continue for 10 to 15 minutes. If it helps, buy a sound-effects tape to increase the reality of the scene. Or imagine a favourite painting or piece of music. You could also try techniques such as meditation (pp. 288-9), yoga (pp 280–3), massage (pp. 268–71), autogenic training (pp. 286–7) or biofeedback (pp. 284–5).

In effective stress reduction, as well as in maintaining more general bodily fitness, exercise, diet and sleep play an enormous part. All too often people become so involved in the serious business of living that they never find the time or energy to play. So make sure that you regularly do things just for fun. This may be taking a walk in the countryside or a park, or going to the cinema, or even doing something you would normally think of as childish, such as jumping in the autumn leaves or splashing in puddles. Life may be a worry, but do try to see the funny side of things. Laughter is a great antidote for stress— and if you can laugh, those around you will feel less stress from being in your company.

A change of routine

Breaking routines helps remove the stress that is bound into our own personal rituals. For example, try coming home by a different route. Pick up a small present for yourself or a loved one on the way home. And when you arrive home, don't always do the same thing. Similarly, at weekends, do not get into a stress-making routine. Vary your activities as much as you can, for the benefit of yourself and the family.

As a rule, increasing your level of activity will be beneficial in reducing stress. The list of possi-

bilities is endless, but why not try walking, singing, window shopping, sunbathing, cooking, painting, gardening or concert going? None is guaranteed to remove all stress, but what is certain is that if you do nothing and change nothing, then stress and its responses will continue as before.

Helping others through voluntary work is a positive approach to stress relief. This is not due to the fact that seeing others with greater problems than your own puts your own life in perspective (although this may be an agreeable bonus), but because helping others involves new social interactions and the use of talents that would otherwise remain untapped. If, however, you start voluntary work but find it competitive or stressful in some other way, you should have no qualms about stopping at once.

Letting off steam is a good way of relieving tension, and it is probably no coincidence that people who bottle things up are often those who suffer most from the physical illnesses associated with stress. But if you *are* going to yell at those around you, always let them know that it is not their fault, just you letting go of your anger and frustration. One of the best, but equally the most difficult, stress-relieving strategies, is to change your responses to the events around you. In a traffic jam, for example, instead of honking your horn and fuming, try leaning back and relaxing. Wind down the window and see if you can catch someone's eye and make them smile. There is no magic solution except to try. And if your first attempt does not work, do not give up—try something different.

Self-talk

When you watch children carrying out tasks such as tying their shoelaces, it is interesting that they talk themselves through the action. Without this chatter, the task is difficult to learn and perform. Recent research has suggested that this approach is also useful to adults, especially when they switch from negative to positive talk.

As you talk to yourself, use the examples in the chart opposite as a guide. Be sure to concentrate on the good, not the bad aspects of the problem in hand. Do not be self-conscious or embarrassed if you find you are talking to yourself aloud. Finding a way to deal with stress is more important than temporary loss of face.

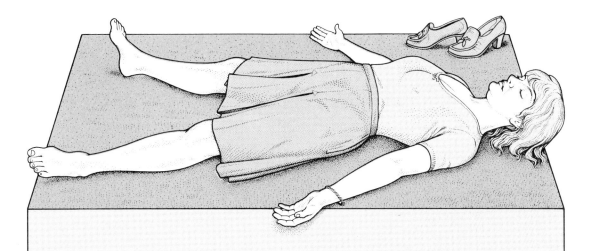

Learning relaxation
1 Do not try to learn relaxation when you are feeling tired. You will learn better and more effectively when you are alert.
2 Try to minimize background sources of stress such as noise and the presence of other people.
3 Do not rush or watch the clock. If you are worried about going on too long, set an alarm to ring after a period of, say, 20 minutes.
4 If you are not succeeding, *do not* try harder. This will only make you more tense. Instead, give yourself a rest for a couple of days and start again, giving most emphasis to the parts of the exercise you found most effective.

Before you begin
1 Choose a quiet, comfortable place.
2 Loosen any tight clothing and take off your shoes.
3 Sit or lie as comfortably as possible.
4 Close your eyes, uncross your legs and hold your hands flat, one on each knee.

Relaxing each body part
Tense each part of the body as described below for a count of 10. Take a deep breath in, feel the tension, then let the tension go as you breathe out, quietly saying the word 'relax' to yourself as you do so to reinforce the message of relaxation.
Toes: curl your toes toward you or down to the floor.
Calves: point your toes toward your face.
Buttocks: push your buttocks hard against your chair or bed, at the same time trying to make your body feel as heavy as possible.

Abdomen: tense your abdomen, as if preparing to receive a punch in the stomach.
Shoulders: shrug your shoulders as high as they can possibly go.
Throat: use your chin to press your throat hard.
Neck and head: press your neck and head against the backs of your shoulders.
Face: tighten as many facial muscles as possible, including forehead, jaw, chin and nose.

Quick relaxation
If there is no time to complete the full procedure, or it is not convenient, use the following actions, tensing and relaxing as above. You can perform such actions unobtrusively in all manner of situations.
1 Tighten and tense the whole of the upper part of your body.
2 Pull in your abdomen or tense your buttocks.
3 Try to force your body off the chair by pressing the soles of your feet hard against the floor and trying to lift your body using your calf and other leg muscles.

Self-talk
Use the following examples to work out some possibilities for yourself:
1 'It may be difficult, but I am going to go through the argument with them again.'
2 'I must turn down that extra work. I can cope now, but with extra I will be snowed under.'
3 'I know I am being yelled at, but she is under stress too and has probably had a bad day.'

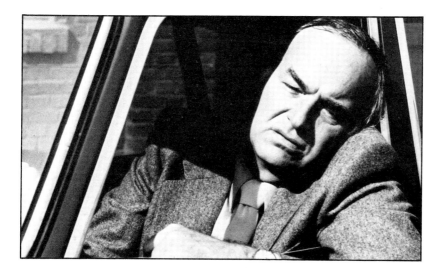

If car travel is a part of your daily routine, be aware of the stress it can involve. If it is impossible to avoid travelling in this way, use delays and traffic jams to advantage by taking the time to relax. Do not become agitated and overstressed by a situation you have no power to change.

Many of the events that we experience produce stress. This is not because of the events themselves, but because of the interpretation we put on those events. The reason for this stems from the mythologies and expectations we have. Some of these we get from our parents, some from our teachers and our peers but most come from the outside world. How many of these can you recognize in yourself?

● I must be competent and win the approval of people I think are significant to me.
● I must please everyone.
● Happiness comes from the outside.
● Life must deal justly with me.
● Others must give me reward and support me whatever I do.
● There is always a clear cut and identifiable solution to any problem.
● I must never make mistakes.
● I must never fail.

Along with the mythologies come the expectations. How many of us think, for example, that people should always be fair and reasonable to us, or never disappoint us?

The consequences of mythologies

Invariably, stress is the consequence of our mythologies. If you feel that you must win the approval of everyone around you, you will spend a great deal of time doing what other people want

— or what you *think* they want. Since it is impossible to please everybody, your actions will be inconsistent and arbitrary. Even more important, you will always be frustrated.

If you believe that happiness comes from the outside, you will waste a lot of time chasing it — and fail to find it. All the evidence suggests that happiness comes from within yourself. You will be similarly disappointed if you believe that justice is always to be expected in life. And you will become stressed almost daily as you bewail your situation. Believing that there is always a clear solution to a problem means that you will often spend a great deal of time seeking non-existent answers.

Never to make mistakes means that you will spend your whole life checking and double-checking. It also means that you cannot admit you are wrong. If you believe that you must never fail, then you are much more likely to do so.

To reduce the stress caused by mythologies and expectations, you must learn to accept the realities of life and to use those realities to best effect. Use a step-by-step approach. First, ask yourself what your own 'shoulds' or 'musts' really are and write them down. Then challenge your own rules, asking yourself, 'Why must I think this way?: Is it so awful if I don't live up to my rule?'

Next, revise the rules to make them more reasonable. Use self-talk methods, saying to yourself things such as, 'It would be nice if others thought well of me. I certainly would feel uncomfortable if everybody did not like me. But if some people do not like me, I think I can live with that. Besides which, I like myself, even if someone else does not.'

Problem solving
The first stage in solving stress-inducing problems is to *define* them clearly. Ask yourself whether a problem is related to a particular situation or is a general reaction — for example, is it all criticism that upsets you, or criticism from particular people? Look, too, for the reasons underlying other people's reactions rather than assuming that it is you who are at fault. You should then think out a wide range of possible solutions, rejecting those which you know from experience do not work. Do not fool yourself into thinking that, if you try hard enough, a chosen solution must work. This is not true. It is trying *well*, in seeking out feasible rather than impossible solutions, not trying *hard* that is important.

Now ask yourself how others might respond if asked to solve a similar problem. This will not only generate more ideas but will help put the problem in perspective. Next, rank each suggested approach in order of desirability and try out the most feasible. Evaluate the results, and use any failures as feedback for attempting a renewed and different approach.

Coping with failure
No one can cheat the laws of chance and win all the time. This is a fact of life. But when some people fail, they sink into a state of 'learned helplessness', in which they lose their ability to believe that they will ever master the situation. People with a keen sense of failure also tend to judge situations as more important to their own self-esteem than they really are. And, unfortunately, they are often afraid to ask others for help or favours, so they do not make the most of the resources available. Remember that it is not whether you fail that determines your success, but how you cope with failure.

If your responses are not resolving your difficulties, then change your response. It is only you who can improve your own performance. You cannot keep blaming past events or other people for your current poor performance. You may get a good deal of sympathy, but you will not achieve the results you want.

Sleep is an activity essential to fitness and well-being. Yet many people have trouble in sleeping well, or worry that the amount of sleep they do get is inadequate for their needs. The massive consumption of sleeping tablets alone is a testament to this fact.

Although you may think you need a certain amount of sleep each night, it is the quality rather than the quantity of sleep that seems to be significant. And too much sleep can make you as irritable and impair your concentration as much as too little.

The amount of sleep that people need varies widely. Some can manage with as little as 5 hours a night, others need 8 or even 9 hours. It does seem, however, that the symptoms resulting from lack of sleep are due as much to feelings of being deprived of sleep, as actually having lost necessary sleeping time.

Sleep and stress

Stress is probably the largest single cause of sleeplessness. What is worse, stress not only leads to insomnia, but insomnia increases stress by producing worries about whether you are getting enough sleep to cope with the next day's problems – and so a vicious circle begins.

People vary in their basic levels of anxiety and this has a bearing on individual sleep patterns. Low arousal people remain calm in most situations and have few if any sleep problems. High arousal people – the worriers – are the ones that lie awake with alert, anxious minds at night. If they fall asleep and then wake up, the anxious thoughts and worries begin again almost immediately, and they find it difficult to drop off to sleep once more.

Most of us fall between these two extremes, and it is only the occasional worry that disturbs our sleep. Unfortunately, the more painful the worry, the more we try to forget it and the more it affects our sleep. When you are under stress, you may, thus, have difficulty in getting to sleep and/or have lengthy periods of wakefulness during the night. In clinical depression, however, it is early morning wakening, rather than getting to sleep, that is the problem.

Temporary insomnia caused by short-term worries, such as moving house or an important business meeting, is not a problem. Long-term worries, however, such as redundancy, emotional upheavals or serious illness in the family, can cause chronic insomnia.

Whenever the mind is unoccupied – as it is immediately before sleep – the 'gap' is filled by worry. This sort of insomnia usually improves

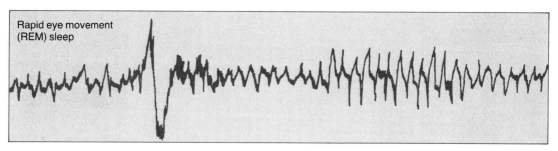

Rapid eye movement (REM) sleep

Sleep consists of several stages, which can be recorded in the brain as electroencephalograms or EEGs. On average, we lie in bed for 15 minutes before falling asleep. Blood pressure, heart rate and body temperature fall. Consciousness shifts from one subject to another. This is Stage 1 sleep. Soon Stage 2 sleep appears. The sleeper is unconscious and heart rate has slowed further. Stage 3 is deeper still, and Stage 4 the deepest.

Some 60 to 90 minutes after the onset of sleep, the heart rate increases, and the eyes dart about beneath closed lids. This is rapid eye movement, or REM, sleep which is associated with dreaming. The sleeper then descends to Stage 2. The next move is to Stages 3 and 4, back through 3 and 2, and into another REM period. The cycle from deep sleep to REM and back again usually repeats itself 4 to 6 times during the night.

It is known that Stages 3 and 4 are essential to avoid feelings of lethargy next day. Loss of REM sleep leads to aggressiveness and irritability. Sleeping pills and other drugs interfere with Stages 3 and 4 and with REM sleep.

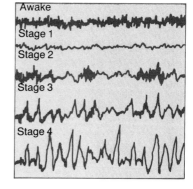

Awake
Stage 1
Stage 2
Stage 3
Stage 4

Getting a better night's sleep

Although the same strategies are not equally successful for everyone, there are some do's and don'ts that should be helpful to most people.

Do:

● Set up and follow pre-sleep routines. A ritual and gradual 'winding down' seems important for many people. This may consist of light exercises followed by a hot bath, a warm milk drink and a short read.

● Take regular exercise.

● Get up earlier in the morning.

● Make your sleep schedule as regular as possible. Go to bed at about the same time each night but, more important, get up at the same time each morning, even if you feel you could do with an extra few minutes or hours in bed.

● Keep warm.

● Drink a glass of milk or a milk drink. Milk contains tryptophan, a substance which promotes sleep.

Don't:

● Eat food that leads to the production of gas in the stomach a few hours before going to bed. Such foods include fruit, beans, nuts and raw vegetables. Don't eat high-fat foods, which keep your digestive system active.

● Drink alcohol. A small amount can help sleep, but too much can rob you of important REM sleep.

with the solution of the problem, but the insomnia may be so ingrained that it persists. Anxiety shifts away from the basic problem to whether or not sleep will arrive. If you do suffer from chronic insomnia, you should discuss the problem with your doctor.

Surprisingly, for some people anxiety or misery can lead to more sleep than usual. In this situation, sleep seems to provide a means of escape from problems.

Sleeping pills

For curing short-term, acute insomnia, pills are useful, but they may impair the quality of sleep and produce feelings of 'hangover' next day. For chronic insomnia they are not advisable because they are drugs of dependence.

If you want to stop using sleeping pills, which is to be recommended, try to cut down gradually and be prepared to experience more restless sleep than you have been used to. Remember that getting back to your normal sleeping pattern will take several weeks and that it will take you time to overcome your physical and psychological dependence on the drugs. Remember, too, that exercise will help, since physical tiredness will help override anxiety.

Dreams and sleep

We all dream, but our dreams are often quickly forgotten. It may be that the dreams that have most meaning to us are the ones we are most likely to recall on awakening. Also, dreams are easiest to remember if we are awoken immediately after a period of REM sleep (see diagram).

Dreams are not now thought to be essential ingredients of sleep. It is REM sleep and not dreams, that is critical to the quality of sleep. Many students of dreams have thought that dreaming helps the mind to sort out problems or reveals hidden feelings, but there is no concrete evidence for this.

Nightmares can be thought of as anxiety dreams – there is no evidence that eating cheese before sleeping causes them, although they may be brought about by alcohol. If you are anxious or depressed and having nightmares unusually often, it would be sensible to try to tackle the underlying problem, perhaps with the initial help of your family doctor.

If you are having difficulties in getting to sleep:

● Avoid taking naps – they aggravate the problem.

● Try relaxation. For most people, muscle relaxation or psychological relaxation (shifting your mind to pleasant events) will help.

● Change your nightly routine. For example, change your bed time, go out in the evening or don't read in bed.

Other strategies

If the above measures do not work, try the following:

● If your mind wanders while you try to accomplish a mental task, change to one that occupies you but does not increase your anxiety. For example, try to take yourself on a guided tour of a house you lived in as a child. Try to imagine a favourite piece of music or plan a holiday. Imagine a favourite walk, step by step.

● Deliberately try to stay awake. If you are sleepless for more than about 15 minutes, get out of bed. You might try attacking a task you have put off, such as writing a letter.

● Don't worry or panic about lack of sleep. You are unlikely to miss so much sleep that your performance will be impaired.

● Don't smoke or drink coffee at bedtime or if you wake during the night. Both are stimulants.

Stress is thought to play a significant part in producing, maintaining or worsening disease. This is particularly so the case in illnesses such as stomach and duodenal ulcers, high blood pressure and hypertension, in which stress is known to be a contributory factor.

It is not difficult to understand why this should be so. If the body is constantly on 'red alert', its chemistry changes, and these changes may well be important in precipitating certain illnesses. Heart and circulatory problems, for example, are commonly accepted as being greatly influenced by the state of stress arousal of the sufferer. And stress is implicated in medical problems such as asthma, rheumatoid arthritis, eczema, migraine and depression.

As well as being a causative factor in chronic disease, stress produces its own, specific set of symptoms associated with the 'fight or flight' reaction (see pp.230-1). People who are under constant stress report frequent indigestion, heartburn, insomnia, a tendency to sweat for no good reason, headaches, cramps and muscle spasms (for example, back pain), nausea, breathlessness and many digestive ills.

This list of illnesses underlines the point that living with stress, and becoming accustomed to the effects it has on you, is potentially extremely harmful. It is much better to try to reduce stressful situations than to force yourself to get used to living with stress.

Hypochondria
Being a hypochondriac usually means that you have an abnormal amount of interest in, and fear about, the state of your health. The typical picture of a hypochondriac is of someone who goes to his doctor for every minor ache and pain, fearful that they may be a sign or symptom of something serious, or of someone who constantly batters family and friends about his illnesses or takes extravagant steps to avoid exposure to health hazards. While the true hypochondriac revels in being ill, the reverse is true of someone with 'illness phobia', who is terrified of contracting a fatal disease.

Many people who go to their doctors to discuss a long series of minor ailments do so, in fact, because they are frightened to reveal a major source of worry. This is particularly so in the case of stress-related disorders and marital and sexual problems. Once the major problem has been identified and solved, the minor ones often disappear. Similarly, many people suffer from psychosomatic pains, which are often stress induced but are no less painful than those associated with organic disease.

Depression
Anxiety and depression are closely related, and reactions to stress can often cause depression. There is no doubt that all of us are depressed from time to time—for periods lasting for a few minutes to days and more. Often we can identify the source of the depression—the loss of a friend or relative or of status, for example. Such depression is a normal part of human existence.

We often become depressed because of our inability to cope with life's demands, or about something that has yet to happen. Anticipation of a crisis, or even an unpleasant reaction from a superior, will often result in both anxiety and depression; but again, this is in no way abnormal.

Depression becomes a problem only when it gets out of proportion. It is accepted as 'normal' if someone becomes completely distraught as a result of grief after the death of a loved one. The loss of employment or health are all reasonable matters to mourn. But if a person is incapacitated for months or even years afterward, then professional help is needed.

As a person tries to cope with life and with his feelings, so depression causes changes in behaviour. Individual perception of the outside world becomes distorted, and events that a person would normally take in his stride become evidence of incompetence and incapability, and a sign that emergence from the 'black pit' is impossible.

The belief that there is no escape is characteristic of depression. Any stress is magnified, and the more frantic the attempts to cope, the worse things get. These attempts are markedly different from the person's normal approach toward problem solving. Thus failure occurs, and the depression deepens.

As concentration and memory become impaired and the situation worsens, sufferers will often cut themselves off from the world completely and stop fighting. They become housebound and, eventually, find it difficult to get out of bed. The feelings of inadequacy are such that

If you are depressed
Try the following:
● Seek out the source of the depression and change things. It may be difficult, for practical reasons, to make large changes, but a small one may be sufficient.

● Seek support. The support of friends and family is important to help overcome depression in its early stages. Make the effort to talk to people. Even if their advice is misguided, social contact will distract you from the problems of the moment. Every minute's respite from the depression helps in your quest for control over life.

● Change your pattern of living. Take up a hobby or start an exercise routine (exercise is a useful antidote to depression).

● Do not try to solve all your problems at once. This approach is doomed to failure, and failure will maintain the depression. Instead, consider your problems one at a time.

● Eat regularly. Depression tends to reduce the appetite. If you are to increase your level of activity, you will need adequate energy supplies.

● Realize that many of the thoughts you have, and the actions you are making, stem from your depression. When you are depressed, it is easy to become trapped into seeing all events as evidence of personal inadequacy.

suicide may be contemplated. (Contrary to popular belief, people who discuss suicide often *do* commit or attempt to commit it.)

Endogenous depression
There is another common form of depression whose source is a complete mystery. This sort of depression seems to come from within the body and is called endogenous depression; it is based on a biochemical change in the brain. It occurs suddenly, and with no obvious cause, unlike reactive depression which usually stems from easily identifiable events.

If you report to your doctor with depression, he will try to find out which type you are suffering from, bearing in mind that endogenous depression is often associated with early morning wakening and weight changes. Antidepressants are drugs that are useful for treating endogenous, but not reactive, depression.

For ways of coping with depression, consult the tips on this page. Most important of all is to seek professional help as soon as possible.

Phobias, obsessions and ruminations
Like many other problems, phobias are related to stress and anxiety. They are irrational fears —accepted as such by the sufferer—which produce disproportionate reactions. These reactions can totally disrupt a normal way of life.

Obsessions are also the result of irrational fears. Someone with an obsession does not avoid a situation but instead performs an action such as washing, cleaning or checking to avoid that distress. Like phobias, obsessions are not bizarre in themselves—they are simply extremes of behaviour that would otherwise be regarded as matter-of-fact. Checking your work carefully once or even twice is conscientious. Checking it four or five times is verging on the obsessional.

Ruminations are similar to obsessions and phobias. They involve anxiety-provoking thoughts such as, 'I am going to jump out of the window', although the action is not carried out. The thought is a touchstone that prevents the deed being committed but is frightening enough to force the sufferer to take avoiding action.

Phobias, obsessions and ruminations are at their worst when the sufferer is anxious, tired or depressed. Trying harder makes the problem worse, and professional help is essential.

If someone you know is depressed
At home or at work, look out for someone who shows a change in behaviour. Remember, when dealing with them:

● Emotional pain is as bad as physical pain.

● Do not tell someone to 'pull themselves together' or to 'snap out of it'.

● Do not report to a person all the features of their life that need improvement.

● The earlier help is sought the better. Encourage anyone who is depressed to seek help from a counsellor or psychologist. It is often the stigma attached to seeking such help that holds people back.

Phobias and obsessions; getting help
It may be time to seek help when one or more of these apply to you:

● The problem is becoming too great to manage.

● Your life is being disrupted by your symptoms.

● Life is becoming unbearable, either because you are fed up or because you know that the cause of your anxiety is unavoidable.

● You have many symptoms of anxiety or depression, such as trembling hands, palpitations and strange aches and pains.

● Others are urging you to seek help.

PRESCRIBED DRUGS

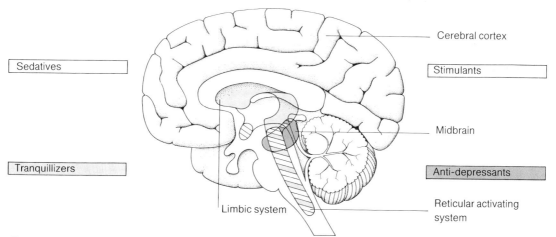

Sedatives

Cerebral cortex

Stimulants

Tranquillizers

Midbrain

Anti-depressants

Limbic system

Reticular activating system

Groups of prescribed drugs alter the activity of many parts of the brain but are designed to have a therapeutic effect by acting principally on the areas indicated. Sedatives lower the level of the conscious experience by acting on the cerebral cortex. Tranquillizers work on the limbic system, which is involved in determining mood and in memory. They also work on the reticular activating system (RAS) whose activities are crucial to the maintenance of consciousness. The RAS is also affected by stimulants and anti-depressants. The latter also act on the midbrain to alter mood.

The taking of drugs is one of man's most ancient ways of dealing with stress. The most recent additions to the list are drugs such as sleeping pills and tranquillizers, which are legally available only on prescription from a doctor.

Up to a point, these drugs are valuable. They can dull the anxiety associated with crisis or help us sleep when we are tense. Used irresponsibly, they produce more problems than they relieve. Dependence, hangover, rebound and side-effects are the hidden costs of drug use. And, most importantly of all, they do not solve problems but only mask their symptoms.

In an ideal world, we would all be able to confront and resolve the elements in our lives that are the cause of stress. We would be able to free ourselves from the vicious circle of anxiety, which, as it continues, diminishes our ability to cope with problems. Drugs are undoubtedly useful in breaking this circle, but after a 'bad patch' is over, they should be given up. All too often people do not, or cannot, do so.

The drugs prescribed

There are three major groups of drugs that your doctor might prescribe to help you cope with anxiety — major and minor tranquillizers and beta blockers. There is no real dividing line between sleeping tablets and tranquillizers. A tranquillizer taken in a high enough dose will induce sleep. A sleeping tablet taken in a low dose will reduce anxiety. Major tranquillizers, such as Largactil, Serenace, Stemetil or Mellaril, are used less frequently than the others and are most often reserved for the treatment of 'major' disorders that need treatment in psychiatric units or hospitals. But about 10 per cent of people being treated with anxiety-reducing drugs take one of the major tranquillizers.

Minor tranquillizers include the most popular drugs prescribed for anxiety such as Valium, Librium, Tranxene, Ativan and Mogadon. They are called 'minor' to distinguish them from the drugs used to treat major psychological illnesses. Of all the people who use drugs to relieve anxiety, 80 per cent take minor tranquillizers. Like the major tranquillizers, they reduce tension and make you feel more relaxed, but possibly a little sleepy.

The beta blockers, which include Inderal and Trasicor, are arguably the most interesting of the drugs prescribed for anxiety. For although they block the action of the nerves that make the heart beat faster and the blood vessels contract, they do not have the side effects of the tranquillizers. They do not cause drowsiness or dependence — that is, they are not habit-forming. Unfortunately, however, many people find that the anxiety from which they suffer is not of the sort that responds well to beta blockers.

Drugs or no drugs?
Taking tablets is not always a bad thing. Using a particular drug to help you get over a major crisis is one of the most useful steps you can take, but it is wise to remember:

● Medication does not help to resolve the underlying problem. It only cures the symptoms of anxiety.

● In taking medication to dull your anxiety, you may lose the impetus to solve the difficulty.

● Drugs can produce side-effects that can diminish your ability to tackle problems effectively.

Coming off tranquillizers
● Talk to your doctor and ask him how best to reduce your intake. If you are severely dependent, you may need treatment in a special clinic.

● Be intelligent about cutting down. Do not be put off your actions because the consequences will be uncomfortable.

● Take it gently. Remember that your body took time to become tolerant to the drug and give it the same time to manage without it.

● Enlist support from those around you. Warn them that you will be irritable and possibly in pain and that you do not blame them.

● Ask your doctor about self-help groups.

● Try to keep involved in distracting activities.

In deciding which drug to prescribe, your doctor will consider your symptoms and their severity, and your past history. His decision will also depend on his familiarity and his experience with prescribing a specific drug.

Another important consideration is side-effects. There is no drug that does not have a multitude of effects on the body. Tranquillizers act on the areas of the brain responsible for arousal. Thus it is logical that they make you feel drowsy, lethargic and weak. They may also affect your concentration and your memory, making you slightly absent-minded. Large doses, taken over a long period, can lead to slurring of the speech and double vision, especially in the elderly. Side-effects may also arise because of your own psychological make-up. We all respond differently to drugs and vary in our sensitivity to them. There is, unfortunately, no way of predicting a person's reactions in advance, so there is bound to be an element of 'trial and error' in your doctor's prescription.

Becoming dependent
All drugs that affect the mind produce dependence. It is this that makes giving up tranquillizers so difficult. There are two types of dependence — psychological and physiological — but the dividing line between them is often hard to define.

Psychological dependence generally means that stopping the drug will bring about withdrawal symptoms, even though your body chemistry shows that you no longer need it. Physical dependence occurs when the body's functions adapt so that they are only efficient in the presence of the drug and are disrupted when the drug is withdrawn. With physical dependence, we also become tolerant to a drug so that larger and larger doses are needed to produce the same effect. Eventually changes occur within the body to compensate for the effects of the drug, so that, as soon as we stop taking it, we find we have developed a craving.

Tranquillizer addiction is a growing problem, and withdrawal symptoms include palpitations, cramps, loss of appetite, insomnia and extreme tension. There is, unfortunately, no knowing how long you have to take tranquillizers for dependence to occur but is likely that if you take them on a regular basis for more than a couple of months, you are at risk.

Using drugs safely
If you need to take drugs, use the following safety rules:

● Discuss with your doctor the actions and possible side-effects of the drugs prescribed for you and how long your treatment should continue.

● Tell a new doctor about any other drugs you are taking in case of harmful interactions.

● Keep to the prescribed dose.

● Tell your doctor at once if any side-effects develop.

● Tell your doctor if you are pregnant or suspect that you may be. Many drugs can damage the developing baby, and all drugs should be avoided in pregnancy if possible.

● Keep all drugs out of the reach of children.

● Do not give in to the idea that drugs can solve everything. If you think you would rather try to do without drugs or try some other drugless form of treatment, such as biofeedback or psychotherapy, discuss this with your doctor.

● If the drugs you have been prescribed make you feel drowsy, avoid drinking alcohol. The effects can be potentially fatal.

● If the drugs you are taking make you feel drowsy or interfere with your vision or muscle tone, do not handle machinery or drive a motor car.

The most widely abused of the drugs acquired without prescription are those that produce euphoria. Even tranquillizers sold on the black market are generally used as part of a cocktail of drugs or alcohol to induce temporary 'highs'. Unfortunately, the price paid for the short-lived pleasure is almost invariably a feeling of depression and, in most cases, drug dependence.

While we consider caffeine, aspirin and tranquillizers innocuously addictive, and others such as cannabis, alcohol and the nicotine in cigarettes more controversial, we would probably all accept that heroin, LSD, amphetamines, cocaine and glue sniffing have more dangerous physical, psychological and legal consequences. Drug taking can lead to criminality as a means of meeting the cost of regular supplies, and injecting drugs on a regular basis can cause fatal infection.

The range of drugs
Caffeine is the stimulant found in coffee, tea and cola drinks. It increases blood pressure, the pulse rate and, when taken in excess, leads to hand tremors, dizzy spells, breathlessness and feelings of anxiety; yet many people drink coffee to calm their nerves. If you drink more than five large cups a day, you are likely to be damaging your health; so if you are at risk, try to cut down or switch to decaffeinated coffee. Reduce the quantities gradually, however, because there may well be some withdrawal symptoms.

It is not unusual for people to become dependent on aspirin, often taking up to 20 tablets a day as a precautionary measure against headaches. This leads to a high risk of bleeding from the stomach and induces withdrawal symptoms.

Individual reactions to cannabis (marijuana, 'grass' or 'pot') seem to be influenced largely by the behaviour of fellow drug-takers. Experiences usually include vivid visual sensations, euphoria and distortions of time, size and distance, often leading to feelings of panic. Cannabis affects short-term memory, concentration, logical thinking and motor performance; but the full extent of its danger is yet to be proved.

Amphetamines stimulate the nervous system to induce wakefulness, a sense of well-being, boundless energy and self-confidence. They also inhibit appetite and have been used in the treatment of obesity. Dependence comes rapidly, with strong side effects, including irritability, anxiety, aggression, tremors, even abnormal thinking and delusions — particularly feelings of persecution.

The stimulating effects of cocaine (coke) are similar to those of the amphetamines, producing a feeling of intense elation, together with a sense of great physical strength and energy and loss of appetite. Tolerance develops rapidly, leading to larger doses; long-term use can damage the mucous membrane lining the nose and cause disturbing feelings of restlessness and over excitability, fear and delusions of threat. In some reported cases, users have imagined the skin reactions to be caused by parasites burrowing into their skin and have literally torn it in a desperate attempt to rout out the parasites.

Heroin, solvent-sniffing and LSD
The drug heroin is derived from morphine, a substance commonly used medically to control severe pain. It gives an almost instant feeling of elation, and a new dose relieves withdrawal symptoms almost immediately on injection.

Solvent- or glue-sniffing is a cheap, accessible way of getting 'high' with a group of friends. The effects, which are similar to drunkeness, include euphoria, confusion, loss of inhibition and alteration in perceptions, leading to hallucinations, aggression, drowsiness, fits and nausea. Death is not uncommon, generally due to heart failure, liver and kidney damage or accident while under the influence of the drug.

LSD produces ecstatic and mystical experiences and sometimes also hallucinations, and, although a large proportion of the experiences are unpleasant, users of psychedelic drugs continue to take them. Long-term use disturbs the concentration, memory and perception.

How drug-taking begins
Simple curiosity leads most people to their first experience with drugs. Social pressure is another significant spur, often arising out of drinking sessions. Some come to drugs in their search for an inner self, but find any truths become meaningless after the 'trip' is over. Escape from everyday problems is another common reason for drug-taking, although personality is also significant. The types of individual thought to be most at risk are those who lack confidence, those who desire instant gratification, delinquents and people who wish to revolt against convention.

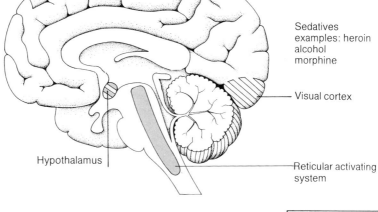

Stimulants
examples: caffeine
amphetamines

Hallucinogens
examples: LSD
cocaine
glue

Cerebral cortex

Sedatives
examples: heroin
alcohol
morphine

Visual cortex

Hypothalamus

Reticular activating
system

What to do if you think you are becoming dependent

● Be sure you want to stop; if you are not convinced, you will find it impossible to deal with withdrawal.

● Ask your doctor for referral to a specialized treatment centre; there you will be told what to expect and given relief from some of the pain of withdrawal.

● If you decide on self-help, take time off and gather: a round-the-clock supply of friends to help you; a small supply of tranquillizers in case the pain is unbearable; a plan for when you are drug free.

● Keep away from old haunts.

● Give yourself substitute rewards through friends not connected with the drug-taking culture.

● The first two weeks are the hardest, but the real difficulties of coping begin *after* two weeks.

Groups of non-prescribed drugs alter the activity of many parts of the brain but are designed to have a therapeutic effect by acting principally on the areas indicated. Stimulants press the reticular activating system, responsible for consciousness, into greater activity. They also act on the hypothalamus to produce typical 'fight or flight' reactions, as occur in stress. Sedatives act on the cerebral cortex to lower conscious awareness. Hallucinogenic drugs produce their bizarre visual effects by interfering with the working of the visual cortex, which is responsible for interpreting signals from the eyes.

Why people continue

The use of drugs, prescribed or non-prescribed, leads to tolerance and thence to dependence. As the dose increases, it becomes less effective at producing the desired response because the body adapts to allow normal functioning despite the pressure of the drug. Soon the adaptation is such that the body is disrupted if the drug is withdrawn, so the user increases the doses to avoid withdrawal symptoms.

Psychological dependence is more complex. The social rewards are often as strong as the physical rewards. Group pressure can be a powerful force, for if the group allows one person to escape drug dependence, it removes from everyone else the excuse that 'no one ever gets better.' Encouragement from others, combined with the ritual pleasure of preparing for a 'fix' (similar to the pleasure of lighting a cigarette without drawing on it) *and* the euphoric effect, amount to a strong incentive to continue.

The real dangers begin when more powerful drugs become available, and the pressure or temptation to try a more sensational drug are too strong to resist.

What to do as a parent
Remember:

● Few children modify their behaviour because we are critical of them; it not only gives them an excuse to continue, but traps them into maintaining such behaviour for fear of admitting they are wrong.

● Nagging, threatening, cajoling, bribery, ignoring, never work.

● The best chance of success is to arrange a meeting between the child and an outside expert, to be carried out as part of a contract in exchange for something the child wants from you. Choose the expert for his personality and track record, not his qualifications.

● Regard your child as an adult in his relationship with his counsellor.

● Remember, however guilty you may feel, you are not to blame.

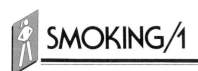

The dangers of smoking

Cigarette smoking is always unsafe. The figures speak for themselves. People who smoke more than 20 cigarettes a day take twice as many days off work each year than non-smokers. Of men now aged 35, the proportion that will die before reaching retiring age is 40 per cent for heavy smokers but only 15 per cent for non-smokers. Smoking causes about 100,000 deaths a year in Britain alone. The illustration shows the parts of the body affected by smoking in both sexes. Women run an additional risk, however. Their unborn babies may be damaged by smoking and smoking increases the risk of cervical cancer.

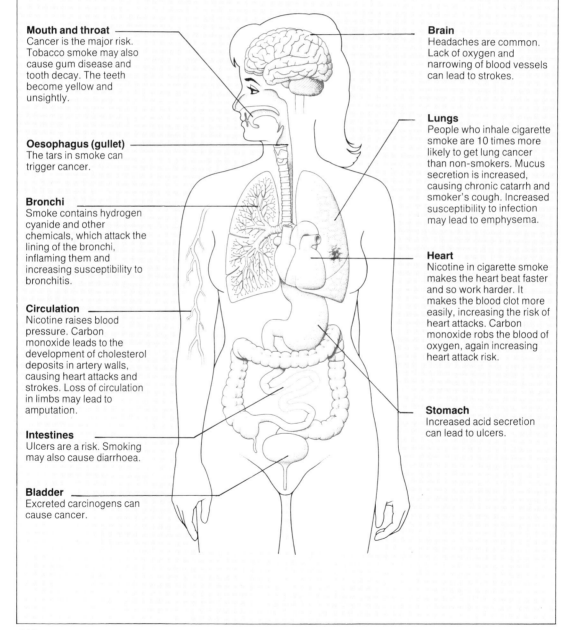

Mouth and throat
Cancer is the major risk. Tobacco smoke may also cause gum disease and tooth decay. The teeth become yellow and unsightly.

Oesophagus (gullet)
The tars in smoke can trigger cancer.

Bronchi
Smoke contains hydrogen cyanide and other chemicals, which attack the lining of the bronchi, inflaming them and increasing susceptibility to bronchitis.

Circulation
Nicotine raises blood pressure. Carbon monoxide leads to the development of cholesterol deposits in artery walls, causing heart attacks and strokes. Loss of circulation in limbs may lead to amputation.

Intestines
Ulcers are a risk. Smoking may also cause diarrhoea.

Bladder
Excreted carcinogens can cause cancer.

Brain
Headaches are common. Lack of oxygen and narrowing of blood vessels can lead to strokes.

Lungs
People who inhale cigarette smoke are 10 times more likely to get lung cancer than non-smokers. Mucus secretion is increased, causing chronic catarrh and smoker's cough. Increased susceptibility to infection may lead to emphysema.

Heart
Nicotine in cigarette smoke makes the heart beat faster and so work harder. It makes the blood clot more easily, increasing the risk of heart attacks. Carbon monoxide robs the blood of oxygen, again increasing heart attack risk.

Stomach
Increased acid secretion can lead to ulcers.

Every cigarette you smoke may shorten your life by an average of five and a half minutes. Cigarette smoking is the major cause of illness and premature death in Western society. Yet people who smoke either cannot believe that such illnesses will afflict them, or are unable or unwilling to give up smoking and thus improve their lives.

Tobacco smoke is dangerous because of the nicotine, carbon monoxide, tars and poisonous substances it contains, as the diagram (*left*) shows. Even 'passive' smokers, who inhale the smoke of others, are at some risk. Exposure to other people's smoke involves, it has been suggested, about a third of the risk associated with smoking a cigarette yourself.

Lung cancer among non-smokers who live with heavy smokers is twice as high as in non-smokers who live in homes where nobody smokes. Non-smoking spouses of cigarettes smokers die, on average, four years younger than the non-smoking spouses of non-smokers. Small children are especially at risk from cigarette smoke: it can cause respiratory infections which leave the lungs damaged for life.

Low tar cigarettes have been marketed as 'safer' than high tar ones, but there is no evidence that reducing tar or nicotine intake per cigarette makes any difference to the development of future difficulties. This is largely because they have no effect on the carbon monoxide that deprives the blood — and thus all body organs, but significantly the heart — of oxygen. And people who smoke 'low dose' cigarettes may smoke more to raise their blood nicotine levels, or because they think such cigarettes are safer.

Changing to a cigar or a pipe can, as long as you do not inhale, reduce the risk of lung cancer. However, the risk of developing cancer of the oesophagus, mouth or throat is just as great.

The reasons why people start smoking are often markedly different from those that sustain the habit. Curiosity, the desire to impress or appear adult, or pressure from others are all common reasons. The first nauseating effects, the dizziness and coughing, soon pass.

Research suggests that people with anxious, or Type A, personalities are more likely to smoke heavily than 'passive' B types (see pp. 226-7). Smokers also associate certain benefits with their actions. Thus, if a smoker truly believes that a cigarette will increase alertness, relaxation, or confidence, then it probably will do so.

Like other drugs, nicotine is addictive, and smoking is a drug addiction. Smokers regulate the dose of nicotine in their blood automatically, and smoke more or less accordingly. Smoking also causes psychological dependence, which makes giving up even harder.

Why do you smoke?
Finding out why you smoke is a good first step toward giving up. Read the statements below, based on research conducted by the US Public Health Service. Score as follows:
Always true: 5 points; Frequently true: 4 points; Occasionally true: 3 points; Seldom true: 2 points; Never true: 1 point.

Stimulation
'Smoking stops me slowing down'.
'Smoking perks me up.'
'Cigarettes give me a lift.'
Stimulation results from the physiological effects of nicotine.

Handling
'Handling a cigarette is enjoyable.'
'I enjoy the lighting-up routine.'
'I like watching the smoke.'
The ritual of smoking is an important, pleasurable element of the habit for some people.

Relaxation
'I find smoking pleasant and relaxing.'
'Smoking is pleasurable.'
'I want a cigarette when I am most comfortable and relaxed.'
One of the paradoxes of smoking is that it can be both calming and stimulating. This may be something to do with the rate and depth of inhalation, but is unproven.

Tension reduction
'I smoke when I am angry.'
'I smoke when I am uncomfortable or upset about something.'
'Cigarettes take my mind off my worries.'
Many people use smoking as a 'crutch' to help them deal with stressful situations. This leads to psychological addiction.

Craving
'I cannot bear to be without cigarettes.'
'I am consciously aware of the times when I am not smoking.'
'I get a gnawing hunger for a cigarette when I haven't smoked for a while.'
Nicotine can cause true physical addiction.

Habit
'I smoke cigarettes automatically without being aware of it.'
'I light up when I already have a cigarette going.'
'I have smoked without remembering lighting up.'
Smoking can become an almost automatic response.

Scoring: A score of 11 or more in any category is high; 7 is low; any score in between is average. A string of high scores means that your reasons for smoking are complex and that it may be hard to give up. For help with giving up smoking see pp. 248-9.

The best way to save yourself from the many illnesses associated with cigarette smoking, and from the difficulty of giving it up, is never to start smoking in the first place. It is, however, extremely difficult to teach children and young adults to say 'no' when so many pressures are on them, from their peers and from the media, to start the smoking habit.

Children are more likely to smoke if their parents smoke. The figures show that a teenager, whose parents or an older brother or sister smoke, is four times as likely to take up smoking as a teenager from a non-smoking family. In smoking families, children are used to absorbing the noxious substances in cigarette smoke passively. They may thus be less powerfully affected by unpleasant side-effects when they smoke their first cigarette.

One effective way of stopping children from smoking is to make a deal with them that provides attractive rewards for not smoking. Children might, for example, be offered a car and driving lessons as a seventeenth birthday present if they do not smoke. A child should be honour-bound to keep to the contract — pressure, suspicion inquisitions and nagging will quickly negate it. Even if a child has smoked occasionally during the period of the contract, this can be ignored. It may be worth giving the child the car or another material possession to boast about at the end of the day, so that he can convince himself and his peers that smoking is not worth while.

Barriers to giving up

The dramatic decrease in deaths from heart disease in the USA since the mid-sixties is almost certainly due to the fall in the number of smokers. But despite the overwhelming evidence that cigarette smoking is harmful (see pp. 246-7), people are, it seems, only likely to give up if they feel that the evidence applies to them.

A reason people often give for continuing to smoke is that giving up will make them put on weight. Most people who give up smoking do put on some weight, largely because their appetite for food increases and because food supplies the oral stimulation once given by cigarettes. Remember that the mortality risks of smoking are more than double those of being overweight, and overweight can be dealt with later.

It is never too late to give up smoking. Even if you have been smoking for 20 or 30 years, it is worth while. From the day you stop smoking, you start improving both your life expectancy and the quality of your life. You will immediately smell better, look better and have more resistance to disease. Your heart and lungs will be more efficient and your risk of heart disease, bronchitis, emphysema and cancers of various kinds, but most significantly lung cancer, will decrease.

How to stop smoking

Motivation is the real key to giving up smoking. You must convince yourself that it is an unhealthy, dirty, expensive habit and unworthy of you. Like giving up any other drug of addiction, there is little chance of success unless you are convinced that you wish to give up. Indeed, the only course of action may be to say to yourself, 'I will never put a lighted cigarette between my lips again.' It may help to decide well in advance on a date on which this will take effect, so that you can prepare yourself mentally, or you could use a heavy cold as an 'excuse' for stopping.

Not everybody is strong willed enough to be able to take, and keep to, such an 'all-or-nothing' decision. If you prefer to try to give up gradually, use the smoker's diary (see right) to see which cigarettes you need least, and cut these out first. Set yourself a target date for stopping completely, and aim to cut down consumption by about a quarter each day or each week.

Whatever method you plan to use, begin by making a smoker's diary. This will warn you of where most difficulties lie. Then consult the questionnaire on pages 246-7 and discover the reasons why you smoke. Your answers will determine your strategy.

If you smoke for pleasure or relaxation, try to do something else instead of smoking. Distract yourself by listening to music or reading a book, or with a relaxation technique (see pp. 234-5). If smoking provides the stimulation you need, try taking up a vigorous exercise or sport to give you a 'high' instead, or find something more interesting to do, if only temporarily.

Doing something with your hands, such as doodling, fiddling with coins, paper clips or pencils can help overcome the problem if handling is important to you. Knitting, sewing and DIY activities can also help. If you are not sure what to do with your hands, watch what other non-smokers do with theirs while you are smoking.

If you smoke to reduce tension, try other means of coping with your problem, including exercise, chewing sugar-free gum or using relaxation techniques. Whenever possible, try to avoid stressful situations. If you cannot, then be aware that these are danger times.

Smokers who crave the 'buzz' that nicotine provides will simply have to bear the trauma of giving up. For such smokers, nicotine chewing gum (available through your doctor) may help, but those smokers who have a real craving for cigarettes are better advised to give up at a single attempt rather than to cut down gradually.

People who smoke out of habit are most helped by changing the routine of their days. They should watch out for 'trigger' events, such as cups of coffee and telephone calls, at which they tend to light up a cigarette automatically.

Smoker's diary

Draw up a diary based on the example given here. In the column headed 'Importance' score as follows:
0: 'I lit up without realizing it.'
1: 'I just felt like it.'
2: 'I wanted a cigarette fairly badly.'
3: 'I was desperate for a cigarette.'
Your answers will give you an idea of how much you smoke and when, and of the relative importance of each cigarette to you. It will provide clues as to which cigarettes will be easy and which difficult to give up.

10 MONDAY AUGUST

Time	Trigger	Importance	Thoughts and emotions
8.15	Having breakfast	3	'I can't start the day without a cigarette.'
8.50	Driving	2	'Aggravated by being stuck in traffic.'
9.30	Cup of coffee	1	'Made me feel more relaxed.'
10.05	Making a telephone call	2	'I needed a cigarette to calm my nerves.'
11.10	Offered a cigarette by a colleague	0	'Accepting made me feel more sociable.'

Motivation

Any technique that can keep you motivated to persist without cigarettes is worth trying. Some of the following may help:

- Tell everyone you are about to give up. This places social pressure on you to keep to your plan. But remember that smokers are likely to be your worst allies — they have a vested interest in your failure. If you can give it up, it means that they may be under pressure to do so.

- Give yourself forfeits for failure, such as carrying out unpleasant but necessary chores. Either way you win — you give up cigarettes or get the chores done.

- Keep reminding yourself of the benefits of giving up and the penalties of continuing. Keep in your mind a picture of someone with lung cancer or chronic bronchitis.

- Think how much money you are saving and promise yourself a present with what you have saved. Put the money you have saved aside in a special jar, marked 'holiday' or 'present'.

- Remember that there will be times when you are tense, feel uneasy and cannot concentrate.

- You may feel dreadful now but always keep in mind that *it does get better*.

Preventing relapses

People relapse into the smoking habit for three main reasons:
1 A negative emotional state such as anxiety, depression, loneliness, boredom, impatience, restlessness, tiredness.
2 Social pressures, particularly those of feeling 'left out'.
3 Personal conflicts.
To help you avoid slipping back into the smoking habit, use the following tips:

- Make sure you are aware of the situations that put you most at risk.

- Do not become complacent.

- If you feel you are at risk, go back to the list of substitutes and pretend that you have just given up.

- Practise saying to yourself and others, 'I have just given up smoking.'

- Get everyone around you to keep congratulating you on having given up.

- Do not fool yourself that, since you have returned to smoking after a period of non-smoking, your body still needs nicotine and that you are a 'hopeless case'. If you have given up once, you can do so again.

- If you make a mistake and smoke a cigarette, try to find out why it happened and practise avoiding the problem in future.

- Go back to being abstinent *now*. Do not say to yourself, 'I will start giving up again this evening or tomorrow.'

Blood alcohol level per 100 ml

30 mg	Light and moderate drinkers feel relaxed Heavy drinkers are unaffected
40 mg	Garrulousness and mild loss of inhibition Increase in accidents
60 mg	Mood change. Judgement impaired. Decision-making capacity affected
80 mg	Physical coordination impared Loss of UK driving licence
100 mg	Deterioration in physical and social control Loss of US driving licence
150 mg	Drunkeness, staggering Double-vision, slurred speech Aggression, vomiting
300 mg	Loss of consciousness Drinker is rousable
400 mg	Coma, possibility of death
600 mg	Breathing stops. Death

600 ml (1 pint) beer or 2 tots of spirits

900 ml (1½ pints) beer or 3 tots of spirits

1.5 L (2½ pints) beer or 5 tots of spirits

3 L (5 pints) beer or 10 tots of spirits

3.6 L (6 pints) beer or 12 tots of spirits

¾ bottle of spirits

1 bottle of spirits

0   100   200   300   400   500   600
mg/100 ml alcohol in blood

Alcohol is generally thought of as a stimulant, because it makes us talkative, aggressive and uninhibited. In truth, however, it depresses the activity of the nervous system and acts as an anaesthetic. At high levels, depression of the respiratory centre in the brain can kill.

People drink for many different reasons. In small doses and for short periods of time, alcohol relieves tension, encourages a sense of well-being and is unlikely to be harmful. However, some people mistakenly use alcohol in an attempt to relieve major problems. This not only leads to alcohol tolerance so that larger and larger doses are needed but, unfortunately, also tends to exacerbate the problems. In large doses, alcohol causes chronic depression, misery and self-doubt.

Social pressures are a subtle spur to drinking because, in small doses, alcohol loosens the tongue and, therefore, convinces us that our social interactions are improved. People also drink to give themselves rewards, to fill in empty hours or to relieve tiredness or lethargy. Consider your own reasons for drinking by keeping a drinker's diary (see p. 292-3).

Two different types of people may be more likely to develop a drinking problem. The first are those who lack self-confidence, have low self-esteem and are often self-punishing. When drunk, the loss of inhibitions provides a welcome lift.

The second type also find it hard to deal with the realities of life, but, unlike the first group, have often been over-indulged in childhood. They shy away from adult responsibilities and resort to alcohol. In both cases, the major problem is the vicious circle created by alcohol abuse.

The effects of drinking
The amount of alcohol in the bloodstream, the blood alcohol concentration (BAC), determines behaviour after drinking. This is the measure that the police use when deciding whether people should be charged with drunken driving, and it is

influenced by three factors. The first is the amount absorbed in milligrams of alcohol (see chart). In this, the type of drink determines the alcohol content and the speed at which the alcohol is absorbed. Spirits are assimilated more quickly than beer, and fizzy mixers increase the rate of absorption. Eating a meal before drinking delays absorption. Secondly, the longer you take to consume the alcohol, the lower your BAC.

The third factor to be considered is body weight. Women, who generally have lower body weight than men, have higher BAC levels if they drink the same amount as men and often have lower tolerance to alcohol. Any drinking that raises the BAC level to above 20 mg increases the chance of accidents. For someone with a light build and small frame, this level can be reached within one hour by having one drink.

A drinking problem
Alcohol tolerance, in which larger and larger amounts are required to produce the same effect, develops rapidly. There is, however, no identifiable point at which someone becomes alcohol dependent. Rather there is a sliding scale from occasional drinking to total dependence, and drinking problems begin well before chronic alcohol dependence sets in.

Like any other drug, alcohol has drastic effects on mental and physical health if taken in excess, and can reduce life expectancy dramatically. Cirrhosis of the liver; disorders of the digestive system; hepatitis; cancer and brain damage are often the result of heavy drinking.

These physical effects of alcohol abuse may or may not precede the behaviourally damaging effects. Thus some heavy drinkers have little behavioural upsets such as decline in memory and intellect, depression, breakdown and notions of suicide before the physical damage takes its toll. In others, the behavioural effects come first.

Family and social relationships are disrupted by alcohol dependence, since alcohol abuse leads to violence, child neglect and, frequently, the break-up of relationships. Even moderate drinkers find themselves increasingly isolated from others, and friendships are soon replaced by alcohol. At work, performance gradually deteriorates and absenteeism increases.

Unfortunately, the effects of alcohol can destroy other people's lives, for fearless behaviour and impaired judgement cause accidents. This is especially so on the roads. In Australia, for example, it has been estimated that at least 50 per cent of deaths on the roads are associated with alcohol consumption.

Are you developing a drink problem?
Ask yourself the following questions, which are based on a questionnaire compiled by the National Council of Alcoholism in the USA.
1 Do you drink heavily after a bad day?
2 Do you drink more heavily when under pressure?
3 Can you drink more than you used to?
4 Do you have twinges of guilt about drinking?
5 Are you impatient for your first drink of the day?
6 Do you often feel uncomfortable without a drink?
7 Do you try to sneak a few extra drinks, secretly?
8 Do you ever have memory black outs after drinking?
9 Do others often discuss your drinking?
10 Have your memory black outs become more frequent?
11 Have you tried to control your drinking?
12 Do you usually drink for an identifiable reason?
13 Do you often regret things you say or do when drunk?
14 Do you want to continue after others stop drinking?
15 Have your good intentions about cutting down failed?
16 Have you ever moved house or job to try to give up drinking?
17 Are you beginning to feel a little persecuted?
18 Have your financial and work problems increased?
19 Do you prefer to drink with strangers?
20 Do you eat irregularly when drinking?
21 Do you drink in the mornings to steady yourself?
22 Do you sometimes feel depressed and hopeless?
23 Are you sometimes drunk for days at a time?
24 Do you find you cannot drink as much as you once used to?
25 Do you see or hear imaginary things after drinking?
26 Do you sometimes feel terribly frightened after you have been drinking?

If you answered 'yes' to any question, you may have a drink problem. 'Yes' replies in each of the following groups indicate the following stages: Questions 1-8 you are entering the risk area; Questions 9-21 you are in the middle stages; Questions 22-26 the final stage is beginning.

Overconsumption of alcohol is a growing problem in many countries. There has, however, been a great deal of argument in scientific circles about whether people who are drinking too much should control the amount they consume or stop drinking altogether. To date, no firm answer has emerged as to which is the better of the two. Early successes with alcohol-dependent drinkers who restricted their intake have been reversed, since many such drinkers have gradually returned to their old levels of drinking.

The weight of evidence suggests that, for most people who are heavily dependent on alcohol, total abstinence is probably the only way in which to achieve success. This is logical, since it is far more useful to learn to do without alcohol altogether and to discover different approaches to underlying problems, than to treat the symptoms by merely cutting down.

Whether you decide to cut down your intake or opt for total abstinence, you must be sure which course of action you are adopting and stick to it. Otherwise your attempts will be doomed to failure. Remember that cutting down is the harder of the two options and that, if you are short on motivation, you will be unsuccessful, whichever path you take.

Total abstinence
Giving up alcohol is similar to giving up other addictive drugs. For a heavily dependent drinker it should not be equated with giving up, say, cigarette smoking. The withdrawal symptoms are unpleasant, and even if they do not amount to delirium tremens, with its symptoms of shaking limbs and hallucinations, may include aching muscles and sweating. This means that, almost certainly, medical help and supervision will be needed. Some people are able to 'dry out' at home under a doctor's supervision, but it is important for them to ask for medical advice before they try to give up, in case of problems.

Many hospitals now provide 'detoxification' centres for alcoholics. Patients are given tranquillizers and vitamins to prevent brain damage and are monitored to chart their condition and progress. Once the withdrawal symptoms have been overcome, a patient may be given drugs, such as Antabuse or Abstem, which induce physical illness if alcohol is drunk. The drugs prescribed in tablet form are effective for only 24 hours after

being swallowed by the patient.

Unfortunately, many patients forget — either deliberately or unintentionally — to take their drugs. The doctor may, therefore, ask another member of the family to supervise drug-taking or may implant a slow-release capsule beneath the patient's skin. This allows a constant dose of the drug to be absorbed directly into the bloodstream of the person in need of help and removes the need for tablet-taking.

Drying-out and drug administration do nothing, however, to help combat the basic problems that lead to alcohol abuse in the first place or to help maintain the state of abstinence. For people to stop or even control their drinking, sobriety must be made rewarding. They need help in developing better work, social and marital relationships, and research suggests that counselling is one of the most important factors in achieving and maintaining abstinence.

Alcoholics Anonymous (AA) and ACCEPT (Alcoholism Community Centres for Education, Prevention and Treatment) are two organizations that help provide support for the ex-drinker. In themselves, they are not magic solutions, but they have the collective experience of thousands of drinkers to fall back on. AA emphasizes self-help, individual motivation and the fact that we are all responsible for our own actions. Al Anon, for spouses, and Alateen, for children of drinkers, are also part of the AA organization and provide valuable support and information for members of an alcoholic's family.

Young people at risk
In helping a young person with a drink problem, it is far better to get help from outside the family. Within the family, there is always a temptation to keep troubles private, but this can do more harm than good. If your child has a problem, try to arrange a visit to an expert chosen for his suitable personality and ability, not for his position. Select someone who will talk to the child unpatronizingly and who will not merely take the unwelcome role of a third parent.

People who drink to excess, whether young or old, usually do so for a reason. Unfortunately, parents are often the last people a child or young adult feel they can talk to. Indeed, poor communication with parents may be *the* problem that is causing the drinking. Whether they are young

Good excuses

The simplest way of refusing a drink is to say, 'No thank you'. There are, however, many social pressures on people to drink. Try some of the following excuses when you have to say 'no'. Present your case firmly and *do not* enter into a debate about the morals of drinking or try to change the drinking habits of another person.

● 'I have given up drinking because the time has come to cut down.' If you repeat this message often enough people will believe you.

● 'I am driving.'

● 'My doctor says I may be getting an ulcer.'

● 'My liver is not in very good condition.'

● 'I am taking antibiotics (or sleeping tablets or any other drugs) and should not drink as well.'

● 'The drink is making me feel unwell.'

● 'I have to watch my weight.'

● 'I've had just about the right amount. If I have any more, I shall feel ill tomorrow.'

● 'Drinking gives me migraine.'

● 'I've stopped drinking at lunchtime, it ruins my concentration in the afternoon.'

Remember, once people realize you are not going to drink, they will stop pressurizing you.

or old, people will not give up drinking unless they can see that it is worthwhile. Parents are often unable to supply the necessary rewards.

Rather than struggling with a situation whose control is beyond their capabilities, parents should aim to talk to a child sympathetically, say that they are enormously worried and upset, and ask the child to make a deal with them to see an outsider. Enlisting the help of a close family friend who can talk to the child as adult-to-adult may also be helpful in this situation.

Cutting down

The 'points' system

Use the 'points' system as an aid if your wish is to cut down your alcohol intake.

Aim for: a maximum of 24 points a week
a maximum of 6 points a day
and no more than 4 'drinking days' a week.

Score as follows:

600 ml (1 pint) beer	= 2 points
1 small sherry or fortified wine	= 1 point
30 ml (1 fl oz) whisky, gin, vodka or brandy	= 1 point
1 small glass of wine	= 1 point

If your weekly score is currently more than 50 points, cut down by 10 points until you reach 40 points. For scores of 40 points a week and below, cut down by 5 points each week.

Helpful strategies

● Make a drinker's diary (see pp.294-5). Note when you are most at risk and which drinks you can cut out with ease.

● Remember that the distribution of your drinking is as important as the quantity. Do not drink to excess on any one occasion.

● Make a list of reasons for not drinking more than your limit. Remember that you will be pressurized into slipping back into old habits.

● Rehearse your excuses and coping skills (*see left and right*).

● Tell everyone you are cutting down because you think you are drinking too much; enlist their support.

● Try exercise or a new hobby to divert your attention from drinking.

● Get professional help to sort out your underlying problems.

Rehearse your coping skills

The first step in adopting skills to cope with cutting out or cutting down on drinking is to identify high-risk situations or cues. Then think of as many ways of coping with them as possible. Rehearse your actions mentally so that you will be assured when the time comes, and not be persuaded into changing your mind.

● At a party, stay for only 20 minutes.

● Drink tonic water or another mixer and pretend that you are drinking alcohol as well.

● Keep moving. If the pressure becomes too great, go to the toilet for a break.

● Rehearse saying 'no' or offering the excuse of your choice.

● Rehearse going into a bar or pub and having just one drink; this is one of the most difficult things to do.

● Rehearse ordering mineral water instead of wine with a meal in a restaurant.

YOUR PLACE IN THE WORLD

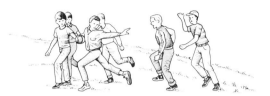

We all feel at times that, somehow, we do not 'fit'. This is natural and normal, for few of us are totally without conflicts, and none of us really qualifies as the *average* person. Nor would many of us be happy to be classed as such, for the average individual may smoke more, drink more, be more violent or less adequate than we are. The years of adolescence are particularly marked by rebellion against conformity, and parents find this hard to cope with.

The idea of conformity

It is often a surprise to realize that the majority of people you see in the street are made uncomfortable by fears, self-doubts, repressed thoughts and drives similar to those we have. Yet we are wrongly led to believe that other people are more perfect, more confident or more acceptable than we are. One survey, for example, suggests that possibly 60 per cent of individuals have sexual difficulties of a significant kind for a substantial period of their lives. Those who have never experienced any sexual problems are, in fact, in the minority. Yet the 'ideal' displayed by the media suggests that you should have a perfect sex life and relationships. We are thus constantly presented with images and standards that we have little chance of living up to.

We all like to be approved of, but this means that, as soon as we join any kind of group, we lose the freedom to behave exactly as we might wish to. Generally, we deliberately avoid doing things that we know will make us unpopular with other members, for if any relationship is to survive, there has to be some agreed way of interacting. The problems begin when we demand too much approval, at the cost of sacrificing our identity.

Many of us fit in well enough, either because we are flexible or because our attitudes or temperaments happen to agree with those of our neighbours and colleagues. For those of us who do not fit easily, there are various choices. If we try desperately to conform, others are usually aware that somehow we are not 'one of them'. Or we can rebel. Adolescence appears to be a period

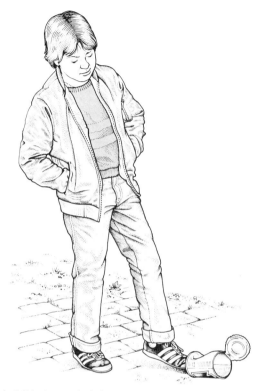

A child who genuinely has a different outlook on life from that of his peers or his parents is likely to be a 'loner'. Any unhappiness experienced will be exaggerated if a child is pressurized to participate in activities he considers worthless.

of rebellion against adult rules, although this is more often conformity to the peer group, which exerts stronger pressure than that applied by the older generation. Outward rebellion is in some ways an easy option, even though it can leave you isolated. Inward rebellion is harder to sustain.

The half-way approach

Another alternative is the half-way approach, which includes conforming to some rules but not others. However, it takes a great deal of self-confidence to carry this through. The wife who is obliged to play hostess at a dinner party for her husband's colleagues may decide, for example, that, since she does not wish to cook, the best compromise is to bring in outside caterers or to invite each guest to provide a course. As a result of this action, she will be regarded by some as an outsider, but she may be surprised to find that others share her feelings and admire her courage, and that she has started a new trend.

The half-way approach must be thought out intelligently. There is no point, for example, in turning up to the firm's annual dinner-dance in a pair of jeans. This is a case in which it may be as stressful to flout the rules as to conform, so it may be better not to attend such a function at all.

Children who do not fit in

A surprising number of people find from early in childhood that they view the world differently from others and face the dilemma: 'Can I be right and 30,000 people wrong, or am I wrong because they are in the majority?' This is neither new nor suspicious, for heroes who have changed history and made major discoveries have often done so by taking a stand against the majority view.

Children who, from an early age, genuinely see things differently from the majority view will suffer if parents pressure them into conformity and participation. As they grow older, they feel that there is something wrong with them. But different does not mean wrong, and these people will often ask questions that make the rest of us feel uncomfortable.

There is no point in trying to force such children to conform, for they are aware of their differences and are usually intelligent enough to realize that attempts to change them will be doomed to failure. All you can do as a parent is to encourage the child and help him explore the world as he sees it.

Another group of children who somehow do not fit are those who lack confidence or are anxious. Again, pressure from parents and other adults is not the answer — although it would appear that this is the most popular course of action. Flooding a child with social interaction, to get him used to situations he fears, is rarely rewarded in practice. Instead, try organizing smaller gatherings or have him invite friends around; try to get him to build up his social confidence steadily and gently.

The third group of children who suffer from 'alienation' are those who are rebelling. Confrontation is unlikely to be successful with such children and will probably lead to intense battles, which force the child to maintain his position.

There comes, for many people, a time when they feel they would like to change their lives. The short answer is to go ahead and do it. Instead of asking 'Can I do it?' ask yourself, 'What is the best way to go about doing what I want to?'

When a crisis occurs, you are usually called upon to play one of two roles. Either you are the recipient of a disaster, or you find yourself in the situation of having to sort out the troubles of others. Matters become somewhat blurred when crises and conflicts involve partnerships (see pp. 258-9) or parents and children, but it is still possible to work out which is your role.

The information in these pages is aimed particularly at helping you to cope with family crises, but much of it is applicable to other kinds of crisis.

1 Your own feelings

If you are the 'recipient' of trouble, try to suspend your own feelings. It is remarkable how much time and effort are lost during a crisis because of reactions such as, 'Why is this happening to me?', 'What will other people think?' or, 'How could they do this to me?'

When someone needs help from you, there is, similarly, little point in indulging your own feelings or dwelling on the way their problems are going to affect you. The priority is to deal with the crisis, not to dither and recriminate.

2 Communicating anxiety

When a crisis arises, whatever your role may be, try not to communicate anxiety. When you are upset, somehow this communicates itself to others, who respond negatively to it. Try to stay calm, even if you do not feel it. If you add your own emotions and fears to the situation, you may well be ensuring that the crisis becomes more serious than it need be.

Keep repeating to yourself, 'What is the problem here?', 'Calm down.' Remember that just as others can 'catch' anxiety from you, they can also 'catch' calmness.

3 Using your intuition

When you are trying to sort out a crisis for someone else, or if you are involved in a crisis that is not of your making, for example, as a parent, remember that intuition is a valuable source of information. Intuition is often thought of as something rather magical, but it is probably no more than an assessment that part of your mind makes of a situation, based on experience.

A thought such as, 'I have a feeling that my son has gone to his friend's house . . .' may be put down to intuition, but, in fact, it is based on previous patterns of events or on clues picked up unconsciously from conversation.

In sorting out a crisis in which you are the 'injured' person, it is also important to follow your intuitive thoughts, despite criticism from others that you are 'giving in' to your feelings. Your actions may not feel logical to you, but if the feeling is strong enough, follow it through.

4 What ought to be done

In a crisis, ignore what you think you 'ought' to do to please other people or to conform with what society expects of you. All too often we are afraid of what others may think and come to a conclusion that pleases them but does nothing to help either ourselves or a person in difficulties.

If a child is abusing drugs or alcohol, parents often feel that one of their priorities is to make sure that other people do not find out — not in the interests of the child, but because it reflects badly on the family to have a child with such problems. Parents of anorexic children will often deny the anorexia, even to themselves, because they feel that it reflects adversely on the way in which the child has been brought up.

If someone is in difficulties, it is important to realize that problems cause pain and that this pain must be resolved. As a rule, it is impossible to cope successfully with a crisis, or to sort one out on behalf of another person, and at the same time to keep up appearances.

5 Gaining valuable insights

When you are the person who is trying to help resolve a crisis, always try to put yourself in the position of the person who is suffering. This not only helps to give you some insight as to why the crisis has occurred in the first place, but will also give you ideas about how to set about achieving a solution. The same is true if you are a passive recipient of trouble.

Take the example of a child who has run away from home. Having discovered the child's whereabouts, there is little point in running angrily to haul the miscreant home. Restrain yourself, however great the temptation, from bombarding the child with questions such as, 'How could you do this to us?', 'Do you know what trouble you have caused?' or 'What will the neighbours think of all this fuss and commotion?' Such questions may seem important to you but are insignificant to the child. Indeed, they may simply make the child feel more wretched than ever and less likely to reveal why he or she ran off in the first place — which is the only thing that matters. They may also make it more likely that the incident will be repeated.

6 Dealing with resentment

If you find yourself mixed up in a crisis because of the actions of another person, do not 'punish' that person. It is all too human to take out your frustration, resentment and anxiety on someone who, in your judgement, is responsible for causing a problem. Thus a child who has run away, or a partner who has left home, often comes back to an angry, not a joyful, welcome. Imagine how you would feel in the circumstances and remember that recrimination solves nothing. Look to the long term and seek solutions that will minimize resentment on all sides.

Because we like to be in control of our lives in as many aspects as possible, we naturally resent people and situations that interfere with this and force us to be problem-solvers. Similarly, we often resent those who are ill because their illness inconveniences us. Again, self-control is an enormously valuable asset in coping with the crisis.

7 Talking and listening

Whatever your role in a crisis, it is worth talking through the situation with a neutral listener. You should also be prepared to listen to the advice of others and to understand what they are saying and why — even though their conclusions may contradict your own interests.

A parent or partner or a good friend may be able to provide the listening ear you need, but often it is better to listen to an outsider with no vested interest in the situation.

When others are offering you advice, it is important to decide whether the advice is worth having. At times of crisis, everyone becomes an 'expert'. We are bombarded with the benefit of their vast experience. You urgently need to decide, however, whether they really do have your interests at heart, or those of the person undergoing the crisis.

Ask yourself, in such a situation, do they *really* know? Why are you being told this? Is their evidence anecdotal or factual? Is the situation being talked about really the same as your own?

Have you good reason to have faith in their opinions and advice?

8 Where to get advice

If you wish to seek outside help in a crisis, whether on your own behalf or on behalf of someone else, try your family doctor as a first resort. He will have access to many resources. You may, however, have to put pressure on him to gain access to those that you need.

Social workers are another valuable source of help. The social services have emergency facilities and can furnish you with immediate aid if necessary. A telephone call to an organization such as the Samaritans could also do some good. Merely talking about a crisis to someone can often help you work out the best solution.

Psychiatrists and psychologists, many of whom are attached to hospitals, may also be of assistance. Psychiatrists are medically qualified doctors who have undergone further training in psychiatry. Many people call themselves psychologists, but those who have been trained to help you with problems and difficulties are described as clinical or counselling psychologists. If you get in touch with a psychologist via your hospital, you can be sure that he is qualified and trained. Qualified counsellors are also available.

9 Judging the 'experts'

As well as judging the advice handed out to you by family, friends and neighbours, it is also important to judge the advice given by outside experts — psychiatrists, psychologists, social workers and counsellors. Does their experience fit in with yours? Do they really understand and evaluate the position you are in? Does their advice sound as if it has come from a textbook, or is it based on experience and sensitivity?

If the advice you get does not sound or feel compatible with your situation or your responses, and those of the other people involved in the crisis, ask yourself why. It may be that the decisions you are making are based upon factors that are not sensible to or understood by outsiders. Or their advice may not take into account important factors that have led to your decisions. 'Experts' do not know everything, but their advice should not be discarded simply because they do not agree with you. So try to negotiate a rational solution with outsiders.

When we enter long-term relationships there is no way of knowing in advance how they will turn out. Yet although no relationship is perfect, it must contain enough 'glue' to keep the partners together, that is, there must be enough in it for both partners to view it as worthwhile. This concept of 'enough' is highly negotiable and is one that all couples should bear in mind.

There are no strict rules that guarantee good relationships or ensure that relationships survive. Nor are there any rules about when relationships should end. In assessing a relationship and its possible future, you can ask yourself certain questions. The most important of these are discussed in detail on these pages.

1 Should I continue?

The very fact that you are asking yourself this question means either that the relationship has considerable flaws or that your expectations are too high. Your first step toward finding an answer to the question is to work out a balance sheet. What are the pros and cons of staying in and getting out? Make a list and see what keeps you in the relationship. Include all the factors and be totally honest with yourself. There is no shame in staying in a relationship because you are economically dependent or are dependent because of disease or alcohol abuse, or because you are worried about how your family and friends will react. Any reason that is recognized and is important enough to you is valid.

The next step is to evaluate the items on this list, that is, to give them a weighting. Again, it is important to consider what matters to you.

We all have different personalities and so will weight matters differently. Many people feel, for example, that their own personal, intellectual or career development has to be compromised or sacrificed for the sake of marriage or a permanent relationship. Others find that they cannot endure the frustration that results from such a situation and will leave a relationship that does not allow them to fulfil their own potential.

For many people, especially those who have already been married and divorced, fear of further failure is given a heavy weighting in the assessment of reasons for staying in any relationship.

Remember, however, that fear of hurting your partner is not the best reason for staying in a relationship that is producing much misery.

2 How can I improve my relationship?

In seeking to improve their relationship, many couples fail to carry out the most obvious and important task — to find out what is actually wrong. Statements, such as 'He always criticizes me in public'. or 'She always nags me', are symptoms of the 'disease' but not its cause. Being criticized may be, for instance, a result of the fact that your partner is threatened by your social performance. Nagging may occur because the nagged partner does not respond *unless* he or she is nagged. Or both types of behaviour may be a symptom of underlying unhappiness with the marriage or the partner.

Another reason for being wary of treating the symptoms of trouble is that most interpersonal actions or themes emerge only after many 'preliminary' exchanges or events. It is no use selecting the end point, to work out where the problem started. Try to think back over events and actions (or lack of them) and to decide the causes for your reactions and those of your partner.

3 What does my partner think?

Many couples attempt to out-guess, out-predict or simply describe what their partner is thinking. This is, however, unreasonable, since you will never be able to see the world as your partner does. Nor, more importantly, will you ever be able to see yourself as your partner sees you.

The best way of surmounting this problem is to offer to discuss your relationship in a way that is likely to produce results and *not* through accusations. If you are not getting the discussion you want, do not blame your partner. If you are failing to get a discussion going, then you are using the wrong approach.

If you have tried one way of communicating in the past, do not keep going on in the same way in the vain hope that somehow, this time, you will be able to have the sort of conversation you want. Instead, change tack and try another approach, taking your cues from your partner's responses to other people.

In any discussion about your relationship, you must give your partner permission to disclose information. The reason for reticence may have been fear of the consequences or of your reactions. Or one partner may feel that there is little point in discussion because the other partner always interrupts to defend their own position.

4 How can I discuss problems effectively?

Many people have discussions as if they were having debates. There is much point-scoring, and neither side will admit being in the wrong. But when trying to sort out a relationship that has gone wrong, it is essential to realize that you are not in a battle to see who is right. Your aim is to resolve the problems and to improve the quality of the relationship.

If you do not allow yourself to be drawn into the 'attack-defend' routine, then your partner will be less inclined to do so. Make concessions freely and acknowledge your partner's point, even if the truth is hurtful. Do not allow a monologue to develop, but try to share your worries.

5 What are our expectations?

In an era when we are regularly exposed to the notion of 'ideal' relationships on television, at the cinema and theatre and in books, it is difficult to be realistic. If we feel that we are entitled to a perfect relationship and that nothing more nor less is to be expected, then, in truth, we are doomed to disappointment. Having accepted that life does not wave a magic wand over us, we must decide how far we can accept the discrepancy between expectation and reality.

Although we may feel disappointed, there is no reason why we cannot attempt to improve things. If improvement is impossible, then the choice between putting up with things as they are or getting out becomes a real one. But do not decide to get out of a relationship without making a concerted effort to improve it.

6 Is it my fault?

Finding fault or blame is not a constructive approach to problem solving. More useful is to ask yourself, 'Is there anything in my performance that might be producing some of the difficulties in the relationship?' If the answer is 'yes', the next question is 'How can I change it?' Follow up your answers with action.

You may, however, be faced with a situation in which your partner is so selfish, self-absorbed, careless or violent that changing your own performance may not be possible. In this instance, you must ask yourself 'Will/can my partner change?' If the answer to this is 'no', then you have the choice of putting up with the situation or not. A good rule of thumb to use is that no one

should put up with violence of any kind. After that, most things are negotiable.

7 How important are sex/affection/fun/intellectual stimulation?

None of these items is an essential ingredient of a relationship, and all are negotiable. The difficulty arises when only one member of the partnership wants one or more of these elements.

It is up to every couple to work out what they want and how — and to what extent — their needs are going to be met. Unfortunately, marriage is a situation in which most people start their negotiations after the contract has been signed. However, this does not mean that you cannot renegotiate, or improve on the contract. When couples marry young, the two members of the partnership often mature differently and find that, as a result, they no longer have a workable relationship. In such a case it may be better for the partners to separate honestly and amicably.

8 Do I need a counsellor?

There are some definite advantages in using the services of an outsider rather than trying to solve all the problems yourself. One is that it breaks the pattern, another is that an outsider can help take the heat out of a situation. And an outsider can often present new alternatives.

You can turn to a marriage guidance counsellor for help, or gain access to a marital therapist through your doctor. Some clinical psychologists and psychiatrists specialize in marital therapy.

9 Are gay relationships different?

The principles in all relationships are the same, and the same processes of negotiation and discussion apply. Most counsellors will just as happily see homosexual as heterosexual couples.

10 What about the children?

Children are remarkably flexible, and it is the experience of many therapists that the upset is no different to the child whether warring parents divorce or not. If anything, the evidence is that children may be less upset by divorce than by being in a situation of constant argument. Furthermore, a child may grow up feeling guilty that the parents stayed together on his or her account. Above all, children should be kept in the picture and discouraged from taking sides.

COPING WITH CRISES/3

The loss of something or someone we love is a crisis we all have to face sooner or later. The words grief and mourning are almost exclusively associated with death, but in fact we feel grief — and mourn our loss — whether we lose a job, a home, our ideals, a treasured possession, a much loved pet, a close friend or a partner. In all such situations we have to make adjustments to new circumstances by means of mourning.

Helping yourself

In coming to terms with the loss — particularly the death — of a loved one, those people best able to cope may be those who come from cultures that have strict, formal and intense mourning rituals. In modern society, we are expected to act as if nothing has happened, but research has shown that mourning is an essential part of coming to terms with a loss. Mourning occurs in three consecutive stages (see chart). But grief should not be used as an excuse for maintaining sympathy or for not changing your life. There comes a time — although its arrival is

ill-defined — at which you have to give up some of your grief and rejoin the mainstream of life.

Mourning is also dangerous to physical and mental health if it does not progress properly through its various stages. Mourning that re-starts after it has apparently finished — often accompanied by other signs of clinical depression (see pp. 240-1) — is another sign that profess-ional psychological help is needed.

Grief is nothing to be ashamed of. It is neither unseemly nor undignified. Certainly those around you may think you are less attractive than usual while you are suffering from grief, and sometimes it is important to try to keep up an appearance of 'normality' for their sake. Remember, too, that you are more likely to escape from your grief for a few minutes if you are talking to someone about a topic other than your loss. Yet it is not your duty to make life easier for those around you if you have sustained a loss. Equally, they should not feel they have to avoid you through embarrass-ment, but should be there to 'hold your hand' during the stages of the mourning process.

Stages of mourning			
Mourning, for whatever reason, takes place in three stages			
	Stage One	Stage Two	Stage Three
Characteristics	Shock and disbelief, a feeling of blank numbness. Inability to accept what has happened. Imagining that nothing has changed — such as expecting the arrival of a loved one at a certain time of day.	Realization that the loss has happened. Feelings of pain sweep over you. Recollection of old emotions and memories. Feelings of guilt. Odd behaviour, difficulty in eating and sleeping. Depression.	Relief from the pain and negative feelings. Return of a positive approach. Acceptance of possible replacements — although you know they can never fully take the place of what has been lost. Acceptance of the loss. Seeking of alternatives.
Comments	It is important not to stay too long in this stage of mourning or your recovery will be delayed.	This stage may last weeks, months or even years. Counselling is enormously helpful in this stage of mourning.	These show that your mourning has begun to be successful. You will not forget what you have lost but are coming to terms with reality.

If you are mourning, do not assume that you have to 'pull yourself together' faster than you feel is necessary. There are no short cuts to the resolution of grief. You will have to go through the mourning process at your own pace and be prepared to entertain thoughts and emotions that are alien to you.

Following bereavement, it takes many people about a year to come to terms with their loss. It is only if grief continues after such a period that you should question whether you are failing to get over that loss. It is at this stage that you may decide to seek outside help to give you that extra 'push' you need to get going again.

Divorce and other types of loss

It is natural to grieve when a marriage ends in divorce, when you lose your job or suffer a loss of similar proportions. In some ways, losses such as these are harder to cope with than death. With death, someone has gone for ever, and although the loss is painful, after the numbness is over, you can and must start to come to terms with it, and begin to create a new life.

With divorce, the 'lost' person is still alive, so beneath all the feelings that exist, there lurks the notion that the relationship might somehow be revived. For this reason, many people find it impossible to start mourning a divorce until long after it has occurred. It may take them many years to realize that the marriage really is over and that the lost partner is not likely to return. Often it is the remarriage of one of the partners that finally spurs the other into proper — and necessary — mourning.

Also important in divorce is the sense of rejection with which it is associated. Although we may feel we could have improved the quality of a dead person's life, death is not usually surrounded by feelings of personal guilt. Divorce, on the other hand, is a situation in which guilt thrives, and this guilt — along with feelings of personal failure — complicate the logical steps of the mourning process.

After someone has died, we often cope with this by building a memorial to them, which can be a physical thing such as a gravestone or a collection of the dead person's prized possessions. Psychologically we also build a memorial, remembering all the good things about them and their actions and forgetting the bad ones. This cannot usually happen with divorce, since the bitterness of the parting and intense awareness of the person's faults prevent it.

Losing your job has many features in common with divorce. The feelings of helplessness, rejection and failure are paramount. And in modern society, it is not considered legitimate to mourn the loss of a job. People may be sympathetic for a short while, but it is not long before you are told to 'pull yourself together'.

Helping others

There are many ways in which you can help someone who has been bereaved. Use the following guidelines to help you act sensibly:

● Let the bereaved person give the lead. Do not make judgments on their behalf about whether they should be 'cheered up', told to pull themselves together or discouraged from mourning.

● Grieve with someone who is bereaved. This gives permission for grief and shows that you, too, valued the person who is being mourned.

● Give practical help. During the early stages — before the funeral or for the first few weeks afterward — practical help is important. After the death of a loved one, people often do not feel capable of carrying out practical day-to-day tasks.

● Remember that, for a bereaved person, practical jobs can help by distracting the mind from the grief. So if the bereaved person shows signs of wanting to accomplish practical tasks, always let them do so.

● Be there. Bereaved people often feel that the existence of help and support — even if they do not use it — is important. Your support should not stop after the first few days of mourning, but will be needed for many months.

● Be reassuring. Gently reassure the bereaved person that they will get over their loss, however much they doubt this at present. See that they understand the mourning process.

● Do not encourage a bereaved person to take drugs such as antidepressants or tranquillizers. It is better to work through the grief without them. Sleeping tablets, taken on a short-term basis, may, however, be useful.

● Be aware. If you are sensitive to the emotions and reactions of a bereaved person, you will see when they are ready to be 'taken out of themselves'. When this time comes, seize the opportunity and make the most of it.

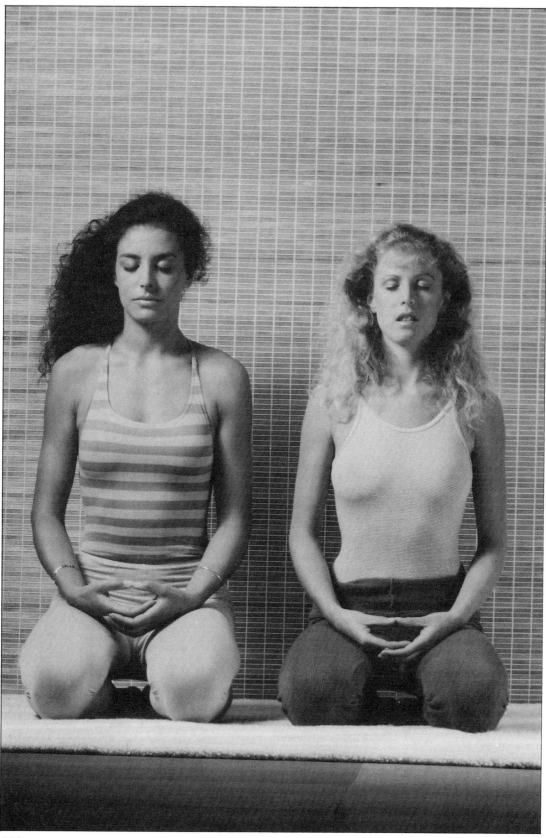

TREATS AND TREATMENTS

In their pursuit of fitness and well-being of body and mind, many people are now turning toward forms of treatment that fall outside conventional medical practice. Indeed, even the medical profession is beginning to accept many of them as valuable alternatives or additions to more usual forms of treatment. Equally, it is becoming widely recognized that the source of many of our physical ills is in the mind. With inner contentment and serenity comes the relief from many troublesome and stress-related symptoms that may range from migraine to backache.

The pages that follow explore a range of the treats and treatments currently available. The emphasis of selection is on variety, safety and self-help. None of the treatments described is harmful, and although there may be no sound medical basis for some of the treatments described, many have their origins in ancient medicine. And there is no doubt that the placebo effect really does work — that is, if you think a certain treatment is doing you good, then it probably is. In these days, when medical therapy may be unpleasant or even potentially dangerous, this could be a distinct advantage.

The possibilities described in this chapter should be readily available to most people. Some, such as herbal remedies, can be self-administered. Many, however, demand the help of expert teachers, at least in the initial stages. These include yoga and the Alexander Technique. Others, including osteopathy, chiropractic and acupuncture, can be administered only by trained personnel. Yet even these treatments may induce an improved attitude of mind, which persists and can be encouraged by self-motivation after the treatment is over. Thus, with experience in biofeedback you should learn how to control your own automatic responses and so be affected less adversely by stress.

Changing ingrained attitudes and behaviour are keys to improved health and happiness. For this reason, the chapter ends with examples of therapies that will help you alter the way you look at yourself. By reassessing your own thoughts and adopting a holistic, or 'whole person', approach to yourself and your problems, you should find yourself well on the way to their solution.

Benefits

Conditions that may be helped by one or more methods of heat therapy include:

● Rheumatism, arthritis and a wide variety of complaints of the musculo-skeletal system.

● Sciatica and many other conditions affecting the nervous system.

● Some skin conditions. Treatments that mimic the radiation contained in sunlight are helpful in treating problems such as acne.

● Respiratory problems, including asthma and bronchitis.

● Success has also been reported in the relief of symptoms caused by inflamation of the kidneys and gall bladder.

Warmth and water are two of the greatest comforts known to the human body. For most people the essence of relaxation is to lie on a beach, breathing the ozone-rich sea air, allowing muscular tiredness and tension to dissolve between warm sand and a benign sun and intermittently enjoying the world's most perfect exercise — a swim in the salubrious saline. It is no wonder that this neat package of heat- light- and hydrotherapies, makes us feel good. Little wonder, too, that winterbound urban dwellers increasingly seek out the surrogate version in the form of jacuzzis, saunas, sun beds, plunge pools and impulse showers at health clubs.

Yet warmth and water provide more than comfort; they induce the conditions for life itself. Life on earth began in the ocean, our own foetal lives take place in fluid, and our bodies are largely composed of water. Although warm blooded creatures, such as man, are able to maintain their body temperature by means of internal regulators, these rely for their integrity on an ambient temperature conducive to life. At extremes of cold and heat, body processes, including the temperature regulation, fail to function.

The uses of heat- and hydrotherapies to promote fitness and well-being, range from the simple hot bath to specific effective therapies used to treat serious ailments. Although particular heat- and hydrotherapies may be carried out separately, the two are often combined for dual benefit in the form of steam cabinets, whirlpool baths and so on. After all heat-therapies it is wise to rest for a period of about 30 minutes in order to allow the body to become restored to its normal resting and balanced condition.

Therapies with dry heat

Dry heat therapies act on the skin and circulation and can bring relief from symptoms of musculo-skeletal problems. These include arthritis and rheumatism, respiratory problems and sciatica. Therapies designed to induce sweating are useful in ridding the body of accumulated toxins. Sweat can act, for example, as a vehicle for the removal of lactic acid, the toxin that causes muscle pain on heavy exertion.

Therapies using dry heat induce a temporary condition called hyperaemia, that is, dilation of the blood vessels, combined with a local temperature rise and an abnormal increase in blood supply to

Warnings

● Avoid heat treatments if you suffer from a heart condition or high blood pressure. After only seven minutes in a sauna, the heart rate almost doubles, imposing a dangerous strain on a weak heart.

● Never take a young baby for heat therapy, since the large surface area of its body will cause it to gain and lose heat extremely rapidly.

● Overheating puts a strain on the heart, and subsequent cooling may result in a chill and respiratory problems.

● Never drink alcohol before heat treatment; you risk dehydration.

Other people at risk include

● Expectant mothers

●Diabetics

●Those suffering from a heavy cold, flu, a heavy menstrual period, glandular obesity and varicose veins.

● Those with low blood pressure.

● Elderly people should use the cooler shelves and limit exposure to extreme heat to 5 minutes.

● Those taking drugs should first consult their doctor

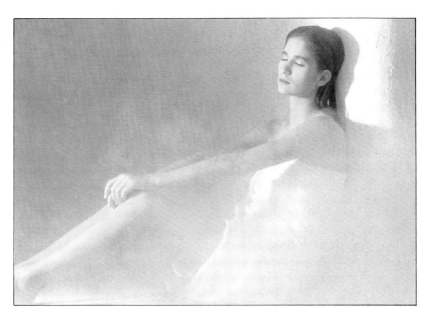

The Russian bath is essentially a steam-filled sauna. As with other types of sauna the benefits are immediate; a glowing complexion, easier respiration, relaxed muscles and a general sense of healthiness and well-being. In modern, electrical versions of this sauna, water ladled over hot stones produces steam to coax impurity-laden sweat out of the pores. The contemporary alternative to the traditional Finnish roll in the snow is a cold shower between bouts in the heat.

the part of the body being treated. Hyperaemia has positive effects, such as increasing the body's response to ultraviolet treatment, but it should be reversed afterward by a brief cold shower. It may also be tempered in progress by applying cold towels to the head and neck.

The principle types of dry heat treatment that are available include:

Infra-red

Any invisible, heat-carrying wavelength of electromagnetic radiation beyond the red end of the visible light spectrum is infra-red. Anything hot emits infra-red, but we can receive it only from sources hotter than ourselves, either luminous or non-luminous. General infra-red treatment is helpful for rheumatic conditions, and local treatment can also relieve lumbago and injuries; treatments last for about 15 minutes in an hour. They should be avoided by diabetics, and people with fair skins need protection with an emollient before treatment.

Radiant heat

Musculo-skeletal pains and the pain of sciatica all respond well to radiant heat. The patient sits or lies beneath a reflective surface lined with light-bulbs. The head is kept well clear and cool during the body's exposure to temperatures of approximately 76°C (200°F).

Cupping

The archaic-looking practice of cupping, used to relieve the symptoms of pleurisy, asthma, bronchitis or pneumonia, is still popular in Europe. A series of heated glass or metal cups is inverted on the skin of the back for respiratory complaints, elsewhere for specific muscles in spasm. As the cups 'cook', they create a partial vacuum, so that the flesh is drawn up into the cups.

Blanket wrap

A purpose-made electric blanket envelops the body to promote intense sweating. A plastic undersheet will increase the effect.

Traditional Turkish bath

The popular misconception that steam is incorporated into the traditional Turkish bath has arisen because steam facilities often are found on the same premises. What is commonly mistaken for a Turkish bath is a Russian bath, which is similar to a steam-filled sauna. In a Turkish bath following the Russian model, there are three phases: first, the cool room, or *frigidarium*; next the *tepidarium*, which is dry with the heat just above 37.8°C (100°F); and, once sweating has begun, the final room of intense dry heat, the *caladarium*, where temperatures may reach 47.8°C (150°F). After approximately 30 minutes of profuse sweating, the session is completed with a cooling shower or plunge and a thorough massage.

Steam cabinet

This is a less strenuous type of sweating bath, since the head is kept cool at all times.

HYDROTHERAPY

In Budapest, one of Europe's traditional 'watering places', the public baths built at the end of the nineteenth century (right) have been adapted with the use of modern technology. In this bath, for instance, a wave machine agitates the water for 10 minutes in every hour.

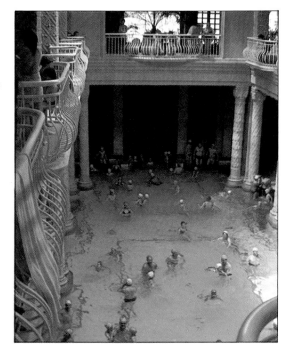

The whole family, including babies (right), can enjoy the benefits of hydrotherapy. As well as immersing the body in natural springs such as these, the water can be drunk. Spring water often contains minerals such as zinc, sulphur and calcium, and have for centuries been regarded as having health-giving properties.

The wide assortment of external and internal hydrotherapies are central to the 'nature cures' offered in modern health farms and spas. These therapies are based on the belief that numerous disorders, from catarrh to cystitis, can be prevented and treated through deep cleansing of the body. To dedicated naturopaths, purification is tantamount to panacea; to others, a simple jacuzzi is a treat to aching muscles and tired skin.

The practice of hydrotherapy dates back at least as far as Roman times and has been credited with curing everything from hangovers to insanity, but sceptics have always coexisted with believers. Spa, the now generic word for health resorts where people 'take the waters', originated from the mineral springs in Belgium, which were among the first to be identified as beneficial by the Roman legions. Bath, in southern England, was the most socially prominent of all spas in the eighteenth century, but its steady decline in popularity in later years reflected the advent of useful drugs and changing attitudes in the medical world. Today, however, hydros are making a well-deserved comeback.

In the modern world of hydrotherapy, the most elementary treatments are cold, hot and alternating hot-and-cold baths. Changing water temperature induces reactions within the body. A cold bath, which is always for a mercifully brief few minutes and at a temperature not less than 16°C (60°F), has a tonic effect. During immersion, the small blood vessels in the skin contract and afterward open up, giving a noticeably warm feeling as the vessels dilate. Hot baths work in the opposite way, initially attracting the blood to the skin and stimulating the sweat glands, after which the body cools.

Alternate stimulation by hot and cold has a pump effect on the blood within the contracting and dilating vessels that helps to reduce congestion and inflammation. With this technique, hot sessions of a couple of minutes are interspersed with 30-second cold dips.

Specific treatments

The sitz bath, derived from the German word for 'sitting', accommodates hot and cold simultaneously. It consists of a chair portion, containing enough water to cover the lower abdomen, and a smaller foot bath. The two sections are filled with water of contrasting temperatures, and after 10 minutes of sitting in hot water, with the feet in cold, the water is changed so that the body is in cold water and the feet in hot, the head and

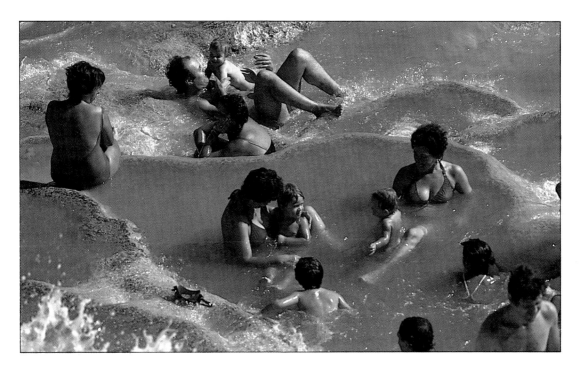

knees being kept clear all the while. The effect is to attract blood flow to the abdomen, and the treatment is prescribed for problems such as pelvic disorders and poor circulation.

A neutral bath, with water at almost exactly blood heat, 36.7°C (98.4°F) is useful in treating tension, insomnia and irritating skin conditions. The addition of Epsom salts (magnesium sulphate) is recommended for aching muscles; it encourages profuse sweating, and a warm shower should follow this treatment.

The fine adjustments of both temperature and pressure possible in water make it a highly adaptable treatment medium. Some hydrotherapy involves water in motion, either gently bubbled with air or pumped powerfully by water jets. Aerated water, which occurs naturally in certain mineral springs and which may be produced artificially, is a pleasant general tonic.

Types of baths
Underwater massage is the most effective and widely used of the pressure/movement therapies. The water is circulated out of the bath, returning as a powerful jet, which can be directed to any part of the body. Since the body is nearly weight-less in water, and the muscles relaxed, a more

intense massage is possible than in the air, so it is important to have a rest afterward.

Whirlpool baths, with their gently swirling currents, are a standard part of physiotherapy for injuries to joints and connective tissue and for some nervous conditions.

Douche refers to treatment with jets of water or sprays of water, from ordinary shower to high pressure hot-and-cold alternating treatment, fine needle sprays and impulse showers. They afford greater latitude than baths for localized treatment but are not advised for the very young or those of a nervously irritable disposition.

Packs and compresses, using lengths of cloth soaked in hot water (to dilate the blood vessels) or cold water (to relieve congestion and swellings) can be applied to large or small areas.

Mineral water is drunk for the reputed qualities of its mineral content, often in gaseous, ionized form, which is easier for the body to assimilate. Sulphur and nitrogen, for example, are thought to relieve rheumatic ailments. The bottled mineral waters are recommended for use during fasting —itself a purifying process.

Steam inhalation is used to treat catarrh and to relieve impaired breathing. Steam, or steam combined with herbal or aromatic oils, may be used.

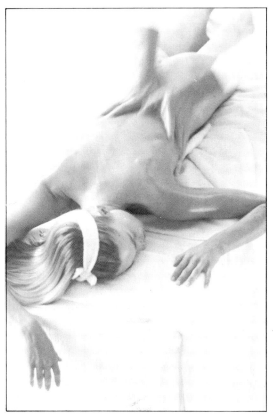

Touching is a means of communication often denied to us because of the taboos imposed by society. Massage is one way in which these taboos can be effectively broken. The giving and receiving of massage help relaxation, reassurance and an improved sense of well-being.

Massage is a class of touch which takes you on a guided tour of your own body and allows you to see more of yourself with your eyes closed than you can in front of a mirror with them open. Massage has existed in virtually every culture throughout history, and its French name, thought to derive from the Portuguese words for knead and dough, aptly expresses its nature.

The principal aim of most massage is to relax the mind and the muscles, promoting the flow of blood and lymph (tissue fluid). The heat generated as the body is massaged promotes the production of sweat and thus helps to remove waste products from the body. Swedish massage, however, is intended to stimulate the mind.

Many people who would benefit from massage never try it, dismissing it as specialist treatment for athletes and disabled people, or an unjustifiable indulgence with lurking sexual overtones. This is not true. You cannot fail to be struck by an elusive sensation of knowledge flowing from and back into the hands of a good practitioner.

The experience of massage

Within the complementary roles of giving and receiving, lies a choice of four experiences: receiving from a professional, receiving from an amateur (partner, friend, or family member); giving as an amateur and self-massage. Professionals offer the benefit of learned skill and experience. Having studied anatomy and physiology, they can readily identify muscles that are in spasm or undesirable connective tissue built up by misuse of the body. Their wide experience of different body types enables them to detect patterns and to choose the appropriate strokes for each individual. Within an hour's session, the routine is timed to build up subtly in intensity, then subside to leave time for relaxation.

Beyond convenience and economy, the value of learning massage yourself, and encouraging someone close to you to learn, is the understanding and well-being gained and comfort shared. Although practice is better than theory, there are books, workshops and courses available, and an introductory series of massages from a professional can be both learning experience and a pleasure. To find someone good, try health clubs, spas and beauty salons or personal recommendations, but do not choose a masseur or masseuse from classified advertisement columns.

The elements of massage

All massage is orchestrated in a series of basic strokes. **Effleurage** *(1)* is a soothing, warming stroke used to establish rapport between giver and receiver. It is moderately light and sweeps the full length of the back or limbs, often during the application of oil or powder. It is traditionally used to begin or end a session.

Pétrissage is useful for locating problem areas. These moderately deep strokes alternate pressure and relaxation, working along a limb or from the buttocks to the neck. For the two-handed method, trace clockwise circles with one hand and counterclockwise circles with the other. For the hand-on-hand method, move in clockwise circles up the left side of the part being massaged and counterclockwise up the right side.

Kneading *(2)* is a deep massage applied at will between other strokes. The thumb and fingers of each hand work on the muscles as if they were dough, alternately grasping and lifting (but not pinching), then releasing the flesh in a smooth motion.

Friction is the strongest of the strokes used in relaxation massage, marking a crescendo from which the massage is wound down. Using the thumbs, fingertips or knuckles *(3)*, deep pressure is applied in tight circles on small areas, to generate heat in the muscle.

The Swedish massage strokes, generally classified as *tapotment*, include hacking, clapping, slapping and pummelling. As an amateur, proceed with caution and remember that, although these strokes are designed to stimulate, the body should never become rigid in self-defence.

To give a facial massage, always smooth upward and outward above the brows *(4)*, ease round beneath the eyelids *(5)* and smooth upward from the chin *(6)* toward the ears. Facial massages cannot get rid of existing wrinkles but may help keep new ones at bay.

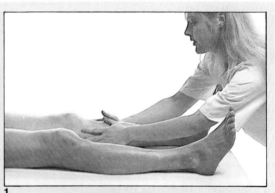

1

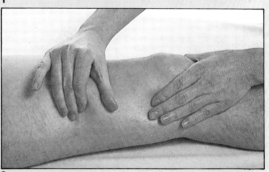

2

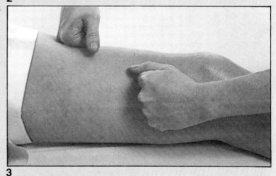

3

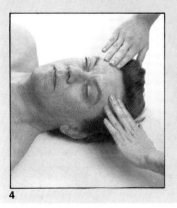

4

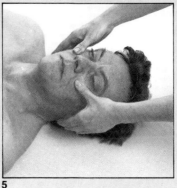

5

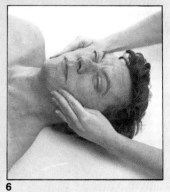

6

Massage is one of the most pleasurable agents of well-being. It improves circulation, relieves pain, enhances body awareness and promotes relaxation, but cannot reduce weight, reverse the ageing process nor improve muscle tone.

The sequence for a complete body massage is a matter of choice, but it is usual to start off with the back and finish with the feet. Begin with the receiver lying in a face down position. Massage the back, shoulders, neck, buttocks, thighs and legs. Then ask the subject to turn over and continue with the arms, hands, head and face, the front of the shoulders, the stomach (with the receiver's knees bent), the legs and ankles and finally the feet.

For self-massage, your own hands are the best aid, but other appliances can also be effective. Wooden rollers, on frames for the feet and on bands for the back; vibrating appliances; and rubber spiked massage sandals are fun to try out and can do no harm.

The full back massage

As a beginner in the art of massage, the back is an ideal learning area, since it is large, flat and emotionally neutral. Use the steps illustrated on these pages to give a full back massage, which should last 20 to 30 minutes. Make sure that you are calm and relaxed before you begin, and that your fingernails are short so that they will not dig into the receiver. Remove your wrist watch and any jewellery that might interfere with the massage. As you work, try to be aware of tense areas in the receiver's body. Apply the strokes evenly — you will adopt your own rhythm as you become more adept. For more information about the strokes see pp.268-9.

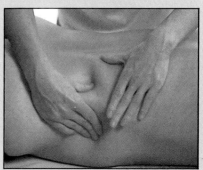

3 Turn sideways on to the receiver. Starting at one side of the lower back, make kneading movements all the way up each side of the back. Seek out tense areas of muscle.

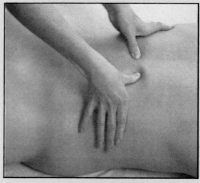

6 With your thumbs on each side of the spine, apply friction. Work up in small, deep circles, searching out knotty areas. Broaden the strokes at the shoulders.

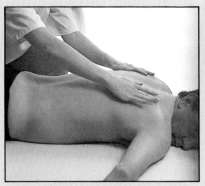

1 **Pour a little oil** into warmed hands and spread it over the back. Make smooth *effleurage* strokes starting at the top of the buttocks and sweeping up each side of the receiver's spine.

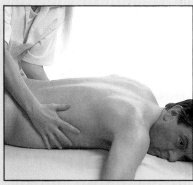

2 **Continue on** up to the neck. Run back down back sides of the body then repeat steps (1) and (2) about a dozen times, gradually increasing the pressure as you do so.

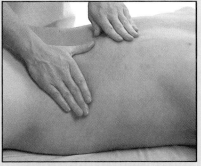

4 **Make alternate** inward- and outward-moving *pétrissage* circles all the way up the back to the shoulders. Repeat for the sides of the body.

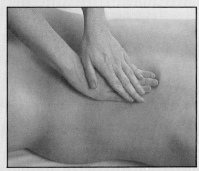

5 **Using the hand-on-hand** method, make further *pétrissage* strokes all the way up the back, working on each side of the spine. Adjust the pressure to suit the receiver.

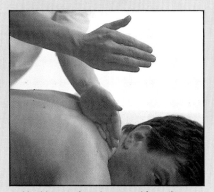

7 **Hacking strokes**, borrowed from the répertoire of Swedish massage, may be applied to areas such as the shoulders and sides if the receiver wishes.

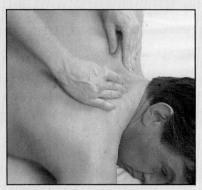

8 **Wind down** by applying more medium-pressure strokes to tense areas. End with a series of flowing *effleurage* strokes. Leave the receiver warmly covered to rest.

Points to remember
● Work on a firm surface — ideally a massage table, but failing that the floor. Beds are too soft, and the giver cannot work around them easily.

● Use a warm room and cover all areas of the body that are not being worked on.

● Always work equally on both sides and stroke in the direction of the heart — upward on arms and legs.

● As giver, exhale to reinforce the outward stroke.

Mistakes to avoid
● Never pour oil directly from the bottle on to the receiver. Do not use cream and lotions absorbed by the upper layers of skin, but keep to plant or mineral oils.

● Do not talk, except to exchange relevant observations, and avoid playing music with any rhythm. Relaxing environmental recordings, such as the sounds of the seashore, can be enjoyable and therapeutic.

● Do not continue for more than an hour.

● Do not press too heavily on bony areas and avoid massaging directly over the spine.

OSTEOPATHY AND CHIROPRACTIC

The back is the 'dark continent' of every body; you need two mirrors to see it comfortably, and still it is a mystery. Yet it has attracted its fair share of explorers, whose enquiries into back pain have led to a variety of manipulative therapies with wide applications. Osteopathy and chiropractic are distinct, but related, drug-free treatments that concentrate primarily on dealing with disorders of the spine.

Hands have been used to heal—particularly the musculo-skeletal system—in countless cultures throughout history; but these two well-known branches of alternative medicine were born in the late nineteenth century in the American Midwest. Within the established medical community, they have met with ambivalence, since they were thought to compete with traditional orthopaedics and physiotherapy. Acceptance of the methods is growing, however, as more people find the treatments effective.

Osteopathy was evolved by Dr Andrew Taylor Still (1828-1917), a Missouri physician motivated by the tragic loss of three of his young sons through meningitis. As a doctor, Still was versed in the art of setting broken bones, but the new treatment he introduced was original, founded on 16 years of meticulous study. He opened the first College of Osteopathy in 1897 and, within 20 years, saw the practice recognized in every state in the Union.

The name osteopathy, from the Greek words for bone and disease, is misleading, since it is not connected with bone disease, but with conditions arising from misuse of the bones and joints, and of the spine in particular. Still's central concept was of the osteopathic lesion. This was how he described structural abnormality that could cause functional or organic disease and pain.

A lesion might be a muscle in spasm or an irritated nerve, manifested as strain, pain, thickening of connective tissue, physical derangement or local swelling. The spinal cord, housed in the spine, is the link between brain and body. Between the vertebrae, spinal nerves emerge from it. These are easily pressurized, causing pain in the parts of the body they serve. The spinal cord also administers and distributes the autonomic nervous system (the controller of automatic respiratory, digestive, circulatory and similar functions), so that seemingly remote organs can suffer when the spine suffers.

Still proposed that disease would not develop if the circulation were free. Thus osteopathic lesions obstructing the system must be located and removed. This is the osteopath's work.

Recent problems, such as a back put out by awkward lifting, are acute and may be cured in one session. Longer-standing conditions, accompanied by tissue damage or structural adaptation by the muscles and ligaments, are chronic and usually a series of treatments is required. Osteopathy has proved particularly successful in treating slipped discs—misplacement of part of the cartilaginous discs between the vertebrae. In badly advanced cases of any kind, the osteopath may, however, advise surgery. The Alexander Technique (pp. 274-5) is a highly recommended form of 'aftercare' to prevent old lesions returning or new ones developing.

Techniques of chiropractic

Chiropractic is the most widely recognized form of alternative, drugless medicine in the world, with more than eight million Americans currently receiving treatment. Unlike osteopathy, which is confined to the treatment of mechanical disorders, it is concerned with a 'system' of disease, and its treatments have a wider scope.

Named from the Greek words for hand/manual and practice, chiropractic was aptly christened by a patient of David Daniel Palmer, who introduced the theory in 1895. Palmer differed from Still in emphasis and terminology more than actual therapy. He discounted Still's notion of osteopathic lesions and referred instead to subluxations—slight displacements or deviations of bony parts, notably the spinal vertebrae.

Compared with Still, Palmer placed greater importance on the nervous system and on the way mechanical disorders of the joints interfere with it. He proposed that mechanical dysfunction was best corrected by mechanical means.

Chiropractic diagnosis is similar to osteopathic, but makes more regular use of X-rays and blood, urine, neurological and orthopaedic tests. Manipulative treatment in chiropractic uses a different type of leverage. Studies have shown that treatment by a trained, registered chiropractor is perfectly safe. It has proved indispensable for many back sufferers but should not be expected to cure advanced complaints, such as serious arthritis, resulting from severe tissue damage.

Visiting an osteopath

On a first visit to an osteopath, the practitioner first takes a full case history and a thorough physical examination follows. Next, the osteopath manipulates each joint through its range of movement to assess how the body rates mechanically; he then feels the joints and soft tissues for diagnostic clues. Where movement is restricted, the osteopath manipulates to open the joint and restore alignment—usually between two vertebrae. Once the bones slip back into place, relief is immediate.

Examination of the lower or lumbar region of the spine is an important part of the osteopath's work. This is a part of the body that is particularly prone to trouble. Backache is prevalent because of the upright human stance, but is also related to stress. The osteopath will check for any indication of muscle spasm, of limited joint movement or of bone disease.

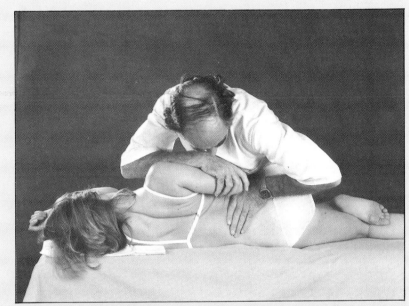

An osteopath will encourage patients to look after all parts of the body, but especially the spine. Positions such as this one mimic the actions of many animals as they yawn and stretch on waking. They allow the bones of the vertebral column to 'mesh' into their correct alignment and exercise the surrounding muscles beneficially. Such actions also alleviate the strain that is put on the spine during daily life.

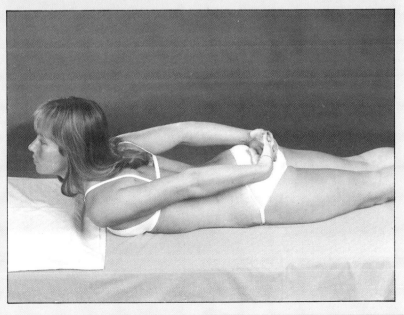

THE ALEXANDER TECHNIQUE

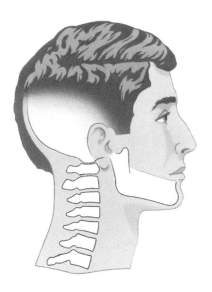

The base of the neck *is the gateway from the brain to the body (above). If the vertebrae move out of alignment or the muscles supporting them go into spasm, through habitual bad posture, the mechanisms of speech and swallowing may be impeded. If blood vessels or nerves are pinched, serious problems may occur in other parts of the body.*

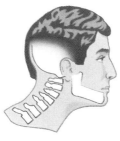

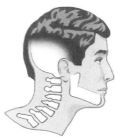

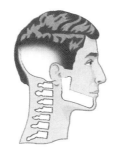

The most common *'bad habit' is to thrust the face forward so that the neck collapses forward, (top). Another familiar problem is a severely arched neck (centre), caused by pulling the head back to correct the forward incline of the neck. Repeated 'wrong' movements may even lead to a slipped vertebra. These contortions can usually be gradually corrected by relearning correct postures (bottom) through the Alexander Technique.*

The Alexander Technique, or Principle, aims to correct damaging habits of posture, which may be affecting your mental and physical efficiency.

An Australian actor, F. Matthias Alexander (1869-1955), stumbled upon the Technique late in the nineteenth century, when he set about discovering what was causing him to lose his voice, and potentially, his career. Through investigating every nuance of his physical behaviour, he established that he shut off his own voice because of the way he drew his head backward and downward. Beginning with this realization, he then pursued a meticulous study of how the human mechanism is designed to operate, and of how modern man frequently interferes with the smooth running of his own machine.

Alexander agreed with the views of osteopathy and chiropractic (see pp. 272-3) on the central role of the spine to fitness and well-being but, unlike them, attributed maladjustment directly to habitual misuse. He also perceived a relationship between physiological and psychological attitudes; that is, a slumping mind or spirit is the likely tenant of a slumping body, and muscular tension probably reflects emotional unease. In this respect, his approach may be described as holistic.

Many of us slouch because 'it comes naturally', but the aggregate product of years of slouching is the misshapen, poorly functioning spine. the greatest challenge raised by the technique is to unlearn old habits.

Demonstration and learning

The Alexander Technique does not consist of exercises, nor can it be learned from a book alone. It must be demonstrated by a qualified teacher, who adapts the instruction to suit the ingrained patterns displayed by the individual pupil. The teacher reveals the correct use of the body by arranging the pupil's body in the correct position so that he or she can feel it is right. Many people are initially confused because postures that feel correct through habit are wrong.

Teaching of the Alexander Technique consists of entirely private lessons or of group sessions supplemented by essential private sessions. The theory alone makes fascinating listening, and many people feel fired with optimism and exhilaration at the end of a class. A typical class might involve a re-enactment of postural evolution, with class members imitating primitive species or babies. The aim is to return people to the state they were in before they began making habitual postural mistakes—induced by tension, trauma, squashy furniture, climate and habitual laziness.

In private sessions, the pupil is subtly adjusted by hand into the deceptively tricky postures of sitting, standing, walking and lying down. Particular emphasis is placed on the transitions between each state. Through painless manipulation, the pupil has the sensation of actually growing.

The gradual re-education of the body involves visualizing oneself moving correctly and auto-suggesting (see pp.286-7) a lengthening of the body. The head has a key role. It is described as a locomotive, pulling the body train, or as suspended from a hook, allowing every part of the body to fall into correct alignment.

Many people have found using the Alexander Technique an enlightening experience. Aldous Huxley, who was one of its most articulate devotees, described it as an ideal form of true physical education, leading to heightened consciousness at all levels, 'and a way to prevent the body from slipping back under the influence of greedy 'end-gaining' into its old habits of mal-coordination.'

The therapy is infinitely subtle and sophisticated and requires perseverance to obtain lasting benefits. Teachers train for 3 to 4 years, and pupils may expect to attend around 30 sessions. People learn the Technique because they feel unexpectedly under par or because they suspect they are not operating at peak capacity. On a physical level, the Technique, which involves neither risk nor exertion, can help reduce the side-effects of stress, help relieve back pain, neuralgia, asthma, indigestion, migraine and high blood pressure, improve sleep and even foster cheerfulness of spirit. On a broader scale, it is supremely liberating and energizing, offering access to full personal potential.

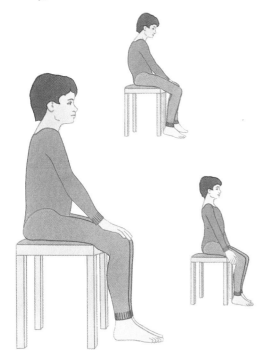

Most of us slouch when we think we are sitting in a relaxed way and over-arch our backs when we think we are sitting correctly. In fact, sitting with a straight back, eyes level, feet firmly on the floor and weight evenly spread demands considerably less effort and is more beneficial than either of the above.

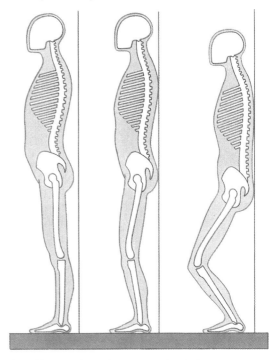

Use this exercise to help you practise the Alexander Technique. Stand with your lower back against a wall, knees bent, head slightly inclined forward,(right).If you find it rapidly tiring, you need to correct your posture. Slowly straighten your knees (centre and (left) and feel how your stance has changed.

HERBALISM AND AROMATHERAPY

Herbalism is the internal and external use of plant-based remedies to treat virtually any human ailment. While these remedies may relieve symptoms effectively, they are also claimed to be of great value in the prevention of illness by keeping the body's systems healthy and able to maintain its natural resistance to disease.

Herbalism makes use of not only the familiar aromatic culinary herbs but also less domestic plants including ferns, trees, lichens and seaweed. The selected part — leaf, stem, root or seed — is used whole, compared with the isolated 'active ingredient' synthesized for conventional drug use.

The history of herbalism is as old as man himself or older, for many animals have always instinctively sought the plants that would cure their ills. All the great ancient civilizations practised herbal medicine — largely because there were no alternatives — and a plant was so closely identified with its healing properties that these were used by the Greeks and, later, for official taxonomic classification. The advent of printing brought forth the great herbals such as Gerard's (1636) and Culpeper's (1653), both still regularly consulted today.

Herbal remedies are inexpensive, effective and free from toxic side effects — all reasons for their current renaissance among people disillusioned with modern drug treatments. Plants contain substances that naturally buffer and enhance their main ingredient, so safeguarding against the harm caused by using strong constituents in isolation.

The huge range of herbal preparations now widely available can be used both for preventive health care and for helping to treat all manner of everyday ills. However, the one that works for you may not be the same one that works for someone else. This is probably due to the 'placebo effect', that is, if you think a preparation is doing you good, then your condition improves. Try herbal preparations in place of coffee and tea to reduce your caffeine intake (see pp. 244-5). There are many common conditions for which they have recorded successes including migraine, catarrh and headaches.

Herbal remedies are safe enough for anyone to experiment with, to derive the most benefit, especially for more serious or long-standing complaints, it is best to consult a qualified herbalist. Herbalists are trained to treat the whole indi-

vidual, not just a disease or its symptoms. Two patients suffering from the same imbalance may require entirely different restorative remedies.

Aromatherapy

The practice of aromatheraphy was given its name by the French cosmetic chemist René Maurice Gattefosse, whose book, the first on the subject, came out in the year 1928. The therapy is comparable to herbalism in that it uses plant substances internally and externally; it treats a wide range of circulatory, respiratory, digestive and neuro-muscular complaints, and remedies are always tailored to the patient. Unlike herbalism, however, it uses highly concentrated, volatile and expensive essential oils. The influence of smell on

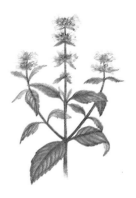

Peppermint (Mentha piperita) *is just one of 700 remedies listed in Egyptian papyri from 1550 BC. Many of these remedies, which include fennel, gentian, juniper, linseed and myrrh, are still in regular use today.*

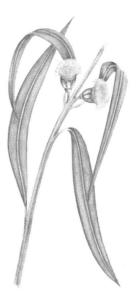

Herbal remedies *are usually prescribed as fluid extracts, tinctures or syrups, but may also be supplied dried, to be taken as infusions or decoctions, or in powdered form as tablets or capsules. External applications can be made with ointments, lotions or poultices. Eucalyptus (Eucalyptus globula), prepared in different ways can treat dozens of ailments, head to toe.*

the mind is such that the remedies aim to treat mental as well as physical ills.

Versions of aromatherapy have been known since before Biblical times. The modern practice ranges from self-help to services offered by health clubs and beauty salons to relieve medical conditions that have failed to respond to conventional treatment. It seems to be most successful with skin problems and in preventing illness.

For both baths and inhalations, a few drops of essential oil are mixed in the water. For massage, the pure oils are diluted considerably and penetrate the skin within minutes. Dosage is critical, since the same oil can act as a sedative or as a stimulant. Teas and medicines, taken internally, are used more rarely.

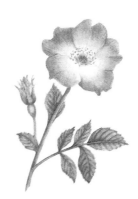

A single pound of rose oil requires 2,000 lb (907 kg) of rose petals, for essences occur naturally in miniscule amounts. They must be extracted with great care, and only the real thing will do, since chemical syntheses are not effective in aroma therapy.

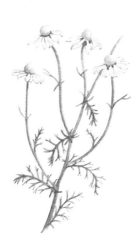

Chamomile (Chamomilla recacita) is a herbal staple used for ailments as diverse as nausea, headaches or boils. But with around 250,000 species of flowering plant yet to be evaluated for medical purposes, it could have equally versatile counterparts.

Bach Flower Remedies

Edward Bach (1880-1936), a fully qualified medical practitioner, pathologist and bacteriologist, became convinced that human illness arose from imbalances caused by negative states of mind. His credo was 'treat the patient, not the disease.' He abandoned London and conventional medicine for the Welsh countryside and an intuitive approach to therapy. He found the cures he sought in 38 species of wild flower, whose vital forces he captured by steeping the flower heads in sun-warmed spring water. The remedies are completely safe, and can be astoundingly, if inconsistently, effective in relieving emotional and personality problems. The remedies are available from specialist homeopathic stockists.

The seven categories of Bach remedies are:
Fear *Rock rose* (terror/panic); *Mimulus* (shyness) *Cherry plum* (fear of mental collapse); *Aspen* (fear of the unknown); *Red chestnut* (fear/anxiety for others).

Uncertainty *Cerato* (self-distrust); *Scleranthus* (indecision); *Gentian* (depression); *Gorse* (despair); *Hornbeam* (inability to cope, tiredness); *Wild oat* (dissatisfaction, lack of direction).

Lack of interest in the present *Clematis* (day-dreaming); *Honeysuckle* (clinging nostalgia); *Wild rose* (resignation, apathy).

Despondency and despair *Larch* (inaction through fear of failure); *Pine* (guilt); *Elm* (temporary despair); *Sweet chestnut* (extreme anguish); *Star of Bethlehem* (all forms of shock and sorrow); *Willow* (resentment, bitterness); *Oak* (despondency through lack of progress); *Crab-apple* (feeling unclean, self-dislike).

Loneliness *Water violet* (pride, aloofness); *Impatiens* (impatience); *Heather* (dislike of being alone, self-concern, poor listener).

Over-sensitivity to influences and ideas *Agrimony* (mental torment hidden behind a brave face); *Centaury* (weak will, exploited easily); *Walnut* (major life changes such as puberty/menopause); *Holly* (jealousy, hatred).

Over-concern for the welfare of others *Chicory* (possessiveness); *Vervain* (stress caused by over-enthusiasm); *Vine* (domination, inflexibility); *Beech* (intolerance, arrogance); *Rock water* (self-denial); *Olive* (post-stress exhaustion); *White chestnut* (persistent worries, mental arguments); *Mustard* (depression for no apparent reason); *Chestnut bud* (slow learner of life's lessons, repeated mistakes).

ACUPUNCTURE AND REFLEXOLOGY

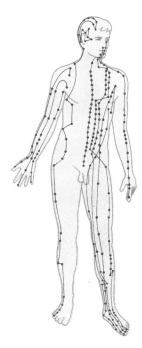

When the acupuncture points *relating to a particular organ or system are joined up, connect-the-dots style, they form meridians. The chi energy is said to flow along these 12 paths so that a needle in the foot, for instance, benefits a migraine headache. The main meridians in the front of the body include circulation/sex; lungs; heart; stomach; liver; kidney; spleen and large intestine.*

Acupuncture is a traditional Chinese therapy used to maintain optimum health and to diagnose and treat a wide range of disorders. In the West it has attracted notice as a drugless analgesic, as an anaesthetic and, less widely, as a treatment for the withdrawal symptoms of drug addiction.

The practice of acupuncture is based on the belief that the body flows with a vital energy, termed *chi*, which must be kept in balance to maintain good health. Orthodox medicine has long been sceptical, since the existence of *chi* has not yet been identified in the same way as, for example, the nervous impulse. Nevertheless, in recent years, acupuncture techniques have been more generally accepted in medical circles as a means of pain control. The theoretical basis for this is that, if a sensory nerve is blocked by simple stimuli, other more serious signals are impeded. Additionally, this nerve stimulation induces the production of endorphins: morphine-related substances which control pain in the body.

The flow of energy

According to the ancient theory, when *chi* becomes blocked or stagnates, it must be stimulated to flow freely. This is done by inserting ultra-fine needles into the skin at designated points — hence Latin *acu* (with a needle) and puncture — or applying an electrical stimulus at these points. Some conventional medical practitioners still find the remote character of the therapy hard to accept, for it treats internal complaints by external means, often using skin areas a puzzling distance from the organ or system undergoing treatment. However, the action of the endorphins may explain how acupuncture has successfully produced anaesthesia.

Yet another alien feature of acupuncture is the preliminary taking of 12 pulses — six in each wrist — compared with just one in ordinary medicine. These are the acupuncturist's chief diagnostic tool and are an invaluable early warning system for any serious ailments that may be developing. The practitioner palpates the radial artery in the wrist to detect fullness, hardness and the degree of activity, and from these and other observations, decides which points to use, and painlessly inserts a sterilized needle.

Many of the same points and meridians that are stimulated by needles in acupuncture may be treated to less powerful, but still beneficial, effect

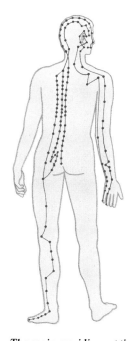

The main meridians *at the back of the body include the bladder; gall bladder; small intestine; large intestine, and triple warmer (a regulating/distributing function). Many acupuncturists advise that you visit 4 times a year at each change of season for a general health tune-up. This ensures your systems are all working well, and any unsuspected problems can be discovered and treated.*

by the related practice of acupressure or Japanese *shiatsu* (literally, finger-pressure) massage, in which the fingers and often the balls of the thumbs are used to press firmly over the points. It is both vigorous and enjoyable.

Shiatsu in Japan and acupuncture in China both have an ancient tradition, and could be described as a case of parallel evolution. The Japanese call the life-energy *ki*. *Shiatsu* is practised regularly and informally among Japanese families to give relief from everyday aches and pains and to prevent the development of illness. There is no fixed order for the massage, but it is considered important that the person giving it should be in good health. It is taught increasingly widely in the West, so the opportunity to learn — or simply to receive — is improving constantly.

The practice of reflexology

Reflexology, also called zone therapy, works on the principle that the entire body is mapped in the feet, and that deep massage of the appropriate areas brings relief to corresponding organs and systems. Like acupuncture and *shiatsu*, reflexology refers to meridians. There are ten of them, all terminating in the toes.

Where there are ailments and problems, tiny crystalline deposits may have formed in the related position in the foot. The reflexologist uses massage to break these down, and although the feet may be sensitive during treatment, the relief obtained may be dramatic.

It is delightful to have professional reflexology treatment, but it is also safe and beneficial to experiment on your own.

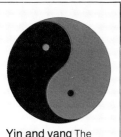

Yin and yang The Chinese symbol for *yin/yang* expresses both the universe's dual nature and ideal balance. For *chi* to flow properly *yin* and *yang* forces must be equalized in the body. Hollow organs which discharge or absorb – intestines, bladders, stomach – are *yin*; regulatory, solid organs – lungs, heart, liver, kidney – are *yang*.

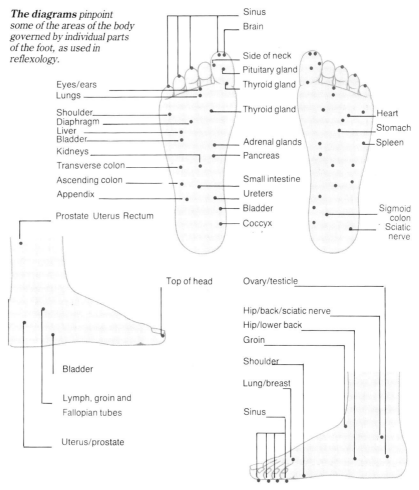

The diagrams pinpoint some of the areas of the body governed by individual parts of the foot, as used in reflexology.

Eyes/ears
Lungs
Shoulder
Diaphragm
Liver
Bladder
Kidneys
Transverse colon
Ascending colon
Appendix
Prostate Uterus Rectum

Sinus
Brain
Side of neck
Pituitary gland
Thyroid gland
Thyroid gland
Adrenal glands
Pancreas
Small intestine
Ureters
Bladder
Coccyx

Heart
Stomach
Spleen
Sigmoid colon
Sciatic nerve

Top of head
Bladder
Lymph, groin and
Fallopian tubes
Uterus/prostate

Ovary/testicle
Hip/back/sciatic nerve
Hip/lower back
Groin
Shoulder
Lung/breast
Sinus

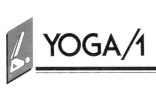

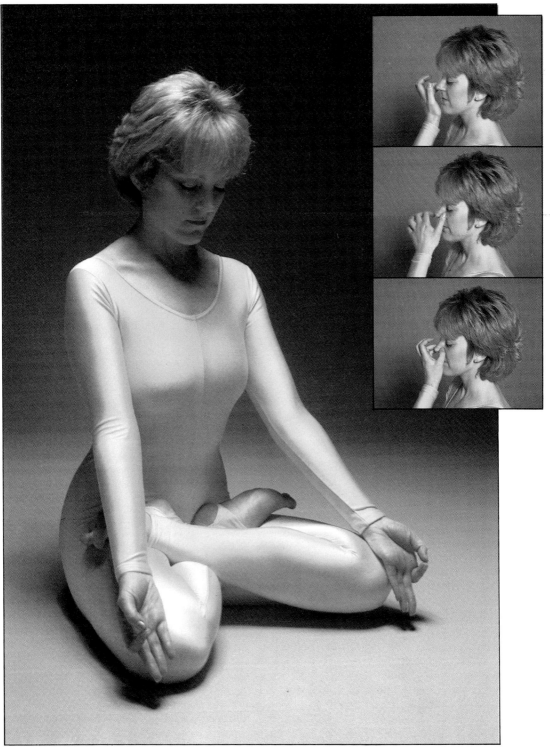

Alternate nostril breathing (left)
has an immediate tranquilizing effect on
the mind. Sit in the lotus position (far
left) *or simply with your back straight,*
and eyes and mouth closed. Shut the
right nostril by pressing the side with
the right thumb. Keep the next two
fingers bent and the last two fingers
together and straight.
1 Breathe in through the left nostril to
the count of 4.
2 Close the nose, using the last two
fingers to press in the left nostril, and
hold your breath for a count of 12.
3 Release the right nostril and exhale
to the count of 8, then immediately
breathe back in to the count of 4.
4 Again close the nose, this time
reapplying the thumb. Hold for a count
of 12.
5 Release the left nostril, breathe out
for 8 counts and immediately in for 4.
Repeat the entire sequence 9 times,
finishing with the final out-breath on the
left side.

The Tadasana, *the mountain or*
standing pose, is the pose from which all
others begin (right). *It helps improve*
posture and so prevents physical and
mental fatigue. With the weight evenly
distributed, the spine stretched,
stomach taut and shoulders relaxed, the
body assumes its natural position. This
frees the body from strain and gives a
feeling of heightened awareness.

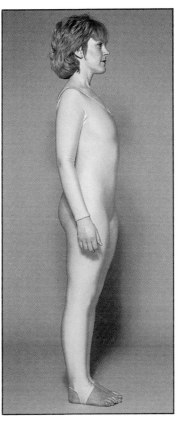

Tips
● Allow your face to relax into a
neutral expression and feel your
throat loosen.

● Imagine the back of your neck is
extending so that your chin tucks in.

● Relax your shoulders until they
slope slightly and your arms hang
limply. As the shoulders incline
backward, your chest comes
forward.

● Stretch your spine and feel
yourself 'grow' several inches.

● Pull your stomach in, without
constricting your breathing.

● Keep your feet together but your
weight evenly distributed.

Traditional yoga offers people of all ages and conditions improved physical flexibility, freedom from stress and a profound sense of well-being. It consists of eight disciplines, of which two are prominent in the yoga most of us experience.

The *asanas* (the postures which form the basis of physical yoga) are more widely taught than the *pranayama* (breathing exercises). However, *pranayama* (from *prana*, the life-giving energy brought in by the breath) is of such value, both in reducing stress and maximizing energy, that it deserves the same attention as the *asanas*. Many yoga teachers combine the two so that breathing control will help in achieving and sustaining the postures. This integration is true to the spirit of yoga, for the harmonious balance of mind, body and spirit is implied in the word *yoga*, which stems from the Sanskrit word for union.

Most of us habitually fail to do justice to our lung capacity and resort to stressful shallow breathing. Bringing breath into control is the first requisite of yoga.

First, become conscious of the lower, middle and upper lobes of your lungs, feel the breath draw deep down into your chest, slowly filling up, without strain, to just under the shoulder blades. Then breathe out fully, from the bottoms of your lungs up. The out-breath is as important as the in-breath and is the only way to clear the lungs of accumulated toxins. While walking, breathe out for double the count that you breathe in. This purges your lungs of stale air and makes room for a good supply of fresh oxygen.

The corpse posture
The Savasana, or corpse posture, can be the kiss of life if you are short of sleep or suffering from nervous exhaustion. It is also a good resting pose between more strenuous postures. Lie flat on your back, with your feet in a V-shape, arms comfortably by your sides. With eyes closed, breathe in for a count of 6, hold for 3, breathe out for 6 and hold out for 3. Repeat the cycle for about 10 minutes, stretch and get up.

The poses on these pages illustrate a range of beneficial yoga poses. The means of achieving these positions must, however, be learned from a qualified yoga teacher, to avoid self-inflicted damage.

The forward bend (Uttanasana) *helps relieve stomach pains and depression and tones the liver, spleen and kidneys. The legs and back are also strengthened* (right).

Child: (below) *is a recuperative pose that stretches the spine, relieves back, shoulder and neck pain, and restores energy.*

Dog (Adho Mukha Svanasana) *is a good pose for runners, since it eases tired legs* (bottom left). *It also strengthens leg and stomach muscles.*

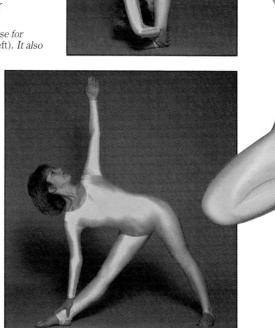

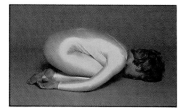

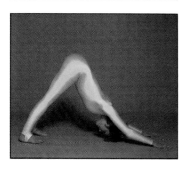

Regular yoga tacitly puts you back in touch with your body and persuades you to take the responsibility for your own well-being.

The *asanas* are the physical poses of yoga, as opposed to breathing exercises. There are hundreds of permutations, but you can devise a useful routine around a dozen, adding and varying poses as you become more adept. You will quickly discover that some poses come to you more easily than others, and that these vary from individual to individual.

The spine, hip joints and hamstrings are the key areas and will become much more flexible by virtue of most of the *asanas*. The spine must be persuaded to go inward and to lengthen; the hip joints need to go outward and loosen; the hamstrings must learn to loosen and stretch. In time, you may experience the yoga ideal — that by gradually freeing yourself of physical blocks, you

Triangle (Uttihita trikonasana) *stretches the legs and hips* (above). *It relieves backache and neck strain.*

Tree (Vrksasana) *gives a sense of poise and tones the leg muscles* (above right).

simultaneously dissolve mental and emotional barriers. You need not be an ascetic in a loin cloth to practise yoga; anyone can do it. Children, pregnant women, the elderly, office workers — all will benefit. Nor is time an obstacle. A thoroughly beneficial routine can be worked through at home in less time than it takes to watch a soap opera on television. Even 10 minutes spent on yoga every day will pay dividends.

Unlike ordinary exercises, yoga poses demand little movement. Once assumed, they are simply held while you continue to breathe normally and strive to perfect the shape. The main groups of *asanas* are standing, seated and recuperative, and

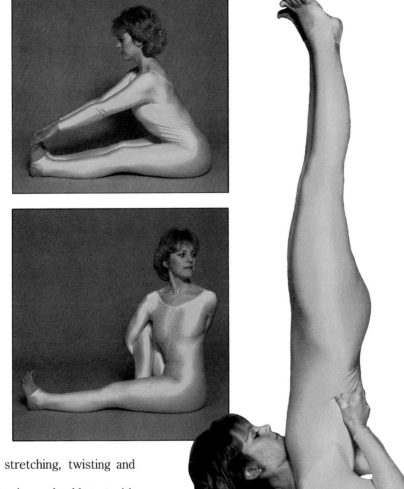

Seated forward bend
*(Paschimottanasana)
tones the abdominal
organs, including the
kidneys, and improves
the digestion. It also
helps to bring
oxygenated blood to the
pelvic area* (right).

Twisting seated pose
*(Ardha Matsyendrasana
1) improves the blood
circulation around the
abdominal organs and
helps backache and stiff
shoulders* (below right).

Shoulder stand
*(Salamba Sarvangasana)
improves the blood
supply to the head,
chest, neck and abdomen*
(far right). *Since it
reverses the strain of
gravity, it relieves
varicose veins and
haemorrhoids and also
helps respiratory
ailments and headaches.
It has a soothing effect on
the nerves, helps relieve
constipation and
menstrual problems and
assists the correct
functioning of the thyroid
gland.*

they involve balancing, stretching, twisting and forward bending.

Any well-intentioned beginner should start with the supervision of a good teacher, to avoid unnecessary injury and frustration. Chance factors, such as cost, location and free time, may dictate your choice of class, but it is worth searching to find a good teacher who inspires confidence but not competition. You will find that your muscles, spine, respiratory, circulatory, endocrine and nervous systems all benefit considerably. Various styles of yoga are taught today, but *hatha* (physical) yoga is the most popular.

After you have learned the basics, it is still valuable to attend open classes or an advanced course to avoid falling into a rut or bad habits. The group atmosphere has a positive effect, and the best way to improve is through the guidance of a good teacher. Meanwhile, practise daily.

The fringe benefits

As you become more skilful at yoga, so you become more graceful. You may suddenly catch yourself floating down the street as buoyant as if you had just had a pay rise (in a way you have). You may realize that your spine is as straight as a ballerina's as you squat to open a cupboard. You will find you use your body more efficiently, treat it with more respect and take more care about how you choose to fuel it. You will not burn many calories in yoga, but once you have learned the secret of breathing more efficiently, you may crave less sugar in your diet.

BIOFEEDBACK

Biofeedback offers people the means to control their own health. It is based on the idea that by feeding information back to a subject, he can learn to control his own physiological responses. As he does so, anxiety, pain and tension can be remarkably modified. A calibrated machine feeds information about factors such as blood pressure, localized muscular tension or skin resistance and temperature back to the individual in the form of light or sound signals. As he learns to relax, and his body responds, he is gradually able to eliminate the signal from the machine.

In the middle of the nineteenth century, various people studying hypnosis, among them Carl Jung (see pp.296-7), discovered that states of anxiety in their subjects caused a marked rise in the electrical resistance of the skin. From the 1930s onward this, and other measurements related to involuntary changes in body physiology, were chiefly used in polygraph or lie detector tests.

It was not until the 1960s that workers in the USA began to realize the potential of such measurements in the detection and control of stress. As a result of extensive work on both humans and laboratory animals a series of devices were developed which, with modifications, are used for biofeedback treatments today.

The benefits
Biofeedback is one of the few medically accepted techniques to demonstrate that the imagination can influence the body. Internal processes, such as pulse rate and skin temperature, which were formally considered beyond voluntary control, are particularly responsive. The debilitating effects of stress in the form of headaches, indigestion, tension, insomnia and so on can be self-regulated. For this reason, biofeedback instruments are now used in some hospitals to treat a wide range of medical problems caused by anxiety; they are also used in some imaginative clinics. This approach has also been used, though less widely, to investigate altered states of consciousness including meditation and hypnosis.

Messages from the skin
The relaxometer is a typical biofeedback machine that measures levels of arousal by recording the electrical conductivity of the skin through electrodes placed on the fingers. When the body is aroused or stressed the sweating increases and the skin becomes moist, so conducting more electricity. The increased current flowing through the electrodes to the machine passes more electrical energy to the light or sound signal and alerts the user to his level of arousal. When the body relaxes, however, the sweating decreases and the skin becomes drier. This reduces the electrical current to the machine, causing the displayed signal to decrease, so informing the user that he is more relaxed. As he learns to reduce the signal by controlling the sweat glands, the individual does indeed become more relaxed.

Another biofeedback instrument in use is the temperature meter, which registers the amount of warmth in the skin. When we are stressed, the 'fight and flight' response of the autonomic nervous system causes blood vessels to contract and to draw blood away from the surface of the skin so that skin temperature drops. When we relax, the blood flows back to the surface of the skin, and the machine indicates the rise in temperature. Many people find that by simply imagining themselves in a warm situation, such as sitting in front of a fire, their hands actually warm up. Yet if one tries to use will-power, rather than imagination to increase skin temperature, the hands are likely to become cold because will-power is governed by the sympathetic nervous stystem that serves the 'fight and flight' response.

Learning to relax
Biofeedback devices do not induce relaxation in themselves but can be used to learn the 'knack'. You are encouraged to allow yourself to become receptive to messages of tension or relaxation, warmth or coldness and so on, given out by your body, usually by imagining a warm and relaxing situation. Subjects report suddenly discovering they can do it, but cannot explain how. With practice, many also learn to relax without the instrument, through auto-suggestion.

Messages from the brain
The electroencephelograph (EEG), which has been used for research into the various levels of brain-wave activity, is one of the best-known biofeedback monitors. Specific wave frequencies have been found to be associated with different states of mind: *beta*, the most common brain wave in a normally active mind, represents the

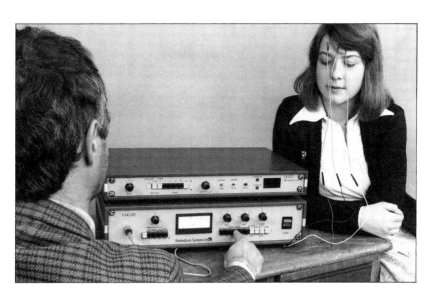

The electrical activity of the brain, which is measured with a type of electroencephalogram (EEG) indicates, to the trained operator, the state of consciousness of the subject. The aim of biofeedback is to teach the subject to control aspects of body physiology that normally occur involuntarily and, in so doing, reduce stress and its associated ills.

fastest level of electrical activity and is associated with active concentration, as when solving a practical problem. *Alpha* is a slower rhythm, usually described as being pleasantly relaxed. The third-slowest is *theta*, which many people experience between waking and falling asleep, and it is often associated with creative or disturbing images. The slowest rhythm is *delta*, which occurs during sleep.

The biofeedback machine gives feedback about the *alpha* waves and is a simpler version of the EEG found in hospitals. The object of the training is to help a person relax into the *alpha* state, which creates a feeling of well-being. More sophisticated practice can help the individual reach higher states of awareness, and, conversely, deeper states of relaxation, which may otherwise take years of meditation to achieve.

Reducing hypertension

Biofeedback has proved effective in easing hypertension—a major cause of heart attacks. The alarm response of the sympathetic nervous system increases blood pressure and mobilizes the whole body into a state of arousal. Many people are unware of living in a semi-permanent state of tension. Through biofeedback and relaxation exercises an individual can learn to create a 'rebound' from a state of arousal to a state of calmness. This involves normalizing the heartbeat and pulsation of blood, and modifying the digestion and muscular tension. Although this process takes longer than, for example, treatment with anti-hypertensive or tranquillizing drugs, it may reduce the risk of drug dependency and allow for a healthier way of life.

Placebos

The effect of placebos suggests how our minds can influence our bodies. A placebo is an innocuous medicament which the individual believes to be a genuine drug prescribed for a specific condition. A variety of research studies has shown that the blood pressure of hypertensive patients could be reduced equally well, whether they were given hypertensive drugs or placebos. The belief that the tablet will help solve a problem often brings about a temporary 'cure', which reflects people's powerful physical response to a conviction.

Although biofeedback instruments are useful in the treatment of physical or psychological problems, they are not essential for the development of self-awareness. If we choose to be attentive, internal and external environments give us continuous feedback about our state of health. A mirror indicates clearly if we are tired, tense overweight or simply looking out of condition. Trusted friends can give valuable feedback as to how one behaves or looks to them. Most important of all, however, is our ability to listen to our own internal messages, for they are the most accurate prompters, advising us as to whether we should be active or should rest.

AUTOGENICS

Graceful living is born of a relaxed body and a sharpened concentration of the mind. Both can be achieved through autogenics — self-generation — which is a method of concentrated relaxation using the power of self-suggestion.

Autogenics was developed in the 1920s by a German neurologist Dr J K Schulz, who used hypnosis to treat his patients. Many of them derived great benefit from the relaxation produced by the hypnotic process, so Dr Schulz experimented to see if they would fall into deep relaxation without hypnosis. He developed the idea of teaching verbal suggestion, which proved highly effective.

The relaxation technique

Autogenic exercises have been used to combat stress headaches, high blood pressure, ulcers and many psychosomatic problems, as well as for improving sports performance. The aim is to try to focus on a specific part of the body and to control experiences within it. We can learn to make parts of the body light or heavy; cool or warm; calm or tense. So, for example, you might begin with saying to yourself: 'My fingers and hands feel warm and heavy.' This is repeated several times before moving on to other parts of the body: the arms, shoulders, head, neck, back, legs and so on until the whole body feels both warm and relaxed.

Autogenic training exercises may also include suggestions that help to slow the breathing and heart rate and so deepen the state of relaxation. Mental alertness is assisted during the process with suggestions such as, 'My forehead is cool and relaxed', which prevents the subject from becoming too drowsy.

Constant practice usually leads to an automatic response when a phrase is repeated, and this can be used effectively during times of stress. For example, saying 'My shoulders feel warm and heavy' to yourself may be sufficient to reduce strain if you are sitting in a traffic jam and worrying about being late for an appointment.

The side-effects

During deep relaxation, long-standing physical aches and pains may surface temporarily because the muscle tissue becomes more sensitive. Similarly, unexpressed emotions, such as anger or sadness, normally held back by muscular tension, may emerge suddenly. For this reason, many people prefer to have a specialist on hand to assist with unpleasant reactions in the early sessions.

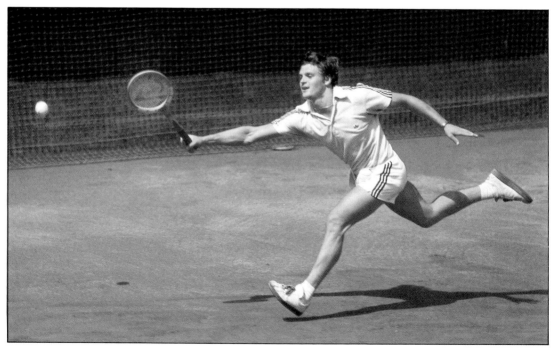

Perfect balance, precise body control and intense concentration are the keys to success in top class gymnastics. Autogenic training helps the mind to block out distractions and improve coordination so that body follows mind in exact harmony.

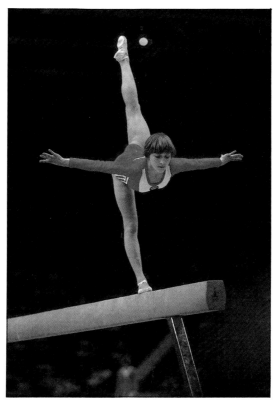

Sustained confidence, control and sharpened reactions are essential qualities for winning at sports such as tennis (below left). Autogenics teaches an athlete to overcome nerves, doubts and self-criticism and to put valuable learning into practice at the most crucial moments.

A training session
A typical autogenic training session starts with the subject seated, with head and shoulders supported, legs uncrossed and arms and legs comfortable. Alternatively, the subject may lie down.

The instructor begins with a series of sentences, which the subject repeats inwardly while concentrating on the message. For example, 'My right arm is heavy and warm' is repeated several times until the arm relaxes.

Other parts of the body are then 'treated' until the sensation of relaxation becomes all-embracing.

These outbursts, however, can help to heal old wounds or reveal new aspects of your personality. Deep relaxation may also induce tiredness, since muscular tension uses a great deal of unnecessary energy, and, when these muscles eventually relax, they feel fatigued.

Mind control
Once the art of relaxation has been mastered, autogenics can be used to improve the powers of concentration — to spectacular effect in the sporting world. Olympic marksmen, for example, have been known to use autogenics during competition to achieve a balance between relaxation and arousal. By repeating sentences such as, 'The target focuses my mind,' they are able to sharpen their attention and block out distractions.

The 'Inner Game'
A recently developed technique for improving sporting performance is called the 'Inner Game'. It claims that the conventional mastery of sport is too concerned with the outer game — with

techniques, such as how to swing a club, bat or racket or how to position the limbs — while it overlooks the player's anxiety, self-doubt, lack of concentration and so on. Exponents of the Inner Game find that the approach encourages the spontaneous interaction of mind and body — an ingredient for success in sport and everyday life. They describe activity in terms of Self 1, who tells us what to do and how to do it, and Self 2, who carries out the action.

The first skill to be developed is non-judgemental awareness. So, when a tennis player says, 'I missed that ball,' he is asked to express this as a simple factual observation, instead of as negative self-criticism.

As Self 1 learns to become less judgemental, so Self 2 is free to become more spontaneously involved in the performance and to rely on the fretful interference of the conscious mind. A key principle in this dynamic relationship is to trust that the innate wisdom of body and mind will lead to more effective performances if you can relax sufficiently for these to occur.

ZEN AND MEDITATION

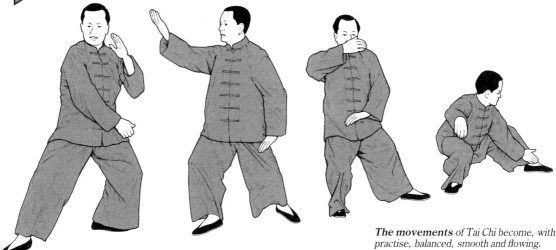

The movements *of Tai Chi become, with practise, balanced, smooth and flowing.*

The aim of meditation is to relax the body and mind and to create a focused awareness in which the 'chatter' within your head gives way to stillness and inner peace. Regular periods of meditation, when carried out in quiet, peaceful surroundings, can provide you with a respite from the hustle and bustle of daily life. They also allow you to find inner peace and reduce stress.

Meditation has been practised for centuries in both East and West. But while in the West it has traditionally been identified with prayer and direct communication with God, in the East its aim has been to free the mind from excessive thought. Simplified forms of many meditation techniques have, in recent times, been incorporated into holistic approaches to mental and physical health.

The means of meditation

One approach common to all forms of meditation is one-pointedness. This means that all your attention is directed to one feature of experience to the exclusion of all else. In Zen meditation, you focus on the inward and outward flow of breath. When your thoughts begin to stray, you merely return your attention to your breathing. In transcendental meditation, the meditator repeats one word, a mantra, over and over again in silence.

A typical meditation involves sitting comfortably but erect and beginning to focus on a mantra, on breathing or on an object such as a picture or a candle flame. By gradually becoming more adept at letting go of conscious thoughts and feelings, the meditator discovers a fresh way of being at the centre of his own experience.

Zen Buddhism is a spiritual tradition that prac-

tises a form of seated meditation. It emphasizes the need for 'emptiness', so that by emptying your mind of all its prejudices and preoccupations you get closer to the true nature of reality. In Zen there is also considerable emphasis on trusting in the natural course of life. From the rhythms and processes of nature, its practitioners argue, you find continual wisdom and simplicity.

All meditative approaches, if performed with full awareness and over a considerable period of time, can have a profound influence on your ordinary life and fitness. By learning how to let go, to enter states of deep relaxation and to develop peace of mind, you can become mentally and physically revitalized. Many people report that they are more sensitive to their surroundings as a result of consistent meditation.

Recent research on the brain has helped us to begin to understand the effects of meditation. Neurophysiologists have discovered that in most people the left hemisphere of the brain is dominant over the right. The left hemisphere is concerned with logical thoughts and ideas, with speech, mathematical concepts and so on. Its dominance is believed to be due, in large part, to your cultural bias toward rationality.

The right hemisphere of the brain deals with artistic appreciation, non-logical thoughts and images and with intuitive methods of understanding. In meditation it has been found that there is a shift in activity away from the dominant left hemisphere and toward the right. This shift of emphasis enables the meditator to attain a higher level of receptivity and awareness than is ordinarily possible in the Western world today.

Other research into the physiological effects of meditation has shown a marked decrease in the 'fight or flight' responses (see pp. 230-1) when people start to meditate. Pulse rate, skin conductivity and muscle tension all show marked decreases during meditation. And a person can learn how to maintain these benefits so that they become permanent. This has obvious value in the treatment of a wide variety of psychosomatic and stress-related disorders, such as high blood pressure, migraine, some digestive disorders and insomnia. It is also one of the reasons why the value of meditation is beginning to be appreciated by the medical profession as part of a holistic drug-free approach to health.

Meditation and spirituality
Many people use meditation as an opportunity to communicate with God, or think about the essence of life. They find that meditation quietens the mind and allows them to listen to God or let the spirit of life enter them. Some people say that listening for the word of God does not mean waiting for some extraordinary revelation, for what they hear or know through meditation is something basic to life that is already known, such as 'be more accepting'.

Meditation, prayer, contemplation or faith can give you a vital sense of transcendence, of being connected to something larger than yourself. On a practical level, they can be enormously useful in helping you to cope with the crises of life and with coming to terms with shattering concepts, such as the fact of your own death. People often speak of 'going' beyond their own minor concerns and worries, when they meditate or pray, to a sense of being unified with others and with the universe.

Peak experiences — those moments at which we are filled with revelation, insight or deep feeling — can also be brought about by physical activity or sport. One woman described recurrent experiences of religious faith while jogging: 'I feel more inspired when I'm jogging than I ever did in church. Sometimes I just have the sense of going beyond myself and being aware of and part of everything around me.'

Meditation can deepen faith, of which trust and love are necessary components. There can be no doubt that in a troubled world any way of reaching a deeper recognition of the value of life and the universe must be important.

HYPNOSIS

Hypnosis is an altered state of consciousness, into which a person enters voluntarily. Usually accompanied by feelings of deep relaxation, it can create physical and psychological changes. These are produced by altering a person's emotions, sensations and imaginings. For many people, hypnosis is a useful means of reducing stress, and the behaviour associated with it, and of coming to terms with deep-seated problems. It can also be valuable in the relief of pain.

The nature of hypnosis

Hypnosis is essentially a 'consent' state. To be susceptible to hypnosis (and most people are), a subject must have a certain degree of trust in the practitioner and a willingness to put aside any resistance. The hypnotist acts primarily as a guide to the subject, giving simple instructions, which, when followed, lead the subject gradually into a trance.

A popular image of the hypnotist at work has the subject looking at a pendulum, a swinging watch or gazing into the hypnotist's eyes. These techniques and others have been used in the past and may still be in use. But what is important about any method is that it should focus the attention and exclude distractions.

Most modern hypnotists use a wide variety of methods. For example, the subject may be asked to count backward from, say, 300 or to gaze at a fixed spot on the ceiling. Often, however, it is sufficient for the subject to sit or lie with closed eyes and listen to the hypnotist's voice—which should be calm and repetitive enough to induce relaxation. By following the suggestions given, the subject allows himself to fall into a state of heaviness and drowsiness that may eventually give access to forgotten memories and experience and, as a result, help with the relief of a wide variety of problems.

The success of hypnosis is a result of the way in which the brain receives and filters information from the environment. At the top of the spinal cord is an area called the reticular activating system (RAS), which regulates the amount of activity in the brain. If the environment is busy and contains many stimuli, the messages reaching the RAS are likely to increase brain activity, leading to arousal and wakefulness. When there is little outside stimulation, the RAS shuts down, brain activity decreases, and the subject relaxes and eventually falls into a deep sleep. The hypnotic state lies somewhere between the two poles of sleep and wakefulness.

When the mind and body are calm and relaxed, the suggestions given by the hypnotist pass directly into the subject's consciousness and are much more likely to be accepted. For this reason, there must be prior agreement between subject and therapist about the nature of the suggestions to be given. It is particularly important for the instructions given to be both calming and positive because in some instances, unpleasant memories and experiences may be brought to the surface of the mind.

It is often much easier to explore disturbing aspects of your life in hypnosis than in the normal waking state because the resistance, or 'critical censor', which the mind normally imposes on such material is in abeyance. In such hypnoanalysis, considerable skill and knowledge is required on the part of the therapist for the treatment to be conducted in a manner that is both safe and effective.

Practical hypnosis

Once their fears have been dispelled with proper explanation and reassurance, most people can be hypnotized, at least into a light trance. It may take a person many sessions to achieve a state of deep trance. However, it is not always necessary to enter a deep trance for much hypnotherapy to be effective. A wide range of problems can be treated with the use of systematic relaxation and suggestion, both of which are important aspects of hypnosis. The relief of general stress and anxiety, eating disorders, smoking, nail-biting, lack of self-confidence and shyness can all be successfully treated, as long as the subject is well motivated and has a good relationship with the therapist.

In solving people's problems, the hypnotist may use one or a combination of strategies. Ego-strengthening is an effective way of building up a person's confidence in his ability to overcome his difficulties. It involves the use of positive suggestion to reinforce motivation and a sense of self-esteem. With some addictive problems, such as smoking, overeating, or the taking of alcohol or other drugs, a type of aversion therapy may be used which emphasizes the unpleasant or damaging aspects of the habit.

Alternatively, or in addition, the therapist may stress the positive aspects of breaking the addiction so that a new set of associations is gradually established that begin to assert themselves in the normal, waking state. For many people, the light trance state may be sufficient for the mind to be receptive to the new associations and for the problem to be surmounted.

As a rule, the greater the ability of a subject to create imaginative ideas or fantasies, the greater the likelihood of success. People who have difficulty in visualizing and creating internal sensory perceptions of smell, taste, touch and so on are likely to prove more resistant to this approach.

Pain relief

The relief of pain during childbirth and in dentistry are two other areas in which hypnosis can be used successfully. These involve the generation of relaxation and local anaesthesia, so that painful sensations in a particular area are reduced or eliminated. For this to be successful, the subject must be adequately trained beforehand, so the hypnotic state can be achieved reasonably quickly when required. Classes in self-hypnosis for childbirth are carried out at some hospitals and by some doctors who find this a valuable approach to drug-free labour.

With this technique, the subject is taught that under hypnosis a particular part of the body will become numb. So, for example, the suggestion is given that no pain or sensation will be perceived in the hand. This is tested, after sufficient repetition, with a small pinprick, which should produce no pain response. The subject is then told that he or she is able to transfer this lack of sensation to any area of the body as required, such as the mouth, in the case of dentistry, or the perineum or lower back in the case of labour.

Many practitioners believe that in using hypnosis for pain relief it is more important to concentrate on the positive aspects of desensitization by avoiding direct references to pain, since this may generate anxiety. Instead, they refer to contractions or to numbness, both of which are more neutral terms.

With practice, many people find that they can teach themselves a type of self- or autohypnosis. This is related to autogenics (see pp. 286-7) and can be a useful tool in helping people to cope with the relief of stress-related symptoms.

BEHAVIOUR THERAPY

Clinical psychologists in USA and Britain practise behaviour therapy more widely than any other form of treatment. In helping yourself to improved fitness and well-being, the behavioural approach can be a way of learning, and of changing habits, even those that are most difficult to break. In this way behaviour therapy can offer a hopeful outlook and new adjustments.

Behaviour therapy focusses directly on external behaviour instead of subtle internal feelings, and asserts that all behaviour — good or bad — is learned through our interaction with other people. This learned behaviour is acquired and sustained as a result of positive or negative feedback.

Positive feedback, or positive reinforcement, produces feelings of pleasure, either physical or psychological, so that an individual is motivated to repeat the approved behaviour. If, for example, a young boy is praised every time he does not cry when he is hurt, he will gradually learn not to do so. Similarly, if a girl receives smiles and compliments every time she sings, she will probably continue to perform.

Negative reinforcement, sometimes supplied in the form of punishment, directs a person away from certain types of behaviour. The office worker whose initiative is always undermined by the boss is likely to think twice about taking initiative on another occasion.

Insights into development
The principles of behaviour therapy are helpful in understanding child development, and are used to good effect when parents have established clearly with their children which types of behaviour should be rewarded. Consistent positive reinforcement is necessary and children who do not receive it often develop problems in later life. Often parents hold up the achievements of the older child, as a standard, for others to follow. If others cannot, and therefore receive insufficient rewards for their own behaviour, they may come to believe that they will never be able to please, whatever they do. This leads to a reduction in a child's self-esteem.

Some parents rely excessively on the use or threat of punishment to produce acceptable behaviour. The child may comply, not because he wants to, but just to keep the peace. This type of negative reinforcement may suppress the old behaviour, but hardly encourages a new and

perhaps more appropriate behaviour to emerge. In the absence of the opportunity to earn reward, the child simply spends his life trying to avoid making mistakes, rather than doing things spontaneously to earn rewards.

New behaviour patterns
When there are a variety of stimuli that provoke an undesirable pattern of behaviour, it can be helpful to narrow down exposure to them. Someone who regularly eats too much, for example, may discover through self-monitoring that being in the kitchen, watching television and reading the newspaper are all activities that encourage eating. In this case, the situation is narrowed down to eating only at the table, staying out of the kitchen when possible and watching television and reading where there are no snacks available. Even the stimulation provided by the food itself can be narrowed by putting extra food out of sight after the portion that is to be eaten at a meal has been put on to the plate.

The problem with most forms of slimming is that the majority of those who try slimming diets return to their original weight. The reason, according to behaviour therapists, is that most people are not learning new eating habits to facilitate dieting and maintain a lower weight. Most slimming diets represent a departure from normal eating which, together with the pain of dieting and being overweight, act as negative reinforcement. Thus it is important to develop new and rewarding habits that provide a distraction and a motivation to continue. Ideally these should be patterns that can continue for life.

These new patterns of behaviour could include going for a walk, calling a friend, cuddling with a partner, doing some breathing exercises and so on. With the resulting positive reinforcement, the individual is more likely to incorporate the new behaviour into his everyday life.

In addition to receiving feedback from the outside, learning is strengthened by self reinforcement: by telling ourselves that what we are doing is good or bad. Research has shown that those who succeed in learning a new habit and weakening an old one, give themselves twice as many positive messages as those who fail; those who do not succeed give themselves twice as much negative reinforcement than the individuals in the other group.

Setting targets

As you change your behaviour, try to set yourself targets to aim for. When dieting, for example, it is important to set up small targets for which you can give yourself approval, instead of having to wait until the end of the week when you weigh yourself. The more immediate the reward, even if it is simply a moment of self-affirmation, the more likely is the new behaviour to be sustained. If you have met your calorie limit for the first half of the day, you might want to reward yourself by thinking of your strong points and congratulating yourself on getting so far.

Negative self-reinforcement is sometimes necessary, but only in small doses. When tempted to eat, for example, you might visualize being unable to fit into your favourite clothes. If you know you have a specific problem, such as drinking, smoking, over-eating or biting your nails, devise a diary such as the one on this page to pinpoint the behaviour and circumstances that provoke the indulgence or the bad habit.

DAY	START	STOP	PLACE	ACTIVITY	MOOD	QUANTITY
MON	18.30	19.00	Bar	Standing; talking	O.K.	2½ pints beer
TUES	13.15	14.00	Bar	Sitting thinking alone	Bored	1 pint beer
	19.00	22.30	Sitting room	Watching TV alone	Depressed	2 gins ½ bottle wine 2 whiskies
WED	18.00	18.30	Cinema	Sitting: (before film)	O.K.	1 pint beer
	22.00	22.30	Friend's house	Talking	O.K.	1 bottle wine
	24.00	01.00	Kitchen at home	Sitting; alone	Tired, emotional	2 whiskies
THURS	20.30	22.20	Dinner party	Talking	Cheerful	3 cocktails 1½ bottles wine 2 brandies
FRI	13.30	14.30	Bar	Sitting; talking	Tired	2 pints beer
	20.30	22.30	Bar	Sitting; talking	Tired	4 pints beer
SAT	13.30	14.30	Bar	Sitting; talking	O.K.	2 pints beer
	18.30	19.30	Party	Sitting; talking	O.K.	5 cocktails
	20.30	22.00	Restaurant	Eating	Fine	1 bottle wine
SUN	13.30	15.00	Lunch party	Eating	O.K.	1 brandy 2 gins ½ bottle wine 4 ports
	22.00	23.00	Kitchen home	sitting alone	Tired	1 bottle wine

Conclusions

Must stop drinking alone, cut down on weekend and lunch-time drinking. If bored or depressed must start a new activity when I feel the impulse to drink.

COGNITIVE THERAPY

Cognitive therapy involves a personal reassessment of fixed, often self-defeating attitudes. It is based on the rationale that our actions are determined by our view of the world and the way we interpret experiences. Cognitions, or the impressions we form of events, develop into an automatic pattern of understanding, which we came to regard as infallible — even though it is not true. Since these habitual thought processes are believable, and since we rarely question their validity, many people spend their entire lives labouring under long-held, sometimes damaging, misconceptions about themselves and others.

Changing your thinking
Take the case of a woman who was recently divorced from a man she relied on to take care of practical household repairs, family accounts and disciplining the children. Not long after the divorce, she realized that she felt depressed and lacked confidence in her ability to manage a household alone. She sought cognitive therapy, and, when she began to analyse her feelings, she realized that the underlying thought that triggered her depressed mood was 'I've never been good at anything in my life.' Gradually, she began to look at herself more realistically and she changed this negative statement to: 'I have some abilities, but I also need help in learning how to cope with my children, with money and loneliness.' Over a period, this reassessment boosted her confidence and resolved her depression.

This example illustrates a common pattern of thinking, which can lead to emotional and behavioural problems. Troublesome thoughts are often simple statements representing absolute beliefs that are never questioned. In contrast to this primitive approach, mature thinking is able to confront situations from different perspectives.

Cognitive therapeutic methods can be applied to people of all ages. An eight-year-old boy, for example, became excessively anxious whenever his mother and father had a difference of opinion, however amicable. The underlying thought that sparked his fear was found to be: 'If Mummy and Daddy disagree, they might get divorced.' Using cognitive therapy, the boy was encouraged to test the reality of his belief by talking to a local shopkeeper, the postman, a teacher and his parents. After learning that a mere disagreement between adults was unlikely to lead to divorce,

the boy changed his view and stopped becoming upset by his parents' differences.

Like adults, children are inclined to see things in black and white. Lacking a varied vocabulary, a child thinks about his feelings in terms of polarities such as happy or sad. If a child is not happy, he may conclude that he is sad. Cognitive therapy aims to open up the many levels of feeling between extremes. If a child's emotional vocabulary is expanded, he will be able to distinguish more subtle nuances of feeling and thus gain measurably in security.

Fixed concepts
Adolescence is a period of life that can be particularly aggravated by misconceptions. Beliefs about physical appearance, masculinity and femininity, for example, are central to the adolescent's identity. In one case, a 15-year-old girl avoided social contact whenever possible. The dominant thought behind her behaviour was found to be: 'No one could really like me because I'm not pretty enough.' With some help, she became aware of her valuable attributes beyond her physical appearance and was soon able to think of herself as an attractive personality.

Our fixed concepts of masculinity and femininity emphasize how unrealistic can be the expectations that we absorb from the media, our parents, and peers. Many unemployed men, for example, have to suffer the pain of re-evaluating their own identities: 'I'm not a man unless I go out to work and earn money.' For many years, women have had to follow the myth that they should not be aggressive or career-minded. At the other extreme, some women suffer from the restrictive view that they should not show any tenderness toward men, attempt to make themselves look attractive to the opposite sex or enjoy heterosexual relationships of any kind.

Unrealistic expectations
Today, many close relationships break down because of unrealistic expectations. From an early age we are taught to have expectations from marriage and life itself. Many of these come from the media or those who try to tell us what relationships *ought* to be like. It is no wonder that we feel our partners let us down. If a couple is experiencing problems, it can help to clarify what each partner expects of the other.

Types of thinking

Our thoughts about ourselves and our own behaviour may be unnecessarily harsh and condemning. Repetition of these negative thoughts over the years may cause significant under-achievement in the long term, unless we realize that the human personality is dynamic and capable of considerable adaption and change in response to more positive thinking. If you find yourself thinking negatively about your character, try to take a more objective view.

Primitive thinking	Mature thinking
Global: 'I'm a bitter person.'	**Many faceted:** 'I'm moderately bitter, generous and fairly intelligent.'
Judgemental: 'I'm a nasty sort.'	**Non-judgemental:** 'I can be more harsh than most people I know.'
Inflexible: 'I always have been and always will be angry.'	**Flexible:** 'My irritations vary in intensity from situation to situation.'
Character judgement: 'I have a defect in my character.'	**Behavioural judgement:** 'I react too assertively in certain situations.'
Unchangeable: 'There's nothing that can be done about it.'	**Changeable:** 'I can learn to respond in other ways.'

Reality testing

What is the evidence for my conclusion? Are there other explanations? How serious is this situation? How much does it actually subtract from my life? Will it really hurt me if a stranger thinks badly of me? What harm will it do me if I try to be more outspoken?

Elderly people frequently fall prey to misconceptions. One woman, who had enjoyed an active, satisfying life up to the age of 60, suddenly became inactive and dejected. After analysing her state, it became clear that she was disturbed by her conviction that life held nothing after retirement, except death. After testing her belief by visiting some organizations for senior citizens and through changing her way of thinking, she became more positive about her future.

If you want to change something that troubles you, try the following approach:

1 Take 15 minutes to write down what you think your belief about your problem is.

2 Identify when an automatic negative thought surfaces.

3 Notice how this thought influences your feelings and actions; try to put it into words.

4 Try talking to other people to see if your belief is really accurate.

5 Check your belief and reword it so that it fits a more realistic and positive perspective.

6 Repeat the newer and more mature thought frequently, particularly when you are in a situation that stimulates the older, habitual thinking.

7 Finally, if your negative thought actually fits the situation accurately, then you may need to explore its importance in your life. Suppose, for example, that it is true that you are not loved by somebody close to you. You may have to face that this is the reality, and that other people who give you love and support can help to compensate.

Example

A young woman who recently divorced feels guilty and depressed about the break-up.

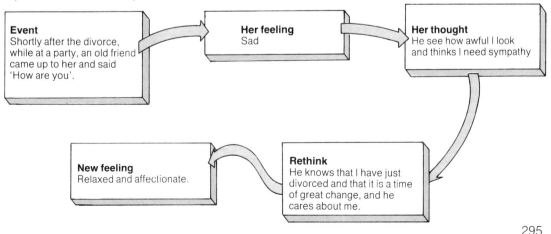

Event
Shortly after the divorce, while at a party, an old friend came up to her and said 'How are you'.

Her feeling
Sad

Her thought
He see how awful I look and thinks I need sympathy

Rethink
He knows that I have just divorced and that it is a time of great change, and he cares about me.

New feeling
Relaxed and affectionate.

PSYCHOANALYSIS

The method of solving problems by psychoanalysis owes its origins to the Austrian physician Sigmund Freud. Near the end of the nineteenth century, Freud was working with people who had nervous disorders. It was then that he first theorized that emotional problems originate in the developmental needs and frustrations of childhood. And, he argued, these remain subconscious for most people because they are concerned with sexual longings of which they were frightened.

Exploring the mind

From the psychoanalytic perspective, problems experienced during childhood are thought to surface in adult life in the form of problems such as marital discord, overeating, alcohol dependence and so on. Unlike many other therapies psychoanalysis is not primarily concerned with the relief of such symptoms but with the gradual uncovering of the underlying cause — which is hidden in repressed memories.

Psychoanalysts assert that unless the original conflict is revealed, the relief of one symptom, such as excessive drinking, will merely be substituted with another, for example, increased anxiety or overeating.

The analytic approach to problem solving involves certain fundamental methods, by which the analyst attempts to get at the conscious mind and to reach into the unconscious desires and memories which, he believes, are determining the subject's life. In classical analysis, the subject attends the analyst up to four times a week. For an hour at each session the subject lies on a couch, while the analyst sits behind him out of direct view. A basic rule of the therapeutic process is that the subject says whatever comes to mind. These spontaneous associations are thought to initiate an unravelling process in the mind. Thus the most intimate and influential attitudes and memories of the subject begin to come to the surface.

It is through the relationship between subject and analyst that repressed needs and conflicts are uncovered. For the most part, the analyst remains aloof, making interpretations designed to break through the subject's resistance to recognizing and dealing with buried emotions and memories. What gradually occurs — at least in theory — is that early feelings, which the subject has repressed from his consciousness, begin to manifest themselves in his developing relationship with the analyst.

Through such a manifestation, which is commonly known as transference, the subject will feel emotions such as love, anger and hate toward the analyst. The many needs and feelings of the transference are discussed between subject and analyst over a long period. When, eventually, the analysis ends, the subject should have integrated these emotions into his consciousness.

Another important way in which the analyst attempts to prise a way into the hidden layers of a subject's mind is through the interpretation of dreams — a method for which Freud is famous. Critics of psychoanalytic theory point out that the interpretation of dream symbols and events are primarily sexual and reflect Freud's belief that it is the sexual desires of the child — whether they be oral, anal or genital — that are at the heart of human conflict. Dream interpretation remains central to many types of psychoanalysis.

Jungian analysis

Carl Jung and Sigmund Freud worked as close colleagues, but Jung broke away from Freud because he believed that there were other dimensions to the individual unconscious than the sexual desires of childhood. Much of Jung's work was based on his extensive knowledge of the religions, myths and philosophies of many different cultures, whose contents and symbols were, he felt, evident in peoples' dreams and fantasies.

Jung based his psychoanalytic theory on a series of archetypes. An example is the archetype of *puer aeternis*, or eternal youth, which often emerges in people's dreams. The *puer aeternis* embodies the freshness and adventurousness of youth. If present in the dream of a depressed person, it may indicate that the subject's liveliness and ability to take risks has been stifled. But if present in the dreams of an immature person, *puer aeternis* may show that the subject needs to become less romantic and more down to earth.

Another common Jungian archetype is the duality of the *animus* and *anima*, or the male and female sides of the personality. Jung emphasized that within every individual are healthy 'male' and 'female' dimensions and that, if these are not acknowledged, imbalance and difficulties with relationships may result. Thus a woman who is out of touch with her *animus* may be drawn to and have a series of unsuccessful relationships with overtly masculine men, who eventually prove too harsh. By getting in touch with the male side of herself, through analysis, she may have less need for this type of man and develop a relationship with someone gentler and less dominant.

Jung believed that his approach to therapy is best used by people in their middle years who need perspective and meaning in their lives. He also felt that it was important to pay attention to the particular phase of life that a person is in and to the seven-year cycles which, in Jung's view, are common to human experience.

Suitable subjects

Psychoanalysis is not a treatment that should be embarked upon by someone who has simple problems that need a quick solution. Nor is it suitable for anyone with severe emotional problems, because of the rigorous, often painful, intellectual and self-critical demands it makes on the subject. Psychoanalysis is most useful for someone who is functioning well in the ordinary world but who values and desires a long-term quest for self-knowledge — and who can afford the high cost of therapy. Regardless of the truth or benefits of any particular theoretical approach, the success of psychoanalysis depends ultimately on the wisdom and sensitivity of the therapist and the commitment and openness of the subject.

When considering possible ways of solving problems, it is important not to confuse formal psychoanalysis and psychotherapy. In psychotherapy, the subject and the therapist sit facing each other. They usually meet about once a week for as long as it takes to remove the problems to the satisfaction of the subject, and the focus is on present relationships, problems and events, rather than on the past. Problems are looked at from a practical point of view, but with a strong emphasis on how they have developed from early relationships and feelings. The therapy may involve other family members if they are willing and the counsellor thinks it necessary and/or helpful. This sort of psychotherapy has a wide range of uses for all types of people and problems.

The chart compares the schools of thought of the two founders of psychoanalysis.

Freud	**Jung**
Sexual desires originating in infancy dominate the unconscious mind.	There is a transcendental and spiritual dimension which expresses itself in our unconscious personal development. This is the 'collective unconscious'.
The unconscious mind is the repository of a person's experience and originates from early relationships between parents and child.	The symbols of dreams may have a universal quality that transcends the culture to which a person belongs.
Dreams contain sexual symbolism. Thus a cave is interpreted as a womb to which a person may be trying to return or which he may be wishing to avoid or penetrate.	Some dream symbols represent universal archetypes which flow into an individual's identity. Thus, if a cave is seen to be womb-like, it is said to reflect the myth of the Great Mother. This is prominent in many cultures throughout the world and which represents the positive life force.
Repressed sexual desires, which emerge in dreams or as 'traumatic' episodes revealed under hypnosis, are commonly the cause of neurotic symptoms in adult life. Therapy aims to uncover these repressed notions.	The personality has many aspects — thinking, feeling, intuitive and sensory. Most people tend to be dominated by one of these characteristics. Therapy aims to create greater balance by enhancing those aspects that are less well developed.
Tends to concentrate on negative thoughts and emotions.	Often a more positive and helpful exploration of the psyche with emphasis on synthesizing life with more universal dimensions.

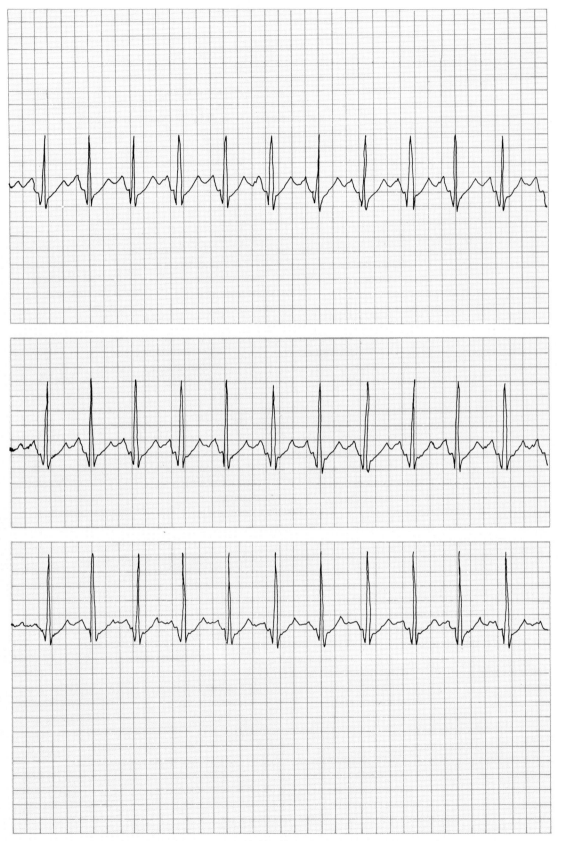

298

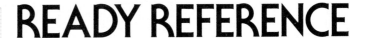

READY REFERENCE

To help you make the fullest possible use of the wealth of information contained in the preceding pages, and to stimulate you to pursue the ideal of fitness and well-being still further, the section that completes this book contains essential reference material.

The pages on health screening detail its assets for both men and women. The significance of each part of the screen is explained in relation to preventive health care. The calorie charts are designed in such a way that you will be able to see at a glance not only the total calorie values of foods but also the percentage of those calories that are provided by carbohydrates, proteins and fats. The charts will, thus, be an invaluable aid in helping you to balance the many nutrients your diet contains in the healthiest possible way.

By using the bibliography, you will be able to pursue further those topics that interest you most. A full index makes the book complete.

ABOUT HEALTH SCREENING

Regular health screening is central to the concept of health maintenance for two reasons. First, because unless certain measurements, such as blood pressure, are taken, the individual does not know whether he is within the normal limits or potentially vulnerable. Second, that the first examination establishes a full series of baseline measurements from which subsequent change — improvement or deterioration — can be charted over a considerable period.

This is important because 'killer diseases', such as heart attack and breast cancer, can produce early and detectable changes long before they cause symptoms, that is, before the individual may become aware of possible hazardous changes in his or her health.

Regular health examinations thus have three benefits, first to measure and record the health status of the individual and to reassure those who are worried; second, to facilitate what is called pre-symptomatic diagnosis, and third, to identify — often with follow-up tests — vulnerable people at, it is hoped, a stage when any problems they may have can be remedied. It is prudent to know your indices.

In the United Kingdom, BUPA have pioneered the development of health screening at their various centres across the country. What you should expect at a BUPA-type health check is outlined below:

Why have a health check?
As has been said, a health check is to measure and monitor your state of health and to pick up any early, pre-symptomatic and possibly harmful changes while they can be treated, usually very simply. It may also reveal other common conditions that need treatment.

This is important because heart disease in men or breast cancer in women are still the biggest single killers for each sex, and both require pre-symptomatic diagnosis if they are to be cured or controlled.

Because health and well-being depend on both mental and physical factors, the check will include a lifestyle assessment, a formal medical listing of any known conditions and symptoms, a clinical examination and various special tests. When all this has been done, there follows a summary and recommendations — or reassurance that all is reasonably well. At this point, the baseline be-

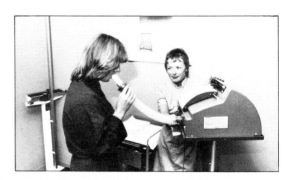

comes established.

Thus in men, it is necessary to know about personal habits, such as exercise, smoking and stress, and to measure weight, blood pressure, lipids and so on. Women require many of the same procedures, particularly if they smoke, plus special attention to the possibilities of breast or pelvic disease.

What's in a BUPA health screen?
A comprehensive screen will take about $2\frac{1}{2}$ hours and for *men* the screen will consist of the following procedures:

1   Personal history
A detailed personal, occupational and medical history is taken. The assessment is made under the headings of work, home and leisure and provides a picture of the individual in relation to his total environment.

This may often be automated on a computer to give a consistent and convenient data base, or it can be by questionnaire. Often more truthful and revealing answers are given to the machine than to a strange interviewer.

2   Tests of hearing and vision
These show any need for glasses or hearing aids and provide a baseline for the future. Many people need better glasses.

3   Measurement of height and weight
To give an accurate assessment of body build and any obesity.

4   Lung function measurement
Pulmonary (lung) function declines with age and prematurely with smoking. It is also critical in assessing exercise tolerance and common conditions such as bronchitis and asthma.

5   Chest X-ray
This is complementary to the lung testing and may reveal early, and possibly treatable, lung

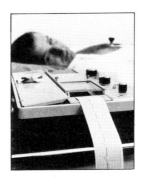

Lung function test (left).

The ECG trace emerging from the electrocardiograph. (right).

cancer. Many centres will also carry out an X-ray of the abdomen, which may show kidney and gall stones, cysts and bowel disease, often unsuspected and worth treating.

6 Blood pressure and electrocardiogram

What is called moderate hypertension, symptomless high blood pressure, often merits treatment to reduce the chances of later stroke, heart attack and heart failure. Thus blood pressure measurement and monitoring are critical. To be known, blood pressure must be measured.

The electrocardiogram (ECG) reveals the state of the heart muscle and internal conducting system of the heart. Minor abnormalities can be significant and provide a baseline measurement valuable in assessing changes over the years.

7 Urine test

Diabetes, kidney disease, infectious and other conditions may be revealed by simple and possibly microscopic and bacteriological urine tests.

8 Blood analysis

This is probably the most important battery of special tests: first for blood disease, such as anaemia or leukaemia; second for a wide range of possible changes concerned with lipids, (blood fats) sugar, liver function, and so on.

Changes in cholesterol are regarded as the best single predictor of coronary vulnerability. Abnormalities may receive more detailed confirmatory tests, which are often done on the same blood sample.

9 The final consultation

The session with the doctor includes detailed discussion of problem areas and abnormal findings and provides an opportunity for an in-depth discussion of any personal lifestyle or work-related problems. The doctor will give guidance and reassurance and advise on any active treatment — personal or medical — required.

Finally, when all the findings have been considered and digested, letters will be written to the individual and his personal doctor stating the results of the health screen.

Health checks for women

In essence, the reasons for women's screening are the same as for men's, and the full screening schedule includes a similar range of tests. But since breast and cervical cancer and pelvic disease are particularly common, extra examinations have to be made for these.

Breast cancer occurs in 1 in every 15 women in the UK, and the incidence is much the same in all Caucasian races. Benign breast lumps are also common but must be regarded as suspicious until proven innocent. Only about 1 in 10 lumps turns out to be malignant. The success of treating cancer with minimal surgery, and thus with minimal effects on the affected breast, depends entirely on the early diagnosis of small lumps.

Properly taught and supervised, a woman can become the best monitor of her breasts, by identifying or reporting on any change. Special X-rays, particularly of large breasts, can detect early cancers which are too small to feel.

Cervical cancer seems to be on the increase in younger women, so regular cervical smears and a pelvic examination are essential.

BUPA offers two types of health check for women; these are:

1 The well woman screen

This focuses on possible breast and pelvic disease and includes a full gynaecological history, special examinations of breast and pelvis and instruction in breast self-examination.

There is also the opportunity to discuss other gynaecological problems and to seek advice about treatment facilities for common problems such as premenstrual tension, the menopause and family planning.

Blood pressure, urine, height and weight are also included as is a cervical smear.

2 Full screening

This includes the 'specials' listed above, the full range of screening tests and a consultation with a doctor. And, as for men, the consultation is lifestyle orientated, providing an opportunity to discuss a wide range of family, personal and work-related problems and their effect on physical and emotional health.

CALORIE CHARTS

The foods selected for these charts contain substantial amounts of nutrients. With a few exceptions, you can eat as many raw fruit and vegetables as you wish without affecting the healthiness of your diet, but as soon as food is cooked with added ingredients such as sugar or fat, the calorie content may change dramatically.

Figures are given for 100g (3.5oz) or 100ml (3.5floz) portions of foods or drinks. Total calories are given, plus total weights of proteins, carbohydrates and fats. To help you calculate the contribution of foods to your recommended daily calorie allowances (see pp. 54–5), the percentage of calories each macronutrient contributes to the calorie total is also given. For alcoholic drinks, figures for alcohol content replace those for fat.

Meat, meat products, offal

	Calories	Protein (g)	Protein as % total cals	Carbohydrate (g)	Carbohydrate as % total cals	Fat (g)	Fat as % total cals
Bacon							
back **g**	405	25.3	25	0	0	33.8	75.1
back **f**	465	24.9	21.4	0	0	40.6	78.6
streaky **g**	422	24.5	28.2	0	0	36.0	76.8
streaky **f**	496	23.1	18.6	0	0	44.8	81.3
Beef							
minced **st**	229	23.1	40.4	0	0	15.2	59.7
rump steak **L/F**	218	27.3	50.1	0	0	12.1	50.0
rump steak **LO**	168	28.6	68.1	0	0	6.0	32.1
sirloin **rst, L/F**	284	23.6	33.2	0	0	21.1	66.9
sirloin **LO**	192	27.6	57.5	0	0	9.1	42.7
stewing steak	223	30.9	55.4	0	0	11.0	44.4
burgers **f**	264	20.4	30.9	7.0	9.9	17.3	59
Chicken b	183	29.2	68.8	0	0	7.3	35.9
rst, MO	148	24.8	67	0	0	5.4	32.8
rst, M/S	216	22.6	41.9	0	0	14.0	58.3
Corned beef **c**	217	26.9	49.6	0	0	12.1	50.2
Duck **rst, MO**	189	25.3	53.6	0	0	9.7	46.2
rst, M/S	339	19.6	23.1	0	0	29.0	77
Frankfurters	274	9.5	13.9	3.0	4.1	25.0	82.1
Ham **b, c**	120	18.4	61.3	0	0	5.1	38.3
Heart, ox **st**	179	31.4	70.2	0	0	5.9	29.7
Kidney, lamb **f**	155	24.6	63.5	0	0	6.3	36.6
Lamb, leg **rst, L/F**	266	26.1	39.3	0	0	17.9	60.6
rst, LO	191	29.4	61.6	0	0	8.1	38.2
loin chop **g, L/F**	355	23.5	26.5	0	0	29.0	73.5
loin chop **g, LO**	222	27.8	50.1	0	0	12.3	49.9
shoulder **rst,L/F**	316	19.9	25.2	0	0	26.3	74.9
shoulder **rst, LO**	196	23.8	48.6	0	0	11.2	51.4
Liver, lamb **f**	232	22.9	39.5	3.9	6.3	14.0	54.3
veal **f**	254	26.9	42.4	7.3	10.8	13.2	46.8
Liver sausage	310	12.9	16.6	4.3	5.2	26.9	78.1
Meat paste	173	15.2	35.2	3.0	6.5	11.2	58.3
Pork, leg **rst, L/F**	286	26.9	37.6	0	0	19.8	62.3

	Calories	Protein (g)	Protein as % total cals	Carbohydrate (g)	Carbohydrate as % total cals	Fat (g)	Fat as % total cals
leg **rst, LO**	185	30.7	66.4	0	0	6.9	33.6
loin chop **g, L/F**	332	28.5	34.3	0	0	24.2	65.6
loin chop **g, LO**	226	32.3	57.2	0	0	10.7	42.6
belly rashers	398	21.1	21.1	0	0	34.8	78.7
Salami	491	19.3	15.7	1.9	1.5	45.2	82.9
Sausages							
beef **g**	265	13.0	19.6	15.2	21.5	17.3	58.8
pork **g**	318	13.3	16.7	11.5	13.6	24.6	69.6
Suet, block	895	0.9	0.4	0	0	99.0	99.6
shredded	826	0		12.1	5.5	86.7	94.5
Sweetbread **f**	230	19.4	33.7	5.6	9.1	14.6	57.1
Tongue **b**	293	19.5	26.6	0	0	23.9	73.4
Turkey **rst, MO**	140	28.8	82.3	0	0	2.7	17.4
rst, M/S	171	28.0	65.5	0	0	6.5	34.2
Veal, cutlet **f**	215	31.4	58.4	4.4	7.7	8.1	33.9
fillet **rst**	230	31.6	55.0	0	0	11.5	45.0
Fish and shellfish							
Cod **f/br**	199	19.6	39.4	7.5	14.3	10.3	46.6
s	83	18.6	89.6	0	0	0.9	9.8
Crab **b**	127	20.1	63.3	0	0	5.2	36.9
b, W/S	25	4.0	64.0	0	0	1.0	36.0
b, c	81	18.1	89.4	0	0	0.9	10.0
Halibut **s**	131	23.8	72.7	0	0	4.0	27.5
Herring **g**	199	20.4	41.0	0	0	13.0	58.8
g, W/B	135	13.9	41.2	0	0	8.8	56.7
Kipper **ba**	205	25.5	49.8	0	0	11.4	50.1
ba, W/B	111	13.8	49.7	0	0	6.2	50.3
Lobster **b**	119	22.1	74.3	0	0	3.4	25.7
b, W/S	42	7.9	75.2	0	0	1.2	25.7
Pilchards **c/ts**	126	18.8	59.7	0.7	2.08	5.4	38.6
Plaice **f/br**	279	15.8	22.7	14.4	19.4	18.0	58.1
f/cr	228	18.0	31.6	8.6	14.2	13.7	54.1
s	93	18.9	81.3	0	0	1.9	18.4
Prawns **b**	107	22.6	84.5	0	0	1.8	15.1
b, W/S	41	8.6	83.9	0	0	0.7	15.4

KEY

b	boiled	**Fr**	fresh	**rst**	roast
ba	baked	**g**	grilled	**s**	steamed
br	in batter	**L/F**	lean and fat	**sd**	shelled
c	canned	**LO**	lean only	**sl**	salted
cr	in crumbs	**MO**	meat only	**st**	stewed
D	dried	**M/S**	meat and skin	**sw**	sweetened
De	desiccated	**o**	in oil	**Sk**	skimmed
f	fried	**p**	poached	**Sm**	smoked
fn	frozen	**P**	peeled	**S/R**	starch reduced
FO	fish only	**r**	raw	**ts**	in tomato sauce

u	undiluted
unsw	unsweetened
Wh	whole
W/B	weighed with bones
W/BS	weighed with bones and skin
W/S	weighed in shells
W/St	weighed with stones

	Calories	Protein (g)	Protein as % total cals	Carbohydrate (g)	Carbohydrate as % total cals	Fat (g)	Fat as % total cals
Salmon c	155	20.3	52.4	0	0	8.2	47.6
p	197	20.1	40.8	0	0	13.0	53.4
p, W/BS	160	16.3	40.8	0	0	10.5	59.1
Sm	142	25.4	71.6	0	0	4.5	28.5
Sardines, c, o, FO	217	23.7	43.7	0	0	13.6	56.4
c, ts	177	17.8	40.2	0.5	1.06	11.6	59.0
Scampi f	316	12.2	15.4	28.9	34.3	17.6	50.1
Shrimps b	117	23.8	81.4	0	0	2.4	18.5
b, W/S	39	7.9	81.0	0	0	0.8	18.5
c	94	20.8	88.5	0	0	1.2	11.5
Sole f	216	16.1	29.8	9.3	16.2	13.0	54.2
s	91	20.6	90.6	0	0	0.9	8.9
Trout s	135	23.5	69.6	0	0	4.5	30.0
s, W/B	89	15.5	69.7	0	0	3.0	30.3
Tuna c, o	289	22.8	31.6	0	0	22.0	68.5
Whitebait f	525	19.5	14.9	5.3	3.8	47.5	81.4
Dairy products							
Butter (salted)	740	0.4	0.2	0	0	82.0	99.7
Cheese							
Camembert	300	22.8	30.4	0	0	23.2	69.6
Cheddar	406	26.0	25.6	0	0	33.5	74.3
cottage	96	13.6	56.7	1.4	5.5	4.0	37.5
cream, full fat	439	3.1	2.8	0	0	47.4	97.2
Danish blue	355	23.0	25.9	0	0	29.2	74.0
Edam	304	24.4	32.1	0	0	22.9	67.8
Parmesan	408	35.1	34.4	0	0	29.7	65.5
processed	311	21.5	27.7	0	0	25.0	72.4
Stilton	462	25.6	22.2	0	0	40.0	77.9
Cream							
double	447	1.5	1.3	2.0	1.7	48.2	97.1
single	212	2.4	4.5	3.2	5.7	21.2	90.0
sterilized c	230	2.6	4.5	2.7	4.4	23.3	91.2
whipping	332	1.9	2.9	2.5	2.8	35.0	94.9
Eggs, whole b	147	12.3	33.5	0	0	10.9	66.7
f	232	14.1	24.3	0	0	19.5	75.7
white r	36	9.0	100.0	0	0	0	0
yolk r	339	16.1	19.0	0	0	30.5	81.0
Milk							
whole	65	3.3	20.3	4.7	27.1	3.8	52.6
skimmed **Fr**	33	3.4	41.2	5.0	56.8	0.1	2.7
condensed **Wh**	322	8.3	10.3	55.5	64.6	9.0	25.2
condensed **Sk**	267	9.9	14.8	60.0	84.9	0.3	1.0
evaporated							
c, usw	158	8.6	21.8	11.3	26.8	9.0	51.3
Yoghurt, low fat	52	5.0	38.5	6.2	44.7	1.0	17.3
flavoured	81	5.0	24.7	14.0	64.8	0.9	10.0
fruit	95	4.8	20.2	17.9	70.7	1.0	9.5
Fruits							
Apricots c	106	0.5	1.9	27.7	98.0	0	0
D	182	4.8	10.6	43.4	89.4	0	0
Avocado pear	223	4.2	7.5	1.8	3.2	22.2	89.6
Banana	79	1.1	5.6	19.2	95.6	0.3	3.4
Dates D	248	2.0	3.2	63.9	96.6	0	0
D, W/St	213	1.7	3.2	54.9	96.7	0	0
Peaches c	87	0.4	1.8	22.9	98.7	0	0
Prunes D	161	2.4	6.0	40.3	93.9	0	0
D, W/St	134	2.0	6.0	33.5	93.8	0	0
Raisins	246	1.1	1.8	64.4	98.2	0	0

	Calories	Protein (g)	Protein as % total cals	Carbohydrate (g)	Carbohydrate as % total cals	Fat (g)	Fat as % total cals
Vegetables							
Beans ba, c/ts	64	5.1	31.9	10.3	60.4	0.5	7.0
haricot r	271	21.4	31.6	45.5	63.0	1.6	5.3
b	93	6.6	28.4	16.6	66.9	0.5	4.8
broad	48	4.1	34.2	7.1	55.5	0.6	11.3
Chickpeas b	144	8.0	22.2	22.0	57.3	3.3	20.6
Lentils r	304	23.8	31.3	53.2	65.6	1.0	3.0
split b	99	7.6	30.7	17.0	64.4	0.5	4.6
Peas D, b	103	6.9	26.8	19.1	69.5	0.4	3.5
fn, b	41	5.4	52.7	4.3	39.3	0.4	8.8
Potatoes ba, Wh	85	2.1	9.9	20.3	89.6	0.1	1.1
old **P, b**	80	1.4	7.0	19.7	92.3	0.1	1.1
new	76	1.6	8.4	18.3	90.3	0.1	1.2
chips f	253	3.8	6.0	37.3	55.3	10.9	38.8
Potato crisps	533	6.3	4.7	49.3	34.7	35.9	60.6
Sweetcorn b	123	4.1	13.3	22.8	69.5	2.3	16.8
kernels c	76	2.9	15.3	16.1	79.4	0	0
Sweet potatoes b	85	1.1	5.2	20.1	88.7	0.6	6.4
Nuts							
Almonds W/S	210	6.3	12.0	1.6	2.9	19.8	84.9
shelled	565	16.9	12.0	4.3	2.9	53.5	85.2
Coconut De	604	5.6	3.7	6.4	4.0	62.0	92.4
Fr	351	3.2	3.7	3.7	4.0	36.0	92.3
Peanuts W/S	394	16.8	17.1	5.9	5.6	33.8	77.2
sl	570	24.3	17.1	8.6	5.7	49.0	77.4
Walnuts Fr	525	10.6	8.1	5.0	3.6	51.5	88.3
W/S	336	6.8	8.1	3.2	3.6	33.0	88.4
Cereals, cereal products							
All Bran	273	15.1	22.1	43.0	59.1	5.7	18.8
Barley, pearl b	120	2.7	9.0	27.6	86.3	0.6	4.5
Bran wheat	206	14.1	27.4	26.8	48.8	5.5	24.0
Bread, white	233	7.8	13.4	49.7	80.0	1.7	6.6
wholemeal	216	8.8	16.3	41.8	72.6	2.7	11.3
Cornflakes	368	8.6	9.4	85.1	86.7	1.6	3.9
Flour, wheat, plain	350	9.8	11.2	80.1	85.8	1.2	3.1
self-raising	339	9.3	11.0	77.5	85.7	1.2	3.2
wholemeal	318	13.2	16.6	65.8	77.6	2.0	5.7
Macaroni b	117	4.3	14.7	25.2	80.8	0.6	4.6
Muesli	368	12.9	14.0	66.2	67.5	7.5	18.3
Pancakes, Scotch	283	6.7	9.5	40.6	53.8	11.6	36.9
other	307	6.1	8.0	36.2	44.2	16.3	47.8
Pastry, flaky	565	5.8	4.1	47.4	31.5	40.5	64.5
shortcrust	527	6.9	5.2	55.8	39.7	32.2	55.0
Porridge	44	1.4	12.7	8.2	69.9	0.9	18.4
Rice, brown r	361	6.5	7.2	86.8	90.2	1.0	2.5
polished b	123	2.2	7.2	29.6	90.2	0.3	2.2
Rice Krispies	372	5.9	6.3	88.1	88.8	2.0	4.8
Rye, flour	335	8.2	9.8	75.9	85.0	2.0	5.4
Shredded Wheat	324	10.6	13.1	67.9	78.6	3.0	8.3
Spaghetti b	117	4.2	14.4	26.0	83.3	0.3	2.3
Sugar Puffs	348	5.9	6.8	84.5	91.1	0.8	2.1
Weetabix	340	11.4	13.4	70.3	77.5	3.4	9.0

CALORIE CHARTS

Cakes, biscuits, desserts	Calories	Protein (g)	Protein as % total cals	Carbohydrate (g)	Carbohydrate as % total cals	Fat (g)	Fat as % total cals
Biscuits							
digestive	471	9.8	8.3	66.0	52.6	20.5	39.2
chocolate	493	6.8	5.5	66.5	50.6	24.1	44.0
gingernuts	456	5.6	4.9	79.1	65.1	15.2	30.0
shortbread	504	6.2	4.9	65.5	48.7	26.0	46.2
wafer (filled)	535	4.7	3.5	66.0	46.3	29.9	52.3
Cake							
rich fruit	332	3.7	4.5	58.3	65.9	11.0	29.8
sponge	464	6.4	5.5	53.2	43.0	26.5	51.4
fatless	301	10.0	13.3	53.6	66.8	6.7	20.0
Cheesecake	421	4.2	4.0	24.0	21.4	34.9	74.6
Crispbread							
rye **S/R**	321	9.4	11.7	70.6	82.5	2.1	5.9
wheat **S/R**	388	45.3	46.7	36.9	35.7	7.6	17.6
Doughnuts	349	6.0	6.9	48.8	52.4	15.8	40.8
Eclairs	376	4.1	4.4	38.2	38.1	24.0	57.5
Ice-cream							
dairy	167	3.7	8.9	24.8	55.7	6.6	35.6
non-dairy	165	3.3	8.0	20.7	47.1	8.2	44.7
Pie							
lemon meringue	323	4.5	5.6	46.4	53.9	14.6	40.7
mince	435	4.3	4.0	61.7	53.2	20.7	42.8
Fruit pie with							
pastry top	180	2.0	4.4	27.6	57.5	7.6	38.0
Soda bread	264	8.0	12.2	56.3	80.0	2.3	7.8
chapatis							
with fat	336	8.1	9.6	50.2	56.0	12.8	34.3
without fat	202	7.3	14.6	43.7	81.1	1.0	4.5

Sugar, sugar products							
Chocolate, milk	529	8.4	6.4	59.4	42.1	30.3	51.6
plain	525	4.7	3.6	64.8	46.3	29.2	50.1
Honey (in jars)	288	0.4	0.6	76.4	99.5	0	0
Jam	261	0.6	0.9	69.0	99.1	0	0
Sugar, demerara	394	0.5	0.5	99.3	99.5	0	0
white	394	0	0	99.9	100	0	0
Sweets **b**	327	0	0	87.3	100	0	0
Syrup, golden	298	0.3	0.4	79.0	99.4	0	0

Oils, spreads, sauces							
Chutney, apple	193	0.7	1.5	50.5	98.1	0.1	0.5
French dressing	658	0.1	0.1	0.2	0.1	73.0	99.9
Horseradish **r**	59	4.5	30.5	11.0	70.0	0	0
Lard	891	0	0	0	0	99.0	100.0
Low-fat spread	366	0	0	0	0	40.7	100.0
Margarine (all)	730	0.1	0.1	0.1	0.1	81.0	99.9
Mayonnaise	718	1.8	1.0	0.1	0.1	78.9	98.9
Oil, vegetable	899	0	0	0	0	99.9	100.0
Peanut butter	623	22.6	14.5	13.1	7.9	53.7	77.6
Pickle, sweet	134	0.6	1.8	34.4	96.3	0.3	2.0
Tomato ketchup	98	2.1	8.6	24.0	91.8	0	0
Marmite	179	41.4	92.5	1.8	3.8	0.7	3.5
Bovril	174	39.1	89.9	2.9	6.3	0.7	3.6
Mustard powder	452	28.9	25.6	20.7	17.2	28.7	57.2

Non-alcoholic drinks							
Blackcurrant **u**	229	0.1	0.2	60.9	99.7	0	0
Coffee, infusion	2	0.2	40.0	0.3	60.0	0	0
Cola	39	0	0	10.5	100	0	0
Lemonade	21	0	0	5.6	100	0	0
Orange juice, unsweetened	33	0.4	4.9	8.5	96.6	0	0
Tea, infusion	1	0.1	100	0	0	0	0
Tomato juice **c**	16	0.7	17.5	3.4	79.7	0	0

Alcoholic drinks	Calories	Protein (g)	Protein as % total cals	Carbohydrate (g)	Carbohydrate as % total cals	Ag	A%
Beer bitter							
draught	32	0.3	3.8	2.3	27.0	3.1	67.8
keg	31	0.3	3.8	2.3	27.8	3.0	67.7
Cider, dry	36	0	0	2.6	27.1	3.8	78.9
sweet	42	0	0	4.3	38.4	3.7	61.7
Liqueurs							
Advocaat	272	4.7	69.6	28.4	39.2	12.8	32.9
Cherry brandy	255	0	0	32.6	47.9	19.0	52.2
Curaçao	311	0	0	28.3	34.1	29.3	66.0
Sherry, dry	116	0.2	0.7	1.4	4.5	15.7	97.7
sweet	136	0.3	0.9	6.9	19.0	15.6	80.3
Spirits 70% proof	222	0	0	0	0	31.7	100
Vermouth, dry	118	0.1	0.3	5.5	17.5	13.9	82.5
sweet	151	0	0	15.9	39.5	13.0	60.3
Wine							
red	68	0.2	1.2	0.3	16.5	9.5	97.8
rosé	71	0.1	0.6	2.5	13.2	8.7	85.8
white, dry	66	0.1	0.6	0.6	3.4	9.1	96.5
medium	75	0.1	0.5	3.4	17.0	8.8	82.1
sweet	94	0.2	0.9	5.9	23.5	10.2	76.0

KEY

Ag	alcohol (g)	**f**	fried	**p**	poached	**Sm**	smoked
A%	alcohol as %	**fn**	frozen	**P**	peeled	**S/R**	starch reduced
	of total calories	**FO**	fish only	**r**	raw	**ts**	in tomato sauce
b	boiled	**Fr**	fresh	**rst**	roast	**u**	undiluted
ba	baked	**g**	grilled	**s**	steamed	**unsw**	unsweetened
br	in batter	**L/F**	lean and fat	**sd**	shelled	**Wh**	whole
c	canned	**LO**	lean only	**sl**	salted	**W/B**	weighed with bones
cr	in crumbs	**MO**	meat only	**st**	stewed	**W/BS**	weighed with bones and skin
D	dried	**M/S**	meat and skin	**sw**	sweetened	**W/S**	weighed in shells
De	desiccated	**o**	in oil	**Sk**	skimmed	**W/St**	weighed with stones

General
The Atlas of the Body and Mind, Mitchell Beazley Publishers Ltd, UK, 1979
The Macmillan Guide to Family Health, Smith, Tony (ed), Macmillan Publishers Ltd, UK, 1982
Man's Body, Corgi Books, UK, 1977
The Sunday Times New Book of Body Maintenance, Gillie, Oliver, Haddon, Celia and Mercer, Derrick, Michael Joseph Ltd, UK 1977
Woman's Body, Corgi Books, UK, 1978

Eating for Health
Cooking for your Heart's Content, Dyson, K., Hutchinson Publishing Group Ltd, UK, 1976
The F-Plan Diet, Eyton, Audrey, Penguin Books Ltd, UK, 1982
Nutrition Cultism, Facts and Fiction, Herbert, Victor, G.F. Stickley, USA, 1980
Vitamins and 'Health' Foods: The Great American Hustle, Herbert, Victor and Barrett, Stephen, G.F. Stickley, USA, 1982
Which? Way to Slim, Consumers Association, UK, 1979

Getting Fit, Staying Fit
The AAA Runners Guide, William Collins & Co Ltd, UK, 1983
Aerobics for Women, Cooper, Kenneth and Mildred, M. Evans & Co, Inc, USA, 1972
The Aerobics Program for Total Well-Being, Cooper, Kenneth, M. Evans & Co, Inc, USA, 1982
Basic Book of Sports Medicine, International Olympic Committee Solidarity 1978
The Bodywork Book, Dunn, Esme Newton, Wm. Collins Sons & Co Ltd, UK, 1982
The Complete Book of Running, Fixx, James F., Random House, USA, 1977; Penguin Books, UK, 1981
Exercise: The Facts, Oxford University Press, UK, 1981
Ischaemic Heart Disease and Exercise, Shephard, R.J., Croom Helm Ltd, UK, 1981
The Lotte Berk Method, Berk, Lotte and Prince, Jean, Quartet Books, UK, 1978
Physical Fitness — 5BX and XBX (Royal Canadian Air Force Manual), Penguin Books Ltd, UK, 1970
The Physiological Basis of P.E. and Athletics, Fox, E.L., and Matthews, D.K., W.B. Saunders, USA, 1981
Sport and Medicine, Sperryn, P., Butterworth & Co, UK, 1983

Head to Toe
The Face and Body Book, Miriam Stoppard (ed), Pan Books Ltd, UK, 1981
Vogue Complete Beauty, Deborah Hutton (ed), Octopus Books Ltd, UK, 1982

Your Sexuality
The Birth Control Book, Shapiro, Howard, Penguin Books Ltd, UK, 1980
The Book of Love, Devlin, David, New English Library, UK, 1975
The Breast, Stanway, Penny, Mayflower Books, UK, 1982
Breast Cancer, Faulder, Carolyn, Virago Press, UK, 1982
Human Sexual Response, Masters, William and Johnson, Virginia E., Bantam Books Ltd, USA, 1980

The Joy of Sex, Comfort, Alex, Quartet Books, UK, 1976
Lifechange, Evans, Barbara, Pan Books Ltd, UK, 1970
The Menopause, Anderson, Mary, Faber & Faber Ltd, UK, 1983
Once A Month, Dalton, Katherina, Fontana Books, UK, 1983
The Pill, Guillebaud, John, Oxford University Press, UK, 1983
Psychology of Women, Bardwick, Judith M., Harper & Row, USA, 1971
Understanding Human Sexual Inadequacy, Belliveau, Fred and Richter, Lin, Hodder & Stoughton, 1971
Understanding Premenstrual Tension, Brush, M., Pan Books Ltd, UK, 1984

Pregnancy and Birth
Birth Without Violence, Le Boyer, Fréderick, Fontana Books, UK, 1977
Breast is Best, Stanway, Andrew and Penny, Pan Books Ltd, UK, 1983
Exercises For Childbirth, Dale, Barbara and Roeber, Johanna, Century Publishing Co Ltd, UK 1982
Jane Fonda's Workout Book for Pregnancy, Birth & Recovery, Delyser, Femmy, Allen Lane, UK, 1983
Multiple Births: Preparation — Birth — Managing Afterwards, Linney, Judi, John Wylie & Sons Ltd, USA, 1983
Pregnancy, Bourne, Gordon, Penguin Books Ltd, UK, 1984
The Twins Handbook, Friedrich, Elizabeth and Rowland, Robson Books, UK, 1983
Your Body, Your Baby, Your Life, Phillips, Angela, Pandora Press, UK, 1983

Growing Old Gracefully
A Good Age, Comfort, Alex, Mitchell Beazley Publishers Ltd, UK, 1977
The Book of Ages, Morris, Desmond, Jonathan Cape Ltd, UK, 1983
How To Plan Your Retirement, Loving, Bill, Woodhead-Faulkner (Publishers) Ltd, UK, 1975

The Whole Person
Coping With Stress, Meichenbaum, Donald, Century Publishing, UK, 1983
Coping With Stress — A Guide to Living, Mills, James W., John Wylie & Sons Ltd, USA, 1982
Dealing with Drink, Davies, Ian, and Raistrick, Duncan, BBC Publications, UK, 1981
Depression — The Way Out of Your Prison, Rowe, Dorothy, Routledge & Kegan Paul Ltd, UK, 1983
Health or Smoking?, Royal College of Physicians Report, Pitman Medical, UK, 1983
Self Help from Your Nerves, Weekes, Claire, Angus & Robertson Ltd, UK, 1979

Treats and Treatments
The Alternative Health Guide, Inglis, Brian and West, Ruth, Michael Joseph Ltd, UK, 1983
Alternative Medicine, a Guide to Natural Therapies, Stanway, Andrew, Macdonald & Jane's Publishers Ltd, UK, 1980
Green Pharmacy, Gibbs, Barbara, Adam Hilger Ltd, UK, 1983
A Visual Encyclopaedia of Unconventional Medicine, Hill, Ann (ed), Triune Books, Ltd, UK, 1978; Crown Publishers Inc, USA, 1979

INDEX

Numerals in bold type refer to main entries.

Acknowledgements

b = bottom, c = centre, l = left, r = right, t = top

Title page Bokelberg/The Image Bank; 52 Berdoy/Elle/Transworld; 58 Leo Mason; 60 D & J Heaton/Colorific!; 68/75 Peter Myers; 78 Paolo Curto/The Image Bank; 79t Michael Yamashita/Colorific!; 79b Weight Watchers (UK) Ltd; 80/85 Peter Myers; 86 Chris Simpson; 88 Michael Yamashita/Colorific!; 95 John Garrett; 96l Tony Duffy/All-Sport; 96r Steve Dunnell/The Image Bank; 97 Owen Franken/Sygma/The John Hillelson Agency; 100/104 John Garrett; 105tl John Garrett; 105tr Woman's Journal/Syndication International; 105t John Garrett; 105b John Garrett; 118 Bokelberg/The Image Bank; 119 Steve Back; 120 Leo Mason; 122 John Kelly/The Image Bank; 123t All-Sport; 123b Terry Hancey/Daily Telegraph Colour Library; 124 Jane Sobel/The Image Bank; 125 Tony Stone Associates; 126 Norbert Schafer/The Image Bank; 127t W. L. Berssenbrugge/Zefa Picture Library; 127b Penny Tweedie/Daily Telegraph Colour Library; 134 Kaldewei; 137 Marshall Editions; 138 U. Seer/The Image Bank; 141t P. Pfander/The Image Bank; 141c David Vance/The Image Bank; 141b Novik/Vital/Transworld; 142 Steve Yarnell; 143 Gerard Champlong/The Image Bank; 145 BUPA; 146 STC Business Systems; 152 Chris Reinhardt/Elle/Transworld; 158 John Garrett; 160/161 Sally & Richard Greenhill; 162 All-Sport; 163 Dave Hogan/Rex Features; 165 Terry Hancey/Daily Telegraph Colour Library; 167 Julian Calder; 168 Robert Farber/The Image Bank; 174 Robin Forbes/The Image Bank; 178 Sally & Richard Greenhill; 183 Chris Bigg; 184 The Press Association; 186 Robin Williams/Science Photo Library; 188 Elizabeth Novick/Gruner & Jahr AG & Co; 191 Val Wilmer/Format Photographers; 192 St. Bartholomew's Hospital; 194/197 John Garrett; 198 Melet/Parents/Transworld; 199 P.L. Constant/Parents/Transworld; 200/201 John Garrett; 202 Sandra Lousada/Susan Griggs Agency; 203 John Garrett; 204 Lawrence Fried/The Image Bank; 206 Robin Forbes/The Image Bank; 208 Sally & Richard Greenhill; 211 Frank Whitney/The Image Bank; 212 W. Maehl/Zefa Picture Library; 213 David Hurn/Magnum/The John Hillelson Agency; 214 Zefa Picture Library; 215 Sally & Richard Greenhill; 216 Rex Features; 219 Western Morning News Co Ltd; 223 J.H. Lartigue/The John Hillelson Agency; 224 Leidmann/Zefa Picture Library; 228 Barry Lewis/Network; 229 Richard Kalvar/Magnum/The John Hillelson Agency; 236 Mohn/Zefa Picture Library; 262 Zao Grimberg/The Image Bank; 264 Feinblatt/Elle/Transworld; 266 de Brantes/Elle/Transworld; 267 Gert von Bassewitz/Susan Griggs Agency; 268 Lange/Elle/Transworld; 269/271 John Garrett; 272 *The Practical Treatment of Backache and Sciatica* by John Barrett and Douglas Golding; 280/283 John Garrett; 285 Biofeedback Systems; 286 Tony Stone Associates; 287 Colorsport; 300/301 BUPA.

Artwork by
John Davies; Tony Graham; Aziz Khan; Jim Robins; Les Smith.
Retouching and make-up Roy Flooks.